NATIONAL ACADEMIES *Sciences Engineering Medicine*

NATIONAL ACADEMIES PRESS
Washington, DC

Newborn Screening in the United States

A Vision for Sustaining and Advancing Excellence

Jewel Mullen, Emily Packard Dawson, and Katherine Bowman, *Editors*

Committee on Newborn Screening: Current Landscape and Future Directions

Board on Health Sciences Policy

Board on Children, Youth, and Families

Health and Medicine Division

Consensus Study Report

NATIONAL ACADEMIES PRESS 500 Fifth Street, NW Washington, DC 20001

This activity was supported by contract no. HHSP233201400020B; task order no. 75P00123F37117 between the National Academy of Sciences and the Office on Women's Health of the Department of Health and Human Services and by grant 2023-332496 from the Chan Zuckerberg Initiative DAF, an advised fund of the Silicon Valley Community Foundation. Any opinions, findings, conclusions, or recommendations expressed in this publication do not necessarily reflect the views of any organization or agency that provided support for the project.

International Standard Book Number-13: 978-0-309-99216-9
International Standard Book Number-10: 0-309-99216-8
Digital Object Identifier: https://doi.org/10.17226/29102
Library of Congress Control Number: 2025938256

This publication is available from the National Academies Press, 500 Fifth Street, NW, Keck 360, Washington, DC 20001; (800) 624-6242 or (202) 334-3313; http://www.nap.edu.

Copyright 2025 by the National Academy of Sciences. National Academies of Sciences, Engineering, and Medicine and National Academies Press and the graphical logos for each are all trademarks of the National Academy of Sciences. All rights reserved.

Printed in the United States of America.

Suggested citation: National Academies of Sciences, Engineering, and Medicine. 2025. *Newborn screening in the United States: A vision for sustaining and advancing excellence.* Washington, DC: National Academies Press. https://doi.org/10.17226/29102.

The **National Academy of Sciences** was established in 1863 by an Act of Congress, signed by President Lincoln, as a private, nongovernmental institution to advise the nation on issues related to science and technology. Members are elected by their peers for outstanding contributions to research. Dr. Marcia McNutt is president.

The **National Academy of Engineering** was established in 1964 under the charter of the National Academy of Sciences to bring the practices of engineering to advising the nation. Members are elected by their peers for extraordinary contributions to engineering. Dr. Tsu-Jae Liu is president.

The **National Academy of Medicine** (formerly the Institute of Medicine) was established in 1970 under the charter of the National Academy of Sciences to advise the nation on medical and health issues. Members are elected by their peers for distinguished contributions to medicine and health. Dr. Victor J. Dzau is president.

The three Academies work together as the **National Academies of Sciences, Engineering, and Medicine** to provide independent, objective analysis and advice to the nation and conduct other activities to solve complex problems and inform public policy decisions. The National Academies also encourage education and research, recognize outstanding contributions to knowledge, and increase public understanding in matters of science, engineering, and medicine.

Learn more about the National Academies of Sciences, Engineering, and Medicine at **www.nationalacademies.org**.

Consensus Study Reports published by the National Academies of Sciences, Engineering, and Medicine document the evidence-based consensus on the study's statement of task by an authoring committee of experts. Reports typically include findings, conclusions, and recommendations based on information gathered by the committee and the committee's deliberations. Each report has been subjected to a rigorous and independent peer-review process, and it represents the position of the National Academies on the statement of task.

Proceedings published by the National Academies of Sciences, Engineering, and Medicine chronicle the presentations and discussions at a workshop, symposium, or other event convened by the National Academies. The statements and opinions contained in proceedings are those of the participants and are not endorsed by other participants, the planning committee, or the National Academies.

Rapid Expert Consultations published by the National Academies of Sciences, Engineering, and Medicine are authored by subject-matter experts on narrowly focused topics that can be supported by a body of evidence. The discussions contained in rapid expert consultations are considered those of the authors and do not contain policy recommendations. Rapid expert consultations are reviewed by the institution before release.

For information about other products and activities of the National Academies, please visit www.nationalacademies.org/about/whatwedo.

COMMITTEE ON NEWBORN SCREENING: CURRENT LANDSCAPE AND FUTURE DIRECTIONS

JEWEL MULLEN (*Chair*), University of Texas at Austin Dell Medical School
DON BAILEY, Genomics and Translational Research Center, RTI International
MEI BAKER, University of Wisconsin School of Medicine and Public Health
WENDY K. CHUNG, Boston Children's Hospital and Harvard Medical School
TITILOPE A. FASIPE, Texas Children's Hospital and Baylor College of Medicine
FAITH FLETCHER, Baylor College of Medicine
MEGHAN HALLEY, Stanford University
AMANDA INGRAM, Tennessee Department of Health
JOSÉ A. PAGÁN, New York University
JOCHEN PROFIT, Stanford University; California Perinatal Quality Care Collaborative; and California Maternal Quality Care Collaborative
SCOTT M. SHONE, North Carolina State Laboratory of Public Health
KAYTE SPECTOR-BAGDADY, University of Michigan Medical School
BETH A. TARINI, Children's National Hospital
KRYSTAL TSOSIE, Arizona State University and Native BioData Consortium

Study Staff

KATHERINE BOWMAN, Study Codirector, Senior Program Officer
EMILY PACKARD DAWSON, Study Codirector, Program Officer
SARAH BEACHY, Senior Program Officer
GAYATRI SOMAIYA, Senior Program Assistant
MICHAEL BERRIOS, Research Associate
EMILY McDOWELL, Research Associate (*March–June 2024*)
EMILY BACKES, Deputy Board Director, Board on Children, Youth, and Families
CLARE STROUD, Senior Board Director, Board on Health Sciences Policy

Consultants

ANNE JOHNSON, Founder and Lead Science Writer, Creative Science Writing, LLC
SUSANNA HAAS LYONS, Civic Engagement Specialist, Susanna Haas Lyons Consulting

Reviewers

This Consensus Study Report was reviewed in draft form by individuals chosen for their diverse perspectives and technical expertise. The purpose of this independent review is to provide candid and critical comments that will assist the National Academies of Sciences, Engineering, and Medicine in making each published report as sound as possible and to ensure that it meets the institutional standards for quality, objectivity, evidence, and responsiveness to the study charge. The review comments and draft manuscript remain confidential to protect the integrity of the deliberative process.

We thank the following individuals for their review of this report:

STANTON L. BERBERICH, The University of Iowa
JOAN M. DUWVE, Indiana University, Indianapolis
ALEX KEMPER, Nationwide Children's Hospital
ANNIE KENNEDY, EveryLife Foundation for Rare Diseases
SYLVIA MANN, Hawaii Department of Health
JELILI OJODU, Association of Public Health Laboratories
NATALIE RAM, University of Maryland
CHARLENE SON RIGBY, Global Genes
LAINIE FRIEDMAN ROSS, University of Rochester
WILLIAM M. SAGE, Texas A&M University
SARAH VIALL, Oregon Health & Science University
AMBROISE WONKAM, Johns Hopkins University

Although the reviewers listed above provided many constructive comments and suggestions, they were not asked to endorse the conclusions or recommendations of this report nor did they see the final draft before its release. The review of this report was overseen by **ELI Y. ADASHI,** Brown University, and **ZULFIQAR A. BHUTTA,** The Hospital for Sick Children, University of Toronto. They were responsible for making certain that an independent examination of this report was carried out in accordance with the standards of the National Academies and that all review comments were carefully considered. Responsibility for the final content rests entirely with the authoring committee and the National Academies.

Acknowledgments

The committee would like to express its sincere gratitude to the speakers and panelists who shared their insights with the committee and those who responded to an online questionnaire and participated in virtual listening sessions as part of the study's call for input, and the many organizations that shared information about the study and opportunities for engagement through their networks.

The committee is grateful to the Susanna Haas Lyons Consulting team, including Susanna Haas Lyons, civic engagement specialist; Anson Ching, civic engagement specialist; and Kiana Alaei, data analyst, for their design, thoughtful facilitation, and careful analysis of the results of the engagement activities, and to the additional National Academies staff members and Mirzayan Science and Technology Policy fellows who served as facilitators and note-takers for the listening sessions: Kathryn Asalone, Constanza Vidal Bustamente, Eva Childers, Rayane Silva Curran, Lotte de Jong, Michelle Drewry, Clara Herrera, Alexis Myers, Wesley Schnapp, Maya Thirkill, and Justin Wang. The committee is also grateful for the many contributions of Anne Johnson, science writer, Eva Childers, assistance with figures, along with the National Academies Research Center for assistance with fact checking.

Contents

PREFACE — xix

ACRONYMS AND ABBREVIATIONS — xxiii

SUMMARY — 1

1 INTRODUCTION — 19
History of Newborn Screening, 20
Concepts Underpinning Public Health Newborn Screening, 23
Emerging Tensions in Public Health Newborn Screening, 25
Study Scope and Approach, 27
Organization of the Report, 30
References, 31

**2 CURRENT LANDSCAPE OF NEWBORN SCREENING
IN THE UNITED STATES** — 35
Overview of Public Health Newborn Screening
  in the United States, 36
Disorders Included in Public Health Newborn Screening, 44
Implementation of NBS Programs, 52
Collection and Use of Blood Spots, 59
Follow-Up Care, 64
Research Programs, 66
Conclusions, 68
References, 69

3 GROUNDING NBS DECISION MAKING IN ETHICAL PRINCIPLES AND VALUES 79

Examining Newborn Screening as a Public Health Service, 79
Establishing a Foundation for Aligned and Consistent
  Decision Making, 81
Understanding Community Views to Inform Ethically Grounded
  Decision Making, 83
A Path Forward for Public Health Newborn Screening
  Grounded in Bioethical Foundations, 90
Examples of Prior Approaches to Ethical Decision Making in
  Newborn Screening, 94
Principles and Values Central to Excellence in Public Health
  Newborn Screening, 96
Public Health Newborn Screening for the Era Ahead:
  This Report's Approach, 101
Conclusions, 108
References, 108

4 SUPPORTING AND SUSTAINING HIGH-PERFORMING NBS PROGRAMS 117

NBS Programs at the Core of the Public Health NBS Effort, 117
Screening and Case Management, 118
NBS Program Data Collection and Performance Management, 123
Ensuring NBS Program Excellence in a Performance
  Framework, 126
Program Sustainability 133
Conclusions, 148
References, 150

5 THE RESPONSIBLE APPLICATION OF EMERGING TECHNOLOGIES IN PUBLIC HEALTH NEWBORN SCREENING 157

Current Landscape of DNA-Based Tests in the
  NBS Ecosystem, 157
Considerations for Incorporating Genomic Sequencing into
  Public Health Newborn Screening, 162
Conclusions, 174
References, 174

6 THE RESEARCH ENTERPRISE RELEVANT TO NEWBORN SCREENING 181

The Importance of Research to Inform Newborn Screening, 182
The Intersection of NBS Research and Rare Disease Research, 188

The Landscape of NBS Research, 190
Challenges in the Evidence-Generation Process, 194
Addressing Unmet Needs in NBS Research, 201
Conclusions, 205
References, 206

7 **ENVISIONING THE FUTURE OF NEWBORN SCREENING** 213
Recommendations, 214
References, 235

APPENDIXES
A Information Sources and Methods 237
B Committee Member and Staff Biographies 243

Boxes, Figures, and Tables

BOXES

S-1 Summary of Recommendations: A Road Map Forward, 4

1-1 Newborn Screening in the United States, 25
1-2 Statement of Task, 28

2-1 Terms Relevant to the Screening and Diagnosis of Conditions, 39
2-2 Key Players Across the Broader NBS Ecoystem, 41
2-3 Federal Partners Involved in Newborn Screening, 42
2-4 Case Study: SCID, 50
2-5 Variability Across State and Territorial NBS Programs, 54

3-1 Criteria Proposed by Wilson and Jungner for Public Health Disease Screening Programs, 94

4-1 State and Territorial-Level Differences in Testing for Cystic Fibrosis Variants and Their Effects on Perpetuating Health Disparities, 121
4-2 Timeliness in Public Health Newborn Screening of Dried Blood Spots, 122
4-3 Two Examples of Models to Support Excellence in Public Health Newborn Screening, 131

5-1 Genomic Sequencing Defined, 158
5-2 Ongoing Newborn Sequencing Studies, 161
5-3 Frameworks for Ethical Genomics Data Use and Sharing, 171
5-4 Selected Questions to Address Before Considering Applying Genomic Sequencing to Public Health Newborn Screening, 173

6-1 Areas of Research for Artificial Intelligence and Machine Learning in Newborn Screening, 186
6-2 Selected Questions to Address as Part of NBS Research, 189
6-3 Examples of NBS-Related Studies Enabled by a Coordinated Research Network, 204

7-1 Goals to Be Addressed with Increased National Vision and Coordination, 216
7-2 Selected Challenges in Public Health Newborn Screening Requiring National Coordination to Address, 216
7-3 Selected Examples of Starting Points and Near-Term Actions, 234

FIGURES

S-1 A summary of recommendations: A road map forward, 4

1-1 Timeline of federal action related to newborn screening, 23

2-1 Basic steps in the NBS process, 37
2-2 Players in the NBS ecosystem, 44
2-3 The process for adding a condition to the Recommended Uniform Screening Panel (RUSP) and the roles of various players involved, 46
2-4 Recommended Uniform Screening Panel decision matrix, 48

5-1 Staged approach to molecular analysis in public health newborn screening, 159
5-2 Composition of ancestral groups included in gnomAD, 168

6-1 NBS iceberg, 183

7-1 Summary of recommendations: A road map forward, 214

TABLES

S-1   An Action Agenda for the NBS Ecosystem, 16

3-1   Several Dimensions of Equity and Their Relevance to Newborn Screening, 100

4-1   Examples of Data NBS Programs Could Commit to Collect to Understand Performance Around Selected Performance Goals, 126

4-2   Support from HRSA and CDC for State and Territorial Public Health NBS Programs, 128

Preface

As a former state and federal public health leader, I always considered participating in National Academies studies a continuation of my public service. When asked to chair the Committee on the Current Landscape and Future Directions of Newborn Screening, I recognized my additional privilege and responsibility to promote the individual contributions of fellow committee members—experts in research, ethics, law, economics, laboratory science, and public health—that also volunteered their time. Equally important to me was to discern and respect the excellence of National Academies staff who are the backbone of our work. Our committee had accepted the charge to accelerate through 12 months of collective learning and deliberation to recommend ways to strengthen newborn screening, one of the nation's greatest twentieth century public health achievements. Great public health achievements, such as early detection of heritable conditions in newborns to reduce their associated morbidity and mortality, should not just be historic. Their beneficial effects must extend to future generations.

That goal informed the congressional directive to the U.S. Department of Health and Human Services Office on Women's Health to commission a National Academies study to make newborn screening programs stronger and more resilient to the challenges the future holds. The Chan Zuckerberg Initiative further supported our work, affording a community engagement component that elucidated viewpoints from people and groups professionally and personally affected by newborn screening and rare diseases. As chair, I especially appreciated that since there is no singular or one-size-fits-all approach to engaging communities, our committee members also amplified perspectives of members of the rare disease community with whom they worked closely. Those perspectives fostered our consistent recognition that to uphold equity, our recommendations must extend to groups with the most common rare conditions and to those with the rarest and still undiagnosed disorders.

Our committee's tasks included recommending an approach to improving current state-run screening programs, adding new conditions to screening panels, modernizing laboratory infrastructure, incorporating and scaling new technologies, and ensuring equitable longitudinal follow-up and quality of life. We also aimed to provide an analysis of potential screening-associated harms and benefits to individuals, families, and society. Informed by longstanding guidance, such as Wilson and Junger's principles for screening, we adhered to principles of public health and research ethics as well as legal policy as we undertook each task. Because of this approach, the committee's considerations on trust, transparency, consent, use of dried blood spots, equity, education, and program quality weave throughout many chapters, rather than residing as single topics.

As we listened to presenters at our three public workshops, our committee quickly determined our imperatives to delineate the functions and future for effective and coordinated governmental public health newborn screening and to differentiate them from newborn screening research, including the application of emerging technologies. We also heard and agreed with the observations and advice of public health, legal, and ethical scholars that it is critical to uphold the current opt-out approach to public health newborn screening so it can remain accessible to every infant born in the United States. The message to uphold trust and transparency to preserve newborn screening as a core public health program also resounded, as did the need to establish additional ways to educate a diverse public about its benefits. We acknowledged the call to support high-quality programs and expertise across all states and to measure their performance and impact. Our committee's recommendation to establish stronger national coordination, leadership, and guidance may help accomplish those goals.

As we valued the current—and anticipated the future—use of new and advanced technologies, the committee was also clear that they are not a replacement for public health newborn screening. Our recommendations for strengthening newborn screening programs are not an effort to maintain the status quo. Increasing the resilience of the system against future challenges, including the application of innovative technologies, entails protecting program integrity by upholding transparency, trust, equity, ethics, and quality across public health programs, research, *and* technological advancement.

In closing, I am grateful for the collegiality and excellent contributions of my fellow committee members. Each one exemplified a commitment to public service, intellectual humility, and collaboration that made my undertaking this work a joy. I also recognize the unflagging support, expertise, and equanimity of our leaders, Katherine Bowman, senior program officer, and Emily Packard Dawson, program officer; the partnering coordination of Gayatri Somaiya, senior program assistant; and the contributions of additional project staff Emily Backes, Sarah Beachy, and Michael Berrios. Lastly, I commend the work of every person and organization that partners to ensure every child can benefit from the promise of newborn screening.

Jewel Mullen, *Chair*
Committee on Newborn Screening: Current Landscape and Future Directions

Acronyms and Abbreviations

ACHDNC	Advisory Committee on Heritable Disorders in Newborns and Children
ACMG	American College of Medical Genetics and Genomics
AHRQ	Agency for Healthcare Research and Quality
APHA	American Public Health Association
APHL	Association of Public Health Laboratories
CDC	Centers for Disease Control and Prevention
CDE	common data element
CF	cystic fibrosis
CFTR	cystic fibrosis transmembrane conductance regulator (protein involved in CF)
DBS	dried blood spot
DCC	data coordination center
eCR	electronic case reporting
ED3N	Enhancing Data-driven Disease Detection in Newborns
EHR	electronic health record
ELC	Epidemiology and Laboratory Capacity
ELSI	ethical, legal, and social issues
ERG	Evidence Review Group
FDA	Food and Drug Administration

GAO	Government Accountability Office
gnomAD	Genome Aggregation Database
HHS	U.S. Department of Health and Human Services
HRSA	Health Resources and Services Administration
ICoNS	International Consortium of Newborn Sequencing
LIMS	laboratory information management system
LPDR	Longitudinal Pediatric Data Resource
NBS	newborn screening
NBS Co-Propel	Cooperative Newborn Screening System Priorities Program
NBS Excel	National Center for Newborn Screening System Excellence
NBS Propel	State Newborn Screening System Priorities Program
NBSTRN	Newborn Screening Translational Research Network
NBSxWGS	Newborn Screening by Whole-Genome Sequencing
NCATS	National Center for Advancing Translational Sciences
NewSTEPs	Newborn Screening Technical assistance and Evaluation Program
NGS	next-generation sequencing
NHGRI	National Human Genetics Research Institute
NICHD	*Eunice Kennedy Shriver* National Institute on Child Health and Human Development
NIH	National Institutes of Health
NSIGHT	Newborn Sequencing in Genomic Medicine and Public Health
NSQAP	Newborn Screening Quality Assurance Program
PAG	patient advocacy group
PCR	polymerase chain reaction
PKU	phenylketonuria
RCDC	Research, Condition, and Disease Categorization
RUSP	Recommended Uniform Screening Panel
SCID	severe combined immunodeficiency
SMA	spinal muscular atrophy
VRDBS	virtual repository of dried blood spots
VUS	variant of uncertain significance (genetic)
WHO	World Health Organization

Summary[1]

Newborn screening (NBS) is a public health service available to approximately 3.6 million infants born in the United States each year. Over 98 percent of those infants receive screening. State and territorial-run NBS programs identify babies at risk of serious but treatable conditions and connect them to a provider for confirmatory testing, treatment, and follow-up care with the goal of providing the best chance at a healthy life. Newborn screening encompasses dried blood spot, hearing loss, and congenital heart defect testing; however, the focus of this report is dried blood spot screening in the United States. The public health impacts of dried blood spot newborn screening are felt across society but perhaps most profoundly by the over 7,000 infants identified annually for timely intervention, along with their families and caregivers. Public health newborn screening is implemented through 56 state- and territorial-run programs and buttressed by the contributions of multiple federal agencies, laboratory and clinical professional communities, health care providers, patient advocacy groups, researchers from academia and industry, and others.

Public health newborn screening faces both longstanding and emerging challenges. Processes for adding conditions to the federal Recommended Uniform Screening Panel (RUSP) and state and territorial NBS panels have come under scrutiny for their limited capacity to keep pace

---

[1] This summary does not include reference citations. References for the information herein are provided in the full report.

with therapeutic developments, and for the burden these processes place on patient advocacy communities and others. NBS programs and professionals need to maintain high-quality services in a resource-constrained environment as screening panels expand. The potential use of genomic sequencing in newborn screening raises scientific and technical questions, as well as social, ethical, legal, and policy questions, including privacy concerns over genomic data. Legal challenges over retaining and reusing residual dried blood spots have led to the destruction of millions of specimens. Ultimately, public health NBS programs must balance their mandate to screen all newborns with the individual needs and rights of each child and their family.

Public health newborn screening also contends with multiple dimensions of variability. Although differences across NBS programs are inevitable and may even be beneficial, variability can be detrimental when driven by insufficient resources or when it negatively affects health outcomes. Insufficient representation of genetic ancestries in databases results in higher rates of false positives and negatives on DNA-based screening assays for infants of non-European descent. Infants from underserved communities experience longer wait times to confirmatory diagnosis and treatment. Issues facing the NBS system intersect with longstanding disparities in the health care system, such as uneven distribution of specialists and differences in insurance coverage or access to new therapies. Although not within the purview of public health newborn screening to address, this landscape impacts the effectiveness of this service in fulfilling its mission.

IMPETUS FOR THE STUDY

Newborn screening as a public heath endeavor is asked to address a complex array of needs, competing priorities, and viewpoints. In response to a congressional request, the Office on Women's Health of the U.S. Department of Health and Human Services (HHS) asked the National Academies of Sciences, Engineering, and Medicine to convene an ad hoc committee to examine the current landscape of newborn screening implementation and research in the United States, recommend options to strengthen public health newborn screening, and establish a vision for the future.[2]

The committee prioritized its efforts toward developing a longer-term vision for newborn screening and a road map to achieve it, recognizing ongoing efforts by federal agencies, state and territorial programs, and

---

[2] Reflecting the complexity of its task, the committee included members with expertise in newborn screening, state and federal public health, lived and parental experience, bioethics and law, existing and emerging screening technologies, health systems, health economics, and clinical care disciplines.

others to address immediate problems within the existing NBS framework. Central to the committee's approach was input from individuals personally and professionally affected by newborn screening. With additional support from the Chan Zuckerberg Initiative, the committee commissioned civic engagement consultants, together with National Academies staff, to hear from multiple sectors of lived and professional experience in newborn screening. The report was also informed by presentations from speakers, published literature, and other sources of evidence.

A ROAD MAP FOR EXCELLENCE IN NEWBORN SCREENING[3]

A central tenet of this report is that a systematic and coordinated approach for public health newborn screening is needed—one that aligns multiple critical partners around shared goals, builds on and enhances connections among the array of efforts and programs already in place, clarifies essential functions and responsibilities, and supports public health NBS excellence now and into the future. The following recommendations reflect priorities to achieve these aims and identify core actors to champion each one within a holistic vision (see Box S-1). Collectively, the recommendations outline a path to navigate the choices facing dried blood spot newborn screening in the United States while preserving and enhancing what is already considered a valuable and effective public health achievement.

The mission of public health newborn screening is to reduce morbidity and mortality for identified infants, and NBS programs are responsible for detecting and connecting those infants with clinical care. Aligning with this mission entails a focus on conditions that are serious, urgent, and have a therapeutic intervention rigorously shown to reduce morbidity and/or mortality in affected infants when delivered in the presymptomatic or early symptomatic period. Public health newborn screening has faced pressures to expand its scope to include conditions that are, for example, later onset or have no available treatment, and to consider benefits beyond reducing morbidity and mortality in the affected infant. However, the parameters guiding routine, universal newborn screening as a public health program are necessarily narrow because of its population-level nature.

Public health newborn screening cannot and should not be the sole or even the primary solution to broader needs in rare disease identification, diagnosis, treatment, and research or to longstanding challenges around access and capacity in the clinical care system. Complementary investments at the nexus of public health, clinical care, and research remain essential.

---

[3] The report focuses on critical functions and actions to strengthen public health newborn screening for the future; descriptions of the roles and structures of federal and nonfederal activities relevant to newborn screening are current as of March 24, 2025.

> **BOX S-1**
> **Summary of Recommendations: A Road Map Forward**
>
> Public health newborn screening requires a systems approach to align multiple parties around shared goals and opportunities. Decision making for public health newborn screening must be aligned with the purpose of universal screening to reduce morbidity and mortality for infants with serious but treatable diseases through connection to diagnosis and care. It must be evidence based as it encompasses technological and therapeutic advances, adds or removes conditions based on clear and consistent criteria, and promulgates national standards and guidance. All 56 state- and territorial-run programs must be equipped to provide excellent, high-quality services to all babies. The following near-term actions and foundational changes can prepare newborn screening for the future.
>
>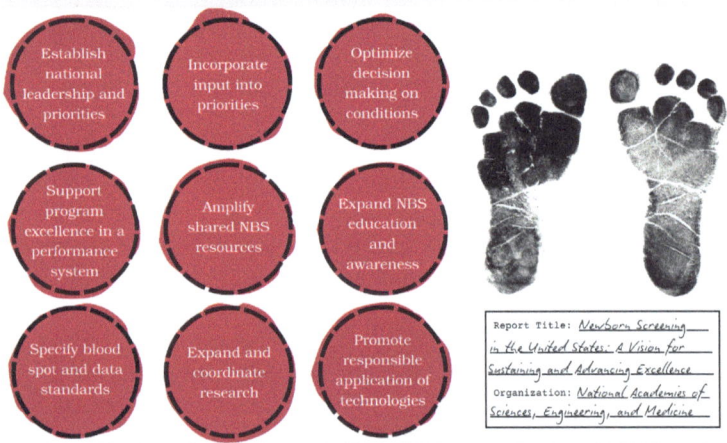
>
> **FIGURE S-1** A summary of recommendations: A road map forward.

This report's recommendations reinforce longstanding calls to address areas such as public awareness of newborn screening, program capacity, continuous quality improvement, evidence generation, and the diagnostic and care impacts experienced by patients with rare diseases, their families, and communities. Efforts supporting NBS excellence already exist among state and territorial NBS programs and state public health services; federal partners such as the Health Resources and Service Administration (HRSA), Centers for Disease Control and Prevention, National Institutes of Health (NIH), Food and Drug Administration, and Agency for Healthcare Research and Quality; and the HHS Advisory Committee for Heritable Disorders in Newborns and Children (ACHDNC). NBS excellence is also being advanced through efforts among disease and community organizations, researchers, and technology developers to enhance the evidence base on which public health newborn screening relies, through professional organizations to collect and analyze data and develop and provide educational resources, and through the activities of many additional organizations and individuals. However, these efforts are subject to variable and often temporary funding, and participation is largely voluntary and ad hoc. Federal programs often require NBS program staff to identify challenges, locate prospective resources, draw on personal networks and contacts, and prepare competitive grant applications, leading to variable participation.

Achieving the report's recommendations will require cooperative action to build on these foundations and extend them to establish a framework in which crucial partners are aligned around a set of shared priorities, supported through sufficient resources and time, and bolstered by infrastructure to support excellence consistently throughout public health newborn screening.

Establish National Vision, Coordination, and Leadership

The lack of a coordinated national approach to public health newborn screening with appropriate resources, accountability, and strategy hampers progress toward an excellent system nationwide. Those involved in newborn screening are committed to its success and work diligently within their spheres, but goals and efforts can misalign. Each of the 56 NBS programs needs to understand whether they are providing high-quality services for all babies born in their jurisdiction while lacking authority over many of their critical NBS partners and contending with varied resources and capacities. The next era of public health newborn screening needs to embrace opportunities for greater national coordination, priority setting, and guidance while leveraging and respecting the autonomy and local expertise of state- and territorial-run programs as well as the unique roles of federal agencies.

Federal leadership, accountability, resources, and coordination are needed to mobilize partners in the NBS ecosystem to implement the actions identified by the set of recommendations in this report, create intentionality within a landscape that is highly fragmented, and ultimately bring resources, authority, and capacity to the national patchwork quilt of public health newborn screening.

Recommendation 1: Establish national leadership and set priorities. The U.S. Department of Health and Human Services (HHS) should provide unified leadership, accountability, and

coordination across government agencies, newborn screening (NBS) programs, and the broader NBS community.

   a. With input from partners (see Recommendation 2), HHS should establish a 10-year strategic plan based on this report's recommendations and begin to implement them.
   b. HHS should designate a mechanism with appropriate authority, accountability, and resources to facilitate realization of this plan.

Newborn screening is experienced by infants and their families and carried out and supported by a large network that spans public health, clinical care, research, government, advocacy, and private companies. Achieving the report's recommendations will also require representation from the full complement of personally and professionally affected groups to provide essential input and galvanize action. Newborn screening touches a complex nexus of federal, state, tribal, and private rights and responsibilities. Additional conversations are needed with tribal nations and leaders to understand these intersecting rights and authorities, to involve tribal communities in the national vision for newborn screening, and to ensure that priorities and solutions meet the needs of Indigenous communities.

Recommendation 2: Incorporate multistakeholder and rightsholder input into newborn screening priorities.[4] The U.S. Department of Health and Human Services should establish a multistakeholder/rightsholder advisory body to provide input to the national leadership identified in Recommendation 1. This advisory body should identify high-level, cross-agency, cross-state, and cross-system challenges; elevate potential solutions to those challenges; inform the development of a strategic plan; and monitor and advise on progress in its implementation. The advisory body should engage wide-ranging expertise and experiences to inform the strategic plan and enable all partners to understand their role in driving it forward.

Currently, the discretionary HHS ACHDNC provides recommendations to the HHS secretary on newborn and childhood screening. The scope of ACHDNC's mandate is theoretically broad, and has encompassed discussions around timeliness, long-term follow up, and

---

[4] The term *rightsholder* is incorporated to recognize use of this term among Native American and Indigenous communities and to reflect their distinct legal and political contexts.

laboratory standards, among other issues. However, its attention and actions are primarily directed toward reviewing conditions for inclusion on the RUSP. This emphasis is responsive to the importance of evidence-based decision making but limits ACHDNC's capacity to focus on overarching strategy, and its current membership does not comprise the full breadth of expertise and experiences that would be necessary for this more strategic advisory mission. As currently designed, ACHDNC and other existing avenues (e.g., state advisory boards, professional society working groups, symposia) are not suitable for this role, which requires broader expertise and connection to national leadership to provide authority, accountability, and resources to enact the vision informed by this advisory body.

The multistakeholder/rightsholder advisory body called for in Recommendation 2 could be established in different ways, including as a formal federal advisory committee realizing the full scope of ACHDNC's mandate or through other federal or nongovernmental convening mechanisms. A wide range of expertise and perspectives will be needed, including

- state and territorial NBS program directors, laboratory experts, and follow-up experts;
- prenatal and birth care providers;
- health care professionals such as genetic counselors, pediatricians, and disease specialists;
- members reflecting family and rare disease community organizations and perspectives;
- representatives from the multiple federal agencies supporting public health newborn screening;
- philanthropic organizations active in this area; and
- the private sector.

Federal guidance on which conditions to include in state NBS panels—the RUSP—was established in 2010. Although not a mandate, the RUSP remains an important source of evidence-based guidance, and striving for RUSP alignment promotes consistency across NBS programs. However, the current process for incorporating new conditions onto the RUSP is long, taking an average of 3 to 4 years (not including additional time at the state NBS level); it is burdensome for advocacy organizations that often shoulder the weight of attracting the attention and funding that drive evidence generation to support consideration for the RUSP; and it is frustrating for all.

Recommendation 3: Optimize decision making on conditions included in newborn screening. The U.S. Department of Health and Human Services (HHS) and state and territorial newborn

screening (NBS) programs should optimize the process of considering conditions in public health newborn screening:

a. HHS leadership should designate a focused committee or mechanism to provide advice on the Recommended Uniform Screening Panel (RUSP), composed of appropriate experts and distinct from the strategic advisory body in Recommendation 2. In addition to advising on nominated conditions, this committee should (1) proactively assess which conditions could meet criteria for inclusion on the RUSP; (2) identify specific gaps in evidence necessary for RUSP decision making for conditions identified in this assessment and highlight what strategic research is needed (see Recommendation 8); and (3) periodically reassess evidence and consider whether RUSP removal is warranted for any condition based on knowledge gained from its implementation in public health newborn screening.
b. HHS leadership should expand the scientific and technical capacity for reviewing evidence for conditions under consideration for addition to the RUSP, including exploring the applicability of rapid review mechanisms.
c. State and territorial NBS programs should have a mechanism to consider implementation of RUSP conditions within a designated time line.

There are no simple answers for streamlining the RUSP evaluation process, and actions in Recommendation 3 represent a starting point. This recommendation could be achieved by focusing and enhancing the ACHDNC's current mission. In the face of genomic sequencing technologies and ongoing therapeutic advances for rare diseases, groundwork needs to be laid for a future when an increased number of conditions that meet the inclusion criteria for newborn screening could be incorporated into the screening process. Exploring the implications of adopting or adapting alternative evidence-review processes may be a promising opportunity. Periodically reexamining the process for adding conditions to the RUSP would provide opportunities to revise it in light of an enhanced NBS system and future developments in platform screening technologies.

The scope of evidence evaluation for optimized RUSP decision making would need to include relevant scientific, clinical, and technical aspects of the condition; the disease's effects and treatments; and implementation in public health screening. Issues related to NBS program operational feasibility are better addressed through supports to state-level programs. As conditions are added to the RUSP, every state or territory needs a mechanism to consider these conditions in a timely manner, even if screening is not ultimately implemented. Successful implementation of high-quality screening across programs—and addressing operational barriers to including conditions on state and territorial NBS panels—will require more robust systems of support (see Recommendations 4 and 5).

Promote High Performance Among All NBS Programs

Variability is innate to any federated system, and state-run newborn screening is no different. States have the authority and knowledge to implement NBS programs to serve their constituents and comply with local requirements. Variability among programs can be beneficial as states are best situated to tailor their approach to the unique needs of their own population and jurisdiction, pilot different approaches and develop best practices, and act as resources among program peers. Other variability is detrimental, however, when it arises from insufficient resources or support and negatively affects health outcomes. All programs must achieve and maintain excellence in the core functions necessary to deliver on the promise of universal newborn screening.

Conclusion 4-1: While respecting the autonomy of each state and territorial NBS public health program to meet the needs of its population, all programs need to be accountable for achieving certain essential functions:

- *Provide every infant born in the state or territory with the opportunity to receive screening for a set of serious, urgent, and treatable conditions.*
- *Provide NBS educational materials to all state/territorial prenatal and birth providers.*
- *Strive for high-quality, timely screening designed to perform accurately for all members of the population.*
- *Ensure high-quality and timely case management for every infant screened. This includes directly communicating out-of-range results for infants to their providers, and ultimately to the family/caregiver, as well as confirming those infants are connected to further evaluation or care by documenting diagnoses. This also includes reporting in-range results such that every infant's results are communicated to their provider, and ultimately to the family/caregiver.*
- *Establish and maintain systems for quality assurance, program excellence, and performance improvement.*

Strengthening the network of NBS programs so all 56 have what they need to achieve high performance requires more systematic data collection and analysis and more strategic alignment of financial and nonfinancial supports and incentives for program participation and quality improvement.

> Recommendation 4: Support newborn screening (NBS) program excellence in performance system. The U.S. Department of Health and Human Services (HHS) leadership (Recommendation 1) and state/territorial NBS program directors should partner to establish a universal performance improvement system. Data collected should enable each program to assess its laboratory and follow-up performance, benchmark with peers, and iteratively improve its processes. To accomplish this the following need to occur:
>
> a. HHS should incentivize participation from all programs.
> b. HHS should collaborate with state and territorial NBS program directors to identify a common set of performance metrics all states will collect to monitor and improve laboratory and follow-up performance.
> c. State- and territorial-run NBS programs should agree to participate and commit to using collected data to close gaps and pursue excellence.
> d. HHS should provide responsive financial investment and technical assistance based on performance assessment.

A universal NBS performance system could build on existing efforts and entities that rely on voluntary submission from NBS programs, such as the Association of Public Health Laboratories' (APHL's) Newborn Screening Technical assistance and Evaluation Program (NewSTEPs) data repository and resource center, supported by a grant from HRSA. These efforts have limited or partial participation, and the data collected are not analyzed or used to inform responsive or strategic improvement and support. This recommendation calls for a more effective approach that will require incentives for broad program participation, alignment on a common set of metrics, and responsive funding and technical assistance based on identified performance improvement opportunities beyond existing ad hoc or grant-based federal resources.

NBS programs vary in their resources, expertise, and capacities for advanced technical analysis of newborn blood spots, development and implementation of new screening assays, establishing connections with specialized genetic counseling and clinical care resources for screened conditions, and other factors. Every NBS program does not need to directly house all such capacities, expertise, and resources, but it is essential for each program to have access to these resources when needed. Establishing cross-network infrastructure would aid programs and ensure that resources, especially scarce ones, are used efficiently to strengthen all programs and benefit all infants born across the United States.

Recommendation 5: Amplify newborn screening (NBS) program excellence through shared resources. The U.S. Department of Health and Human Services (HHS) leadership (Recommendation 1) should foster NBS programs' ability to efficiently access and use specialized resources and expertise. To achieve this, HHS should survey NBS program directors to identify each program's capacities, strengths, and sources of specialized expertise in both laboratory and follow-up performance; assess this resulting landscape; and establish infrastructure for more systematic and efficient use of shared resources among programs.

By analyzing the landscape of program capacities and developing a centralized repository of information, the unique strengths, specialized resources, and expertise of different NBS programs can be efficiently used throughout the system to facilitate connections between programs.

Fulfilling Recommendations 4 and 5 would require establishing an implementing mechanism with overall guidance and accountability provided by HHS leadership established in Recommendation 1. Additional strategies to implement this recommendation could include establishing or designating formal or informal centers for expertise providing technical assistance or direct services to partner programs in specific areas. This could include, for example, laboratory testing and implementation, expert clinical management guidance, clinical care handoff, or long-term follow-up. Partnership and resource-sharing agreements may need to be established to enable broad participation in a networked system. HHS would need to provide guidance and support, working in collaboration with NBS program directors.

Strengthen the Trustworthiness of NBS Programs

Limited public awareness about what newborn screening is and why it is undertaken, coupled with recent lawsuits over the storage and use of residual newborn dried blood spots, threaten to undermine trust in newborn screening. Transparency and engagement are needed so programs can continue to earn the trust of the public and provide newborn screening as an essential public health service. To build trust, longstanding calls for more systematic information for parents and caregivers about newborn screening during the perinatal period must be met.

Recommendation 6: Expand public and professional newborn screening (NBS) education and awareness. Engagement with

pregnant individuals, parents, and caregivers should occur at multiple points during the perinatal period. This education should start in the prenatal period and cover the purpose of newborn screening, when and how it will happen, what to expect after blood spot collection, parental options, and communication of the infant's results.

a. All professional associations involved in perinatal and infant care should issue recommendations for communicating about newborn screening with pregnant patients, parents, and/or caregivers and support accurate communication through professional education.
b. The multistakeholder/rightsholder advisory body described in Recommendation 2 should work with relevant professional societies, patient/family organizations, and experts in effective public communication to design goals and communication approaches that can be adapted to local contexts, drawing on existing materials and research.

After NBS tests are completed, residual, or leftover, dried blood spots may remain. These residual dried blood spots are essential for program quality control and assurance efforts. Dried blood spots can also be useful for research. Few consistent policies at the federal, state, tribal,[5] or laboratory level exist for retention and use of dried blood spots and derived data, and parental disclosure or consent policies also vary. The fact that some states have allowed law enforcement access to NBS dried blood spots for criminal or civil liability also raises legal and public trust concerns. This is a controversial area, subject to recent and ongoing litigation. Developing clear and transparent federal and state protections for dried blood spot and derived data retention, sharing, and use is necessary to act in trustworthy ways and avoid federal constitutional challenge.

Recommendation 7: Specify standards for the retention, sharing, and use of newborn dried blood spots and derived data.

a. State legislatures should set law and policy for the retention, sharing, and use of newborn dried blood spots and any derived data. These policies and laws should do the following:
   i. Protect the retention of newborn screening (NBS) dried blood spots for at least a limited period for primary

---

[5] Additional clarifications may be needed to understand legal authorities over newborn dried blood spots collected in tribal health care settings, jurisdiction of tribal data sovereignty, and applicable state laws governing NBS programs.

public health screening goals including, but not limited to, retesting samples, quality assessment, and quality improvement.
ii. Set transparent practices for the retention, sharing, and use of dried blood spots for purposes other than those described above, including research.
iii. Allow parents the option to request the destruction of their child's specimen after the limited time period of retention for primary public health screening goals, and allow the dried blood spot contributor the option to request the destruction of their own specimen when they reach the age of 18.
iv. Prohibit the sharing or use of NBS dried blood spots and derived data to conduct criminal, civil, or administrative investigations and/or impose criminal, civil, or administrative liability on the NBS contributor or blood relatives.
b. The U.S. Department of Health and Human Services (HHS) leadership (Recommendation 1) should provide national guidance or recommendations on these standards.
c. HHS leadership and state legislatures should establish additional guidance if NBS programs begin implementing genomic sequencing methods that increase the generation and identifiability of sensitive data.

Preparing Newborn Screening for the Future

Evidence is needed to guide decision making about NBS policies and practice. However, research providing such evidence is often funded and completed too late to inform programmatic and policy decision making, not responsive to the most pressing needs of the system, or comprised of multiple small studies limiting the ability to draw clear conclusions and hindering the impact of NBS research investments. Indexing newborn screening in the NIH Research, Condition, and Disease Categorization system would also improve assessment of the federal government's investment in NBS research, particularly for investigator-initiated funding.

A national plan with associated research infrastructure would help ensure that research informing newborn screening is more strategic, coordinated, nimble, and has allocated sufficient resources to provide the evidence needed for newborn screening to adapt to a rapidly changing landscape.

Recommendation 8: Expand and coordinate research to inform newborn screening (NBS) policy and practice. The U.S. Department of Health and Human Services should establish an NBS research network with centers that address system-level research priorities in a coordinated and nimble manner. This network of research centers should operate in partnership with state/territorial NBS public health programs as appropriate to carry out research in the following areas:

a. Defining diseases to guide screening, diagnosis, and treatment.
b. Developing laboratory tests and applying emerging technologies.
c. Understanding ethical, legal, and social issues.
d. Investigating public health practice, feasibility, and impact.

Involving patient advocacy groups in an NBS research network would facilitate bidirectional communication to inform responsive research. Centers in the network would work together to generate evidence to address high-priority issues, improve the process of conducting NBS research, and inform analyses around delivery, quality, cost, and outcomes. Investing more systematically and strategically in NBS research would also help advance rare disease research by informing the development of treatments and other related priorities. This recommendation is not meant to replace all federally funded investigator-initiated NBS research, which remains important in promoting creativity and elevating questions identified by investigators throughout the community. In addition, the network resources need to be accessible to outside investigators.

The application of new technologies to newborn screening has garnered significant attention and investment. The use of emerging technologies by NBS programs must be considered through the lens of achieving, rather than changing, the goals of universal, public health newborn screening. Therefore, decisions on the inclusion and role of emerging technologies require the same level of scrutiny, analysis, and alignment with public health values and principles as any other decision affecting the practice of public health newborn screening.

One of the technologies currently attracting the greatest interest, research attention, and momentum is DNA sequencing, which is already used in limited ways in some NBS programs. New approaches for genomic sequencing could facilitate screening for all genetic conditions that meet the inclusion criteria for newborn screening using a single platform as a first step.[6] Such approaches could generate a tremendous amount of data—much of which would not be relevant to newborn screening as

---

[6] DNA sequencing across the entire genome is often referred to as *whole genome sequencing* (WGS). This term can be misinterpreted as it suggests that the genome is fully sequenced, analyzed, and reported in its entirety. WGS may generate data across the genome, but not all the sequencing data are typically analyzed and interpreted into reportable results. This report uses the term *genomic sequencing* to avoid this confusion.

a public health initiative. The use of genomic sequencing for panels of conditions that align with the goals of public health newborn screening has promise, but technical, ethical, psychosocial, and implementation questions would need to be addressed before this technology could be implemented as a primary NBS approach outside of consented study contexts. Key questions can guide the investments and activities of funders and investigators across government, academia, nonprofit organizations, and industry.

> **Recommendation 9: Promote the responsible application of technologies to newborn screening (NBS).** Funders and investigators of feasibility studies should address the following key scientific, technical, ethical, and implementation questions before considering genomic sequencing for public health newborn screening:
>
> a. What sequence should be generated, what sequence/variants should be analyzed and interpreted, and what results should be returned?
> b. What strategies are necessary to ensure the accuracy of variant interpretation across ancestral populations?
> c. What are public attitudes concerning the application of genomic sequencing into public health newborn screening as a first-tier screening tool?
> d. What data should be stored after screening, if any, and how will the privacy of genomic data be protected given its risk of reidentification?
> e. Is genomic sequencing as a first-tier screening methodology cost-effective?
> f. What funding, resource sharing, and/or distributed system of clinical expertise would be necessary and effective to support employing population-based genomic sequencing as a first-tier tool across NBS programs?

FINAL THOUGHTS

The future of public health newborn screening needs to remain rooted in its fundamental purpose to screen all infants for conditions that are serious, urgent, and treatable, and connect those at risk with diagnosis and care. Delivering on this promise across all states and for all infants will require greater national coordination to align the many partners that support newborn screening and drive forward the recommendations proposed in this report. Table S-1 provides a high-level summary of opportunities for actors throughout the NBS ecosystem to help translate these recommendations into practice.

TABLE S-1 An Action Agenda for the NBS Ecosystem

Actor	Select Action
U.S. Department of Health and Human Services (HHS)	• Provide leadership, accountability, and coordination. • Establish 10-year strategic plan and mechanism to realize this plan. • Establish a multistakeholder/rightsholder advisory body. • Analyze the landscape of conditions that could meet RUSP inclusion, and identify key evidence gaps. • Partner with NBS programs to establish a universal performance improvement system and metrics. • Provide targeted funding for NBS program support based on performance gaps and needs. • Develop a centralized repository of program capacities, strengths, and sources of specialized expertise. • Recommend standards for transparency and trustworthiness in the retention and use of newborn dried blood spots and derived data. • Establish a newborn screening research network.
Federal agency partners	• Participate on the multistakeholder/rightsholder advisory body. • Participate in establishing a universal performance improvement system and metrics. • Participate in providing funding that supports NBS program excellence and advances NBS research priorities.
NBS programs	• Participate on the multistakeholder/rightsholder advisory body. • Be accountable for achieving high performance in essential functions. • Participate in establishing a universal performance improvement system and metrics. • Collect and use metrics to close gaps and pursue excellence. • Identify capacities, strengths, and sources of expertise in laboratory and follow-up performance.
State legislatures	• Establish clear standards and policies for the storage and reuse of residual dried blood spots and derived data. • Support state-run programs to achieve excellence as described in the report's recommendations.
Patient and family organizations	• Participate on the multistakeholder/rightsholder advisory body. • Partner to implement goals and communication approaches around newborn screening. • Inform research priorities through the newborn screening research network.

TABLE S-1 Continued

Actor	Select Action
Health providers and care settings	• Participate on the multistakeholder/rightsholder advisory body. • Partner to implement goals and communication approaches. • Require communication about newborn screening. • Communicate NBS results with parents and caregivers. • Partner to ensure a handoff between public health and clinical care for infants identified as being at risk in screening.
Professional associations and societies	• Participate on the multistakeholder/rightsholder advisory body. • Partner with HHS leadership and NBS programs to help advance report recommendations. • Contribute to the infrastructure and resources available to implement areas such as data collection, performance and quality improvement systems, provider and parent education and training materials, and other priorities.
Researchers in areas relevant to newborn screening	• Participate on the multistakeholder/rightsholder advisory body. • Address high-priority issues for defining diseases; developing assays; understanding ethical, legal, and social issues; and addressing public health impact and feasibility. • Address key questions on the application of emerging technologies.

NOTE: NBS = newborn screening; RUSP = Recommended Uniform Screening Panel.

1

Introduction

Newborn screening (NBS) programs in the United States provide a public health service available to all infants regardless of geographic, ethnic, or socioeconomic differences (Boyle et al., 2014; CDC, 2011). State- and territorial-run NBS public health programs identify babies at risk of serious but treatable conditions, and connect them to follow-up care with the goal of providing the best chance at a healthy life (HRSA, 2023a). Public health newborn screening encompasses dried blood spot, hearing loss, and congenital heart defect testing. Hearing loss and congenital heart defect screening are often referred to as point-of-care testing because these tests are both administered and interpreted at the site of clinical care for the newborn, rather than in a laboratory. Dried blood spot screening, on the other hand, involves collection at the point of clinical care but testing in a designated laboratory (Kemper et al., 2012). This report is focused on U.S. public health newborn screening using dried blood spots.

As a population health initiative, nearly every infant in the United States is screened at birth—by collecting blood from the baby's heel on a special card, typically within the first 24–48 hours—and a small proportion of babies will be identified as at risk for a condition that benefits from early medical intervention (CDC, 2012; HRSA, 2023b). States and territories have authority over the policies and operations of NBS programs within their jurisdictions, while the federal government provides national guidance and some support and coordination. Although each state or territory independently determines what conditions their program will screen, a recommended set of conditions is provided by the secretary of the U.S. Department of Health and Human Services (HHS) with the support of a federal advisory committee. Ultimately, states and territories choose which conditions to screen to address the needs of their populations and comply with factors such as legislative requirements, budgets, workforce availability, technological resources, and the influence of advocacy (Grosse et al., 2016). Among those in public health, newborn screening is considered a great achievement based on its identification of infants with serious, urgent conditions who can receive life-saving treatment and intervention (CDC, 2011).

NBS programs provide a public health service to infants that extends beyond the screening test. Public health professionals play key roles in informing and educating parents of affected newborns and connecting these infants with confirmatory testing and follow-up care in the health care system. Further, NBS programs work with partners in a larger ecosystem that supports identification, follow-up, and treatment of babies. These partners include regulatory agencies, researchers, care providers, payors, advocacy groups, patients, and parents, among others.

HISTORY OF NEWBORN SCREENING

Early Roots in Advocacy

Public health newborn screening was built on a bedrock of advocacy and personal experience, with no clearer example than Robert Guthrie himself—whose work in the 1960s provided the scientific basis for newborn screening. As the father and uncle of children with intellectual disabilities, Guthrie applied his expertise as a medical microbiologist studying cancer toward developing an inexpensive bacterial inhibition assay that allowed for early detection of phenylketonuria (PKU) in newborns (Levy, 2021). PKU is a rare disorder in which buildup of the amino acid phenylalanine leads to brain damage and intellectual disability; early reports suggested that a low phenylalanine diet prevented intellectual disability in children with PKU (Bickel et al., 1953; NHGRI, 2014). The knowledge that intellectual disability from PKU could be prevented hit close to home for Guthrie, whose niece was diagnosed with the rare condition, influencing him to envision universal PKU screening. As a result, the concept of newborn screening was born—with the initial goal of population screening to identify infants at risk of PKU and connect them with prompt diagnosis and treatment (Levy, 2021).

Mandated screening for PKU, performed without parental consent, quickly became widespread, despite calls for further research on the disease pathology, test validity, and treatment outcomes and more cautious implementation (AAP, 1967; Paul, 1998; Rule, 1965). Ultimately, PKU screening prevented intellectual disability for many infants identified with PKU who received treatment; however, there were several unintended consequences including malnutrition for infants with PKU with inappropriate diet management, PKU anxiety syndrome,[1] and the phenomenon of maternal PKU (Brosco et al., 2008; Lenke and Levy, 1980; Paul and Brosco, 2013; Rothenberg and Sills, 1968).[2]

Tandem Mass Spectrometry and the Expansion of Newborn Screening

Following PKU screening, researchers began developing and implementing tests for other conditions (Watson et al., 2022). For decades, the number of conditions that could be screened was limited by the amount of blood available for testing. However, the application of tandem mass spectrometry to newborn screening in the 1990s opened the door to screening for exponentially more conditions. Using this biochemical technology, the levels and patterns of numerous metabolites can be analyzed from a single dried blood spot, enabling more accurate detection of risk for more conditions than previously possible (Chace et al., 2003). Tandem mass spectrometry was incorporated into public health newborn screening by some programs, leading to an increase in both the number of disorders screened and variability across NBS programs in the United States (Tarini, 2007; Tarini et al., 2006).

American Federalism and the Creation of Federal Guidance on Public Health Newborn Screening

State and territorial health policy decisions, including those for public health newborn screening, are made in the context of American federalism—the division of power and responsibilities between national and state roles (Turnock and Atchison, 2002). The relationship between state and federal roles in public health newborn screening has evolved over time. Under the U.S. system, states and territories establish health care practice standards unless Congress determines a significant national

---

[1] In the 1960s, PKU anxiety syndrome was used to describe parents presenting with acute and chronic anxiety after their child received a false-positive screening result. These parents "persisted in their belief" that their infants may have intellectual delays "despite repeat [PKU] negative tests and considerable reassurance and support from physicians" (Rothenberg and Sills, 1968).

[2] Maternal PKU occurs when a pregnant woman with PKU does not have appropriate diet management before and during pregnancy. High levels of phenylalanine in the mother's blood can harm the developing baby and lead to intellectual disability, behavioral problems, and seizures in the baby (Lenke and Levy, 1980; Paul and Brosco, 2013).

policy warrants preemption of these standards (Kraszewski et al., 2006). From the inception of public health newborn screening, states and territories have had the authority to establish and implement NBS programs with the earliest statutes enacted in the 1960s (Levy, 2021). For nearly four decades, state and territorial laws on newborn screening were developed, and this decentralized approach led to variation in policies and practices for NBS programs across the United States.

In the early 2000s, several actions were taken at the federal level to address the variability across state and territorial programs that had developed in the absence of national guidance (HRSA, 2021). First, the federal Advisory Committee on Heritable Disorders in Newborns and Children (ACHDNC) was formed in 2003 as a provision of the Public Health Service Act to advise the secretary of HHS about newborn and childhood screening.[3] Then, in 2005, the American College of Medical Genetics released a report commissioned by the Health Resources and Services Administration (HRSA) with recommendations to strengthen newborn screening nationally, including a proposed uniform panel of 29 conditions (ACMG Newborn Screening Expert Group, 2006). This report laid the foundation for the Recommended Uniform Screening Panel (RUSP), a list of disorders that the secretary of HHS recommends be included as part of every NBS program—established in 2010 (HRSA, 2021).

The Newborn Screening Saves Lives Act was enacted in 2008 to expand federal support for state and territorial NBS programs and develop national guidance, including requiring ACHDNC to make recommendations on conditions for newborn screening. This legislation, which was reauthorized in 2014, expired on September 30, 2019 (Figure 1-1). Since then, attempts to reauthorize, and thereby reinstate, grant programs and other initiatives to support newborn screening, have been unsuccessful, at least in part due to concerns about the retention and reuse of newborn dried blood spots without informed consent (Sterman and Molina, 2023). Despite this, ACHDNC continues to operate as a discretionary committee and advise the secretary concerning conditions to include on the RUSP and improvements to public health NBS delivery (HRSA, 2021).

States and territories continue to have authority over the policy and practice of NBS programs in their jurisdiction, whereas the federal government provides support for state and territorial programs, offers national guidance—such as the RUSP, and coordinates some cross-state activities. Some states have also instituted RUSP alignment laws, which require a state's NBS program to screen for conditions added to the RUSP within a certain time frame (EveryLife Foundation for Rare Diseases, n.d.).

---

[3] Section 1111 of the Public Health Service Act, 42 U.S.C. 300B-10.

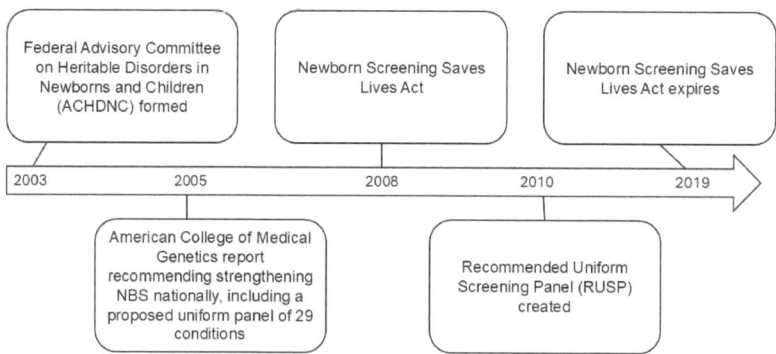

FIGURE 1-1 Timeline of federal action related to newborn screening.
NOTE: NBS = newborn screening.

The federal guidance provided by the RUSP thus plays a greater role in such states than in those that use other processes to establish their set of screened conditions. Overall, this combination of state and territorial-based approaches with federal guidance and support allows states and territories to consider the needs of their population and their available resources but can produce variation in the ability of NBS programs to achieve and maintain excellence.

CONCEPTS UNDERPINNING PUBLIC HEALTH NEWBORN SCREENING

Principles for Population-Based Screening

Early NBS programs were heavily influenced by a 1968 report published by the World Health Organization titled the *Principles and Practice of Screening for Disease*, which recommends 10 principles, commonly known as the Wilson and Jungner principles, to guide screening for chronic conditions (Crowe, 2008; Wilson and Jungner, 1968). When applied to newborn screening, these principles have influenced inclusion of conditions based on the criteria of severity, urgency, and treatability— and with an emphasis on direct benefits to the child (Crowe, 2008). This report also discussed characteristics that screening tests should have to be employed at a population level (i.e., validity, reliability, yield, and cost). Wilson and Jungner proposed that tests should accurately, reliably, and efficiently identify individuals who have a condition and those who do not with high sensitivity and specificity, and they should do so relatively cheaply (Wilson and Jungner, 1968). These principles continue to guide the delivery of public health newborn screening and choices concerning which conditions should be added to screening, although there are pushes to expand programs to include both conditions and screening technologies that may not fulfill these criteria (Currier, 2022; King et al., 2021).

Many jurisdictions in the United States operate public health newborn screening without a requirement for formal informed consent, meaning that parents do not have to give permission but may opt out for religious or other reasons (King and Smith, 2016).[4] Although parents are generally permitted to refuse screening, many may not be aware of public health newborn screening or that they have the right to refuse (Rothwell et al., 2010). Different aspects of governmental authority are referenced when discussing nonconsented public health newborn screening, including the concept of *parens patriae* in which states have a role in defending the interests of those who are unable to protect themselves, including assuming parental rights to protect a child's health and welfare when the parents are unable or unwilling to do so (Gostin, 2000; King and Smith, 2016). The ethical justification for nonconsented public health newborn screening was first articulated by Faden, Holtzman, and Chwalow. In their paper, the authors argue that PKU screening has a clear net benefit and parental refusal poses a serious, if unlikely, risk of harm to the baby; therefore, a lack of explicit consent is appropriate in this specific circumstance (Faden et al., 1982). Although not necessarily the authors' original intent, the justification for nonconsented screening for PKU has been extended as other conditions have been added to public health newborn screening based on the criteria of urgency, severity, and treatability (Currier, 2022; Faden et al., 1982). Bioethical frameworks and principles underpinning public health newborn screening are explored further in Chapter 3.

Documenting the Public Health Achievements of Newborn Screening

As reflected in Box 1-1, those involved with and affected by newborn screening in the United States attribute several important successes to these programs. However, demonstrating the impact of newborn screening at a national level and its benefit to the public is complicated by limited coordinated data collection efforts for screening, short-term follow-up, and longitudinal monitoring of health outcomes (Watson et al., 2022). For example, it is difficult to draw clear lines between receipt of newborn screening and metrics of long-term benefits or cost savings at the population level from available data, although some evidence is

---

[4] Consent and opt-out requirements vary across the 56 state and territorial NBS programs. These practices are discussed further in Chapter 2 and more information about individual programs can be found at https://www.newsteps.org/data-center/state-profiles (accessed January 30, 2025).

BOX 1-1
Newborn Screening in the United States

Newborn screening is considered an achievement by those involved in public health (CDC, 2011), but quantitatively documenting its successes can be difficult. Nevertheless, there are several features that indicate the value of newborn screening and the tremendous investment that has been made to identify infants at risk of serious, congenital conditions.

- All infants born in the United States have access to newborn screening.
- Of the ~3.6 million infants born annually, approximately 98 percent receive newborn screening (CDC, 2012; NCHS, 2024).
- Approximately 7,000 infants are identified with a disorder annually via dried blood spot screening (~20 per 10,000 infants) (Gaviglio et al., 2023).
- The United States provides global leadership in quality and accuracy of newborn screening through CDC's Newborn Screening Quality Assurance Program (NSQAP), which offers quality assurance services to more than 670 laboratories worldwide, including all laboratories in the United States, laboratories in more than 86 countries, and 32 NBS test manufacturers (CDC, 2024b).
- The United States has led technology and assay development for newborn screening, including the incorporation of tandem mass spectrometry and molecular methods (Furnier et al., 2020; Therell and Adams, 2007; Watson et al., 2022).

---

available for a subset of conditions (Grosse, 2015; Van Vliet and Grosse, 2021). Even the most recent national statistic on the percentage of infants screened annually (over 98 percent) was published by the Centers for Disease Control and Prevention (CDC) in 2012—more than a decade prior to the publication of this report (CDC, 2012), although more recent statistics are available for birth prevalence (Gaviglio et al., 2023). Instead, these NBS achievements are most often illustrated through individual stories (APHL, 2013).

EMERGING TENSIONS IN PUBLIC HEALTH NEWBORN SCREENING

This report envisions a path forward to navigate the mounting tensions, challenges, and pressures facing newborn screening in the United States, while preserving and strengthening what is already considered a public health achievement. Tensions arise in public health newborn screening between population health needs and individual autonomy, challenging the ability of the system to address these often-competing priorities (Bayefsky et al., 2015). Public health NBS programs, for example, must balance their mandate to screen all newborns with the individual needs and rights of each child and their family, including rising concerns about data privacy, as well as wavering trust (Grant, 2022). Public health newborn screening must also contend with opportunities and challenges posed by transformative therapies and genomic sequencing, which open the door to expanding the conditions screened within an already resource-constrained environment (Andrews et al., 2022; CDC, 2012; GAO, 2016). The process for adding conditions to the RUSP ensures a rigorous evaluation of evidence but struggles to keep pace with medical advances and places a burden on advocacy communities and others (Andrews et al., 2022; Bailey et al., 2021; Kemper et al., 2014). Furthermore, well-resourced advocacy communities are better positioned to engage in research and advocate for inclusion of their condition on the RUSP and state panels, whereas conditions with less funding and advocacy support face challenges gaining recognition and prioritization (Halley et al., 2022; Largent and Pearson, 2012). These tensions are often highest among those deeply interested in or affected by newborn screening. If unaddressed, the tensions, challenges, and pressures described, among others, may imperil this public health service (Currier, 2022; McCandless and Wright, 2020).

Ongoing Efforts by Partners in the NBS Ecosystem[5]

Partners across the NBS ecosystem recognize these complex, ongoing challenges and are taking actions to address them. Reflecting the scope of public health newborn screening, partners involved in these activities include federal agencies, state and territorial public health departments, researchers, professional societies and consortia, advocacy groups, individuals, and others. To strengthen NBS programs and harmonize across states and territories, the Association of Public Health Laboratories (APHL) entered a cooperative agreement in 2012 with the Genetic Services Branch of HRSA to coordinate the Newborn Screening Technical assistance and Evaluation Program (NewSTEPs), which provides quality improvement tools, an innovative data repository, and technical resources (Ojodu et al., 2017). APHL has received new funding from HRSA through a cooperative agreement titled National Center for Newborn Screening System Excellence (NBS Excel).[6] Initial steps have also been taken by different partners to build a more robust data infrastructure, including the NewSTEPs data repository for programmatic data, quality indicators, and short-term follow-up data, established in 2013, and then more recently, CDC's creation

---

[5] The report focuses on critical functions and actions to strengthen public health newborn screening for the future; descriptions of the roles and structures of federal and nonfederal activities relevant to newborn screening are current as of March 24, 2025.

[6] See the NBS Excel and NBS Propel notice of funding opportunity, https://www.hrsa.gov/grants/find-funding/HRSA-23-077 (accessed February 3, 2025).

in 2021 of a national laboratory data platform, Enhancing Data-driven Disease Detection in Newborns (ED3N) (CDC, 2024a; Ojodu et al., 2017).

HRSA launched a series of grants in 2023 to fund activities to improve and expand the NBS system, address timely collection and reporting of NBS specimens to improve early diagnosis and treatment for individuals with heritable conditions, improve short-term follow-up through long-term follow-up, and help families understand and navigate the process from confirmation of a diagnosis to treatment (HRSA, 2024).[7] In lieu of passing the NBS Saves Lives Act, Congress increased funding for CDC's NSQAP and HRSA's Heritable Disorders Program.[8] Rare disease patients, their families, and advocacy groups, such as the National Organization for Rare Disorders, EveryLife Foundation for Rare Diseases, and Expecting Health, have created influential resources (e.g., Newborn Screening State Report Card and the Newborn Screening Family Education Program) to help reduce gaps in the NBS ecosystem, built nomination packages, developed disease-specific registries to inform research, and raised their voices for changes to better support the needs of their communities (Andrews et al., 2022; Expecting Health, 2024).

A vision forward could help foster and integrate these parallel efforts and address challenges to public health newborn screening that still loom on the horizon. To build upon these ongoing efforts, Congress included a mandate in the 2023 appropriations process for a National Academies of Sciences, Engineering, and Medicine study "to examine the current status of Newborn Screening systems, processes, and research and make recommendations for future improvements."[9]

STUDY SCOPE AND APPROACH

In recognition of these challenges and to help inform the future of U.S. newborn screening, the Office on Women's Health in the Department of Health and Human Services asked the National Academies of Sciences, Engineering and Medicine to convene an ad hoc committee of experts to provide short-term options to strengthen existing NBS programs and a vision for the future. The committee's statement of task is presented in Box 1-2.

---

[7] See the NBS Excel and NBS Propel notice of funding opportunity, https://www.hrsa.gov/grants/find-funding/HRSA-23-077 (accessed February 3, 2025), and the NBS Co-Propel notice of funding opportunity, https://www.grants.gov/search-results-detail/349438 (accessed February 3, 2025).

[8] *Consolidated Appropriations Act of 2023*, Public Law 117-328, 117th Congress (December 28, 2022); House of Representatives Report No. 117-403 (2022).

[9] *Consolidated Appropriations Act of 2023*, Public Law 117-328, 117th Congress (December 28, 2022); House of Representatives Report No. 117-403 (2022).

BOX 1-2
Statement of Task

An ad hoc committee of the National Academies of Sciences, Engineering, and Medicine will examine the current landscape of newborn screening (NBS) systems, processes, and research in the United States. The committee will make recommendations for future improvements that help modernize newborn screening to be adaptable, flexible, coordinated, communicative, capable of efficient and sustainable adoption of screening for new conditions using new technologies, and a public health program from which all infants benefit. The committee's work will focus on the following tasks:

1. Examine state and federal capacities to strengthen current screening processes and implement screening for new conditions, including considerations for future conditions added to the Recommended Uniform Screening Panel (RUSP).
2. Review existing and emerging technologies that would permit screening for new categories of conditions and describe
   - how these new technologies may impact states;
   - changes to public health infrastructure needed to incorporate new technologies while upholding and implementing the required components of newborn screening;
   - options for incorporating new technologies to allow for screening of additional conditions; and
   - research, technological, and infrastructure needs to improve diagnosis, follow-up, and public health surveillance.
3. Review NBS data collection processes for tracking disease prevalence, improving health outcomes, conducting longitudinal follow-up, defining the natural history of conditions that can be screened for, and measuring quality of life.
4. Examine the RUSP review and recommendation processes, including the process of selecting new conditions that could be added to the RUSP; conducting review of the evidence to support adding new conditions; scaling up these review and recommendation processes to efficiently handle the review of potentially hundreds of conditions; and considering whether additional factors should be included in the analysis of harms and benefits (e.g., societal harms such as financial cost or opportunity costs, and family benefits such as avoiding the "diagnostic odyssey").

The committee's final report will describe (a) short-term options that could be implemented at the state and/or federal level over the next 2 to 3 years to help strengthen existing NBS programs and address the current challenges facing state programs, and (b) a vision for the future of NBS and a road map for how to implement and achieve that vision over the next 5 to 15 years. The report will include options for how to implement longitudinal follow-up data collection to improve understanding of the impact of NBS on infant health outcomes (including morbidity and mortality, and quality of life for screen-positive infants). The committee will consider the resources required for implementation, such as changes to the current NBS system that will need to occur; the feasibility of implementing the future vision; and the challenges and barriers that may arise when trying to implement the road map.

The committee's charge focuses on newborn screening through blood spot testing. During the newborn period, babies receive other types of testing, including hearing screening and pulse oximetry screening for potential heart disease; these other forms of newborn assessment were out of scope for this study. Similarly, the study focuses on the NBS program as implemented in the United States, and the strategies set forth in this report are targeted to partners within the U.S. NBS ecosystem. The United States has long been at the forefront of newborn screening, influencing and supporting initiatives and programs worldwide (APHL, 2013; CDC, 2024b). Therefore, this report's guidance may also help inform other countries and international bodies including the World Health Organization and the International Society for Neonatal Screening as they encounter challenges and opportunities similar to the ones this study addresses.

Committee's Interpretation of the Charge

Although the statement of task asks for both near-term operational solutions and a long-term vision for the future, the committee quickly realized that no single study could fully attend to both duties with the given scope and time line. A number of partners supporting public health newborn screening, including such federal agencies as HRSA and CDC, are actively working to address more immediate problems within the existing framework. With the encouragement of these partners, the committee prioritized its efforts toward developing a longer-term vision for building a more modern, sustainable, and adaptable NBS ecosystem and a road map to accomplish this vision after first reviewing and examining the current state and ongoing efforts to address challenges in public health newborn screening.

A future for public health newborn screening in which all infants can benefit needs to be grounded in clear goals and ethical principles. Public health newborn screening plays an important role in detecting disease and connecting affected infants and families to the clinical care system to improve health outcomes. However, disparities in access and quality can affect babies' and families' experience of public health and health care systems and affect these outcomes. The report focuses on recommendations to strengthen the excellence and support the quality of public health newborn screening, while recognizing that systemic issues in the larger U.S. clinical care system are likely to present ongoing and important areas of work but are outside of this study's scope.

Study Approach

Reflecting the complexity of its task, the committee included 14 members with expertise in public health newborn screening, state and federal public health, lived and parental experience, bioethical and legal issues, existing and emerging screening technologies, health systems, health economics, and clinical care disciplines. The committee met multiple times over the course of the study for public virtual and hybrid workshop sessions with speakers who generously shared their research, evidence-based observations, expertise, and experiences with the committee, as well as in committee and working group discussions to analyze the available evidence and develop the conclusions and recommendations presented in this report. See Appendix A for further information on how the committee conducted its work and Appendix B for brief biographies of committee members and staff.

Central to the committee's approach was soliciting input from individuals interested in or affected by newborn screening in the United States to support ethical decision making; enhance legitimacy, transparency, and justice; and build trust (APHA, 2019). With additional support from the Chan Zuckerberg Initiative, the committee commissioned a team of consultants, together with National Academies staff, to engage with groups and individuals across multiple sectors with lived or professional experience in newborn screening through a series of listening sessions and a virtual questionnaire available in both English and Spanish. More than 600 people participated in these activities, including parents, members of the rare disease community, health care providers, researchers, NBS laboratory and follow-up professionals, public health professionals, payors, industry representatives, privacy advocates, and members of the public.

While responsive to outside needs, concerns, and preferences, the committee recognized that different groups have varied desires and interests and it examined ideas and suggestions in the context of the available scientific evidence. An overview of this engagement process is available in Appendix A with further details on who participated (demographics and sector/group affiliations) and a paper summarizing input is publicly available and titled *What We Heard: Engagement Summary on Newborn Screening in the United States*.[10]

ORGANIZATION OF THE REPORT

Following this introduction, Chapter 2 reviews the history and current implementation of public health newborn screening in the United States, including the landscape of partners involved in the broader NBS ecosystem. Chapter 3 discusses the importance of grounding decision making for public health programs such as newborn screening in ethical principles,

---

[10] Susanna Haas Lyons Engagement Consulting, 2024. Available on the study website at https://www.nationalacademies.org/our-work/newborn-screening-current-landscape-and-future-directions (accessed October 8, 2024).

concepts, and values. It articulates the approach this report takes to the focus of newborn screening and types of diseases it includes, providing a foundation for analyses and recommendations made in subsequent chapters. Chapter 4 focuses on NBS programs implemented at the state and territorial levels as central actors in achieving the aims of newborn screening, discussing how to support and enhance program excellence. Chapter 5 considers how public health newborn screening can responsibly apply emerging technologies, particularly opportunities and challenges associated with the use of genomic sequencing. Chapter 6 describes the research enterprise relevant to newborn screening. Such research is essential for generating and expanding the evidence base informing public health newborn screening; better understanding and addressing ethical, legal, and social issues; and addressing public health impacts and implementation. Finally, Chapter 7 describes how all parties in the NBS ecosystem can take actions to enable a future vision for newborn screening, through both strategic coordination and optimization of existing processes.

REFERENCES

AAP (American Academy of Pediatrics). 1967. Statement on compulsory testing of newborn infants for hereditary metabolic disorders. *Pediatrics* 39(4):623-624.

ACMG Newborn Screening Expert Group. 2006. Newborn screening: Toward a uniform screening panel and system. *Genetics in Medicine* 8(Suppl 1):1S-252S.

Andrews, S. M., K. A. Porter, D. B. Bailey, and H. L. Peay. 2022. Preparing newborn screening for the future: A collaborative stakeholder engagement exploring challenges and opportunities to modernizing the newborn screening system. *BMC Pediatrics* 22(1):90.

APHA (American Public Health Association). 2019. *Public health code of ethics*. https://www.apha.org/-/media/files/pdf/membergroups/ethics/code_of_ethics.ashx (accessed December 30, 2024).

APHL (Association of Public Health Laboratories). 2013. *The newborn screening story: How one simple test changed lives, science, and health in America*. https://www.aphl.org/aboutAPHL/publications/Documents/NBS_2013May_The-Newborn-Screening-Story_How-One-Simple-Test-Changed-Lives-Science-and-Health-in-America.pdf (accessed December 30, 2024).

Bailey, D. B., K. A. Porter, S. M. Andrews, M. Raspa, A. Y. Gwaltney, and H. L. Peay. 2021. Expert evaluation of strategies to modernize newborn screening in the United States. *JAMA Network Open* 4(12):e2140998.

Bayefsky, M. J., K. W. Saylor, and B. E. Berkman. 2015. Parental consent for the use of residual newborn screening bloodspots. *JAMA* 314(1):21.

Bickel, H., J. Gerrard, and E. Hickmans. 1953. Preliminary communication: Influence of phenylalanine intake on phenylketonuria. *Lancet* 262(6790):812-813.

Boyle, C. A., J. A. Bocchini, and J. Kelly. 2014. Reflections on 50 years of newborn screening. *Pediatrics* 133(6):961-963.

Brosco, J. P., L. M. Sanders, M. I. Seider, and A. C. Dunn. 2008. Adverse medical outcomes of early newborn screening programs for phenylketonuria. *Pediatrics* 122(1):192-197.

CDC (Centers for Disease Control and Prevention). 2011. Ten great public health achievements - United States, 2001-2010. *Morbidity and Mortality Weekly Report* 60(19):619-623.

CDC. 2012. CDC grand rounds: Newborn screening and improved outcomes. *Morbidity and Mortality Weekly Report* 61(21):390-393.

CDC. 2024a. *Enhancing data-driven disease detection in newborns.* https://www.cdc.gov/newborn-screening/php/about/ed3n-project.html (accessed September 20, 2024).

CDC. 2024b. *Newborn screening quality assurance program.* https://www.cdc.gov/laboratory-quality-assurance/php/newborn-screening/index.html (accessed July 31, 2024).

Chace, D. H., T. A. Kalas, and E. W. Naylor. 2003. Use of tandem mass spectrometry for multianalyte screening of dried blood specimens from newborns. *Clinical Chemistry* 49(11):1797-1817.

Crowe, S. 2008. *A brief history of newborn screening in the United States.* Staff discussusion paper (President's Council on Bioethics). https://bioethicsarchive.georgetown.edu/pcbe/background/newborn_screening_crowe.html (accessed January 14, 2025).

Currier, R. J. 2022. Newborn screening is on a collision course with public health ethics. *International Journal of Neonatal Screening* 8(4):51.

EveryLife Foundation for Rare Diseases. n.d. *RUSP alignment legislation.* https://everylifefoundation.org/newborn-screening-take-action/support-legislation/ (accessed February 21, 2024).

Expecting Health. 2024. *The newborn screening family education program: Learn. Connect. Advocate.* https://expectinghealth.org/programs/newborn-screening-family-education-program (accessed August 21, 2024).

Faden, R. R., N. A. Holtzman, and A. J. Chwalow. 1982. Parental rights, child welfare, and public health: The case of PKU screening. *American Journal of Public Health* 72(12):1396-1400.

Furnier, S. M., M. S. Durkin, and M. W. Baker. 2020. Translating molecular technologies into routine newborn screening practice. *International Journal of Neonatal Screening* 6(4):80.

GAO (Government Accountability Office). 2016. *Newborn screening timeliness: Most states had not met screening goals, but some are developing strategies to address barriers.* GAO 17-196. https://www.gao.gov/assets/gao-17-196.pdf (accessed January 10, 2025).

Gaviglio, A., S. McKasson, S. Singh, and J. Ojodu. 2023. Infants with congenital diseases identified through newborn screening—United States, 2018–2020. *International Journal of Neonatal Screening* 9(2):23.

Gostin, L. O. 2000. *Public health law: Power, duty, restraint* (vol. 3). Oakland, CA: University of California Press.

Grant, C. 2022. *Police are using newborn genetic screening to search for suspects, threatening privacy and public health.* https://www.aclu.org/news/privacy-technology/police-are-using-newborn-genetic-screening (accessed July 23, 2024).

Grosse, S. 2015. Showing value in newborn screening: Challenges in quantifying the effectiveness and cost-effectiveness of early detection of phenylketonuria and cystic fibrosis. *Healthcare* 3(4):1133-1157.

Grosse, S. D., J. D. Thompson, Y. Ding, and M. Glass. 2016. The use of economic evaluation to inform newborn screening policy decisions: The Washington state experience. *Milbank Quarterly* 94(2):366-391.

Halley, M. C., H. S. Smith, E. A. Ashley, A. J. Goldenberg, and H. K. Tabor. 2022. A call for an integrated approach to improve efficiency, equity and sustainability in rare disease research in the United States. *Nature* 54:219-222.

HRSA (Health Resources and Services Administration). 2021. *History of the ACHDNC.* https://www.hrsa.gov/advisory-committees/heritable-disorders/timeline (accessed July 31, 2024).

HRSA. 2023a. *About newborn screening.* https://newbornscreening.hrsa.gov/about-newborn-screening (accessed July 29, 2024).

HRSA. 2023b. *Newborn screening process.* https://newbornscreening.hrsa.gov/newborn-screening-process (accessed July 29, 2024).

HRSA. 2024. *Cooperative newborn screening system priorities (NBS Co-Propel) program.* https://mchb.hrsa.gov/programs/cooperative-newborn-screening-system-priorities (accessed September 26, 2024).

Kemper, A. R., C. A. Kus, R. J. Ostrander, A. M. Comeau, C. A. Boyle, D. Dougherty, M. Y. Mann, J. R. Botkin, and N. S. Green. 2012. A framework for key considerations regarding point-of-care screening of newborns. *Genetics in Medicine* 14: 951-954.

Kemper, A. R., N. S. Green, N. Calonge, W. K. K. Lam, A. M. Comeau, A. J. Goldenberg, J. Ojodu, L. A. Prosser, S. Tanksley, and J. A. Bocchini, Jr. 2014. Decision-making process for conditions nominated to the Recommended Uniform Screening Panel: Statement of the US Department of Health and Human Services Secretary's Advisory Committee on Heritable Disorders in Newborns and Children. *Genetics in Medicine* 16(2):183-187.

King, J. R., L. D. Notarangelo, and L. Hammarström. 2021. An appraisal of the Wilson & Jungner criteria in the context of genomic-based newborn screening for inborn errors of immunity. *Journal of Allergy and Clinical Immunology* 147(2):428-438.

King, J. S., and M. E. Smith. 2016. Whole-genome screening of newborns? The constitutional boundaries of state newborn screening programs. *Pediatrics* 137(Suppl 1):S8-S15.

Kraszewski, J., T. Burke, and S. Rosenbaum. 2006. Legal issues in newborn screening: Implications for public health practice and policy. *Public Health Reports* 121(1):92-94.

Largent, E. A., and S. D. Pearson. 2012. Which orphans will find a home? The rule of rescue in resource allocation for rare diseases. *Hastings Center Report* 42(1):27-34.

Lenke, R. R., and H. L. Levy. 1980. Maternal phenylketonuria and hyperphenylalaninemia. *New England Journal of Medicine* 303(21):1202-1208.

Levy, H. L. 2021. Robert Guthrie and the trials and tribulations of newborn screening. *International Journal of Neonatal Screening* 7(1):5.

McCandless, S. E., and E. J. Wright. 2020. Mandatory newborn screening in the United States: History, current status, and existential challenges. *Birth Defects Research* 112(4):350-366.

NCHS (National Center for Health Statistics). 2024. *Birth data.* https://www.cdc.gov/nchs/nvss/births.htm (accessed July 31, 2024).

NHGRI (National Human Genome Research Institute). 2014. *About phenylketonuria.* https://www.genome.gov/Genetic-Disorders/Phenylketonuria#al-1 (accessed July 25, 2024).

Ojodu, J., S. Singh, Y. Kellar-Guenther, C. Yusuf, E. Jones, T. Wood, M. Baker, and M. K. Sontag. 2017. NewSTEPs: The establishment of a national newborn screening technical assistance resource center. *International Journal of Neonatal Screening* 4(1):1.

Paul, D. B. 1998. The history of newborn phenylketonuria screening in the US. In *Promoting safe and effective genetic testing in the United States*, edited by N. A. Holtzman and M. S. Watson. Baltimore, MD: Johns Hopkins University Press.

Paul, D. B., and J. P. Brosco. 2013. *The PKU paradox: A short history of a genetic disease.* Baltimore, MD: John Hopkins University Press.

Rothenberg, M. B., and E. M. Sills. 1968. Iatrogenesis: The PKU anxiety syndrome. *Journal of the American Academy of Child Psychiatry* 7(4):689-692.

Rothwell, E., R. Anderson, and J. Botkin. 2010. Policy issues and stakeholder concerns regarding the storage and use of residual newborn dried blood samples for research. *Policy, Politics, & Nursing Practice* 11(1):5-12.

Rule, J. 1965. Screening of newborn infants for metabolic disease: Committee on fetus and newborn. *Pediatrics* 35:499-501.

Sterman, J., and D. Molina. 2023. *Tasked with critical testing, newborn screening programs feel pinch of funding struggles.* InvestigateTV. https://www.investigatetv.com/2023/05/22/tasked-with-critical-testing-newborn-screening-programs-feel-pinch-funding-struggles/ (accessed August 2024).

Susanna Haas Lyons Engagement Consulting. 2024. *What we heard: Engagement summary for committee on newborn screening: Current landscape and future directions*. Washington, DC: National Academies of Sciences, Engineering, and Medicine.

Tarini, B. A. 2007. The current revolution in newborn screening. *Archives of Pediatrics & Adolescent Medicine* 161(8):767-772.

Tarini, B. A., D. A. Christakis, and H. G. Welch. 2006. State newborn screening in the tandem mass spectrometry era: More tests, more false-positive results. *Pediatrics* 118(2):448-456.

Therell, B. L., and J. Adams. 2007. Newborn screening in North America. *Journal of Inherited Metabolic Disease* 30(4):447-465.

Turnock, B. J., and C. Atchison. 2002. Governmental public health in the United States: The implications of federalism. *Health Affairs* 21(6): 68-78.

Van Vliet, G., and S. D. Grosse. 2021. Newborn screening for congenital hypothyroidism and congenital adrenal hyperplasia: Benefits and costs of a successful public health program. *Médecine Sciences* 37(5):528-534.

Watson, M. S., M. A. Lloyd-Puryear, and R. R. Howell. 2022. The progress and future of US newborn screening. *International Journal of Neonatal Screening* 8(3):41.

Wilson, J. M. G., and G. Jungner. 1968. Principles and practice of screening for disease. *Public Health Papers* 34. Geneva: World Health Organization.

2

Current Landscape of Newborn Screening in the United States

"Our daughter's newborn screen changed the entire course of our lives . . . The support and education we have received since the positive result has been a blessing. It is knowledge that every family deserves." – Parent

For more than 60 years, public health newborn screening (NBS) has directly touched the lives of essentially all babies born in the United States. The public health impacts of newborn screening are felt across society, but perhaps most profoundly by infants born with serious conditions screened for at birth, along with their families and caregivers. These achievements are made possible by a vast array of individuals, organizations, infrastructure, processes, and funding mechanisms that compose an informal NBS system that supports public health newborn screening for approximately 3.6 million babies born across the country each year.

Before considering the future for public health newborn screening, understanding the current landscape is critical. This chapter provides context on the history, goals, and implementation of public health newborn screening using dried blood spots in the United States;[1] discusses the roles of key players in newborn screening; and identifies developments that may bring new opportunities and raise new questions.[2]

---

[1] As reflected in Chapter 1, newborn screening encompasses dried blood spot, hearing loss, and congenital heart defect testing. The scope of this report is limited to dried blood spot screening in the United States.

[2] Descriptions of the roles and structures of federal and nonfederal activities relevant to newborn screening are current as of March 24, 2025, including the Advisory Committee on Heritable Disorders in Newborns and Children.

OVERVIEW OF PUBLIC HEALTH NEWBORN SCREENING IN THE UNITED STATES

Public health newborn screening is intended to support both the health of individuals and that of the U.S. population overall (Brosco et al., 2015). It is carried out and supported by a large and varied network of public health and private laboratories, public health follow-up programs, clinics, research organizations, private companies, and government entities, yet unlike many other sprawling bureaucratic systems, it is experienced by each family individually during what many consider to be among the most momentous occasions of their lives—the birth of a child.

Terminology Used in this Report

This report distinguishes three distinct, yet interrelated domains related to newborn screening: public health NBS programs, the public health NBS system, and the broader NBS ecosystem. These distinctions help clarify roles, responsibilities, and the scope of activities involved in the screening, identification, and treatment of newborns.

NBS programs: Public health newborn screening is implemented by 56 separate public health NBS programs covering individual U.S. states and territories with the goal of identifying babies at risk of certain conditions and connecting them to clinical care.[3]

Public health NBS system: The successful delivery of newborn screening as a public health service depends on partnerships beyond individual NBS programs. The public health NBS system refers to all the partners directly involved in implementing public heath newborn screening. This public health NBS system includes state- and territorial-run NBS programs; state and territorial entities that oversee and support the operations of NBS programs; offices, advisory committees, and programs within federal agencies that provide guidance and support to NBS programs; clinical care providers and infrastructure involved in executing newborn screening for all infants and follow-up to confirm and connect those identified as at risk; partnerships with patient and family organizations, nonprofit entities, and professional associations tied directly to policy and practice of public health NBS; and others.

Broader NBS ecosystem: The report uses the term NBS ecosystem to represent the broadest scope of activities related to newborn screening. This ecosystem includes the NBS system and all sectors that interact with and influence newborn screening beyond the public health framework.

---

[3] There are 56 newborn screening programs, including all 50 states, the District of Columbia, Puerto Rico, Guam, American Samoa, Commonwealth of the Northern Mariana Islands, and the U.S. Virgin Islands. Programs are run by states and territories, but for brevity, the report will refer to these as state-run programs.

This includes activities providing long-term clinical care and support for affected infants and families, research to better understand the genetic basis, natural history, and detection of diseases in newborns and develop new tools, technologies and treatments, additional or complementary forms of screening carried out in clinical settings (separate from the sample collection and screening carried out through public health NBS), and the broader array of public- and private-sector efforts and organizations that support relevant research and clinical care.

By delineating these three domains, this report aims to provide a more structured understanding of the NBS landscape. Recognizing these distinctions enables more precise discussions to enhance the effectiveness and sustainability of public health NBS efforts.

The next section provides an overview of the NBS process as families experience it. This section also expands on the descriptions above to describe the array of processes and players involved in implementation of the public health NBS system and the broader NBS ecosystem.

How Families Experience Public Health Newborn Screening

Although there is wide variation in how public health newborn screening on dried blood spots is carried out across the United States, in general, the process can be broken down into three main steps (Figure 2-1) (HRSA, 2023b; NICHD, n.d.).

Families may learn about newborn screening before the birth of their child, or they may not know of its existence until a nurse comes to collect a blood spot from their newborn, or they may never know (Botkin et al., 2016). In most programs, there is no formal opt-in process, although families do

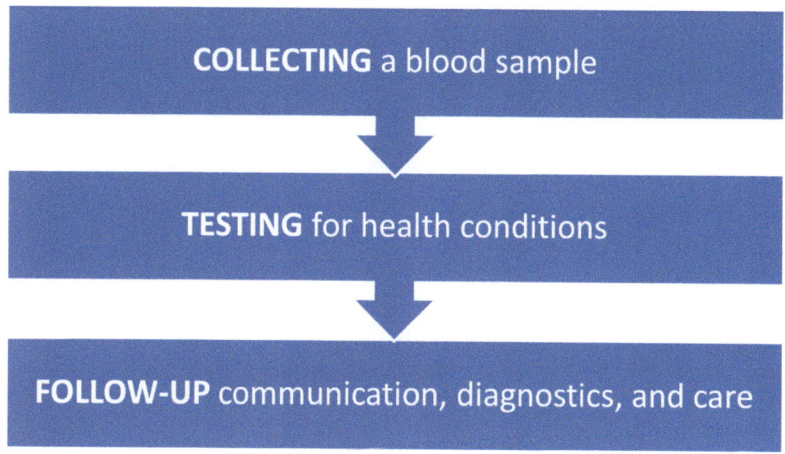

FIGURE 2-1 Basic steps in the NBS process.
NOTE: NBS = newborn screening.

have the option of opting out in most jurisdictions (President's Council on Bioethics, 2008).[4] To collect the blood spot, a nurse, midwife, or technician pricks the baby's foot with a small needle, a procedure known as a "heel stick." A few drops of blood are then extracted from the baby's foot and applied to a filter paper card. A nurse, midwife, technician, or hospital or birth center clerk records additional details about the infant on the card (such as name, sex, weight, race and/or ethnicity, and contact information for the baby's parents and primary care provider). The blood spot is then transported to a laboratory for testing. Results from testing are transmitted to state- or territorial-run follow-up programs that then communicate findings with the baby's health care provider, either directly or through office personnel, and in some cases, directly with the family. If the results suggest that the baby may have a health condition the screening process is intended to detect, health care providers and NBS program personnel work together with the family to refer the infant for further retesting as needed, diagnostic evaluation and confirmatory testing, and clinical care (HRSA, 2023b; NICHD, n.d.).

This process is intended to happen quickly. According to timeliness goals established in 2015, the blood spot should be collected within 48 hours after birth, the blood spot should arrive at the laboratory for testing within 24 hours of collection, and all tests should be completed within the infant's first 7 days of life (HRSA, 2017). For certain time-critical health conditions (e.g., maple syrup urine disease), the laboratory aims to communicate any presumptive positive results to the baby's health care provider by the time the baby is no more than 5 days old (HRSA, 2017).

Box 2-1 includes definitions of terms relevant to the screening and diagnosis of conditions in infants.

Players and Processes Involved in NBS Program Implementation

NBS programs are implemented at the state or territorial level with decision making and operations largely under state or territorial authority (Andrews et al., 2022; HRSA, 2023a; Watson et al., 2022). There is no central or integrated system for laboratory testing of newborn blood spots, and the 56 NBS programs use the services of an array of NBS public health laboratories and privately run laboratories (Dubay and Zach, 2023).[5]

---

[4] Two exceptions are Wyoming, which requires parental informed consent (see https://health.wyo.gov/wp-content/uploads/2020/01/Updated-Newborn-Screening-Rules-12-2019.pdf), and Nebraska, which does not permit parents to opt out of screening (see https://law.justia.com/cases/nebraska/supreme-court/2008/1136.html).

[5] See https://www.newsteps.org/data-center/state-profiles?q=data-resources/state-profiles (accessed September 26, 2024) for up-to-date information on each state or territory's newborn screening program, including their responsible laboratory.

> **BOX 2-1**
> **Terms Relevant to the Screening and Diagnosis of Conditions**
>
> **Screening test:** The systematic application of determinations (i.e., measurement procedures, physiological evaluations, or assessments) among a defined population (e.g., newborns) with the goal of detecting individuals at sufficient risk for a specific disease, group of diseases, or phenotypic difference to merit additional investigation or guide preventive action.
>
> **Diagnostic testing:** Also called confirmatory testing. A test to prove or disprove the presence of a specific disease, group of diseases, or phenotypic difference suspected based on screening results. For newborn screening and identity confirmation, confirmatory testing must be performed on a new specimen, rather than on any existing screening specimen.
>
> **First-tier screen:** A single test, combination of tests, physiological measurement, or assessment performed on all newborns to screen for a disease, group of diseases, or phenotypic difference as the first step in the laboratory screening algorithm.
>
> **Second-tier screen:** Also called reflex testing. Additional test, physiological measurement, or assessment, performed as a second step in a laboratory screening algorithm on a subset of newborns, that uses the initial screening specimen (i.e., specimen recollection not necessary) when first-tier screening results are out of range.
>
> **In-range screening result:** Also called expected range. The range of values for a measure in a typical healthy population.
>
> **Out-of-range screening result:** Test result that is outside the expected range of testing results.
>
> **Borderline result:** A term sometimes used for an out-of-range screening result that is close to a program-established screen-positive cutoff value and that indicates moderate risk/possible disease, rather than high risk/probable disease.
>
> **Screen negative:** A final, reportable result for a disease, group of diseases, or phenotypic difference, based on the NBS result(s) and laboratory screening algorithm, indicating that the risk for that disease, group of diseases, or phenotypic difference is low and that no additional NBS follow-up is needed
>
> **Screen positive:** A final, reportable result for a disease, group of diseases, or phenotypic difference, based on the NBS result(s) and laboratory screening algorithm, indicating that the risk for that disease, group of diseases, or phenotypic difference is higher and that additional follow-up is needed.
>
> **Screen inconclusive:** A final, reportable result based on the NBS result(s) and laboratory screening algorithm for a screened disease, group of diseases, or phenotypic difference, indicating the inability to accurately interpret the screening result, typically leading to a request for a repeat dried blood spot specimen.
>
> **False-positive result:** Screen-positive result in an unaffected newborn.
>
> **False-negative result:** Screen-negative result in an affected newborn.
>
> SOURCE: CLSI, 2023.

Although the federal government provides guidance and some support for these programs, the federated nature of NBS programs across the United States has led to substantial variation in how screening is implemented in different places, which is discussed in greater detail below.

Looking behind the scenes at the three main steps in the public health NBS process reveals a complex array of processes and players that make the NBS system run (Kanungo et al., 2018). During the *blood spot collection step*, the main players involved include newborns and their families; personnel who take and handle the blood spot at the hospital, birth center, or home birth setting; and those involved in transporting the sample to a laboratory for testing (Kanungo et al., 2018). The specific processes determining where, when, and how samples are collected, processed, and transported may be influenced by legal mandates and rules, funding mechanisms, and various state and institutional policies (HRSA, 2023b).

During the *testing step*, key considerations include what conditions are tested, what assays are performed, and cutoff values for what is considered in or out of range. Laboratories and NBS programs are the groups most directly involved in this step day to day. However, the practices and processes they use are determined by a wide range of additional partners and factors across the NBS ecosystem, including the advisors, advocates, and lawmakers involved in determining what conditions are included and how laboratories operate; scientific research enterprise, which contributes to the evidence about conditions that may be selected for screening; and the research, industry, and government entities involved in test technology development and capacity.

The results of laboratory testing determine the next steps of follow-up communication, diagnostics, and care. Results can be categorized as screen positive, screen negative, screen inconclusive, false positive, or false negative (see Box 2-1) (CLSI, 2023). If the results are in range for all tests performed, no further testing is done, and the results are made available to the baby's primary care provider who may share them with the family. If the results are out of range, this triggers additional testing and follow-up, a process that can involve NBS program personnel, primary care providers, specialty clinicians, and families (HRSA, 2023b). If a diagnosis is confirmed for a condition, health care providers may recommend intervention or monitoring (HRSA, 2023b). Health care systems and policies, payors, patient advocates, and families can all play a role in determining the follow-up care received by people born with serious conditions. Box 2-2 briefly summarizes the roles of key players in the broader NBS ecosystem. Box 2-3 summarizes the roles of federal partners involved in newborn screening. Figure 2-2 provides further detail on the many players involved in implementing and supporting newborn screening.

BOX 2-2
Key Players Across the Broader NBS Ecosystem

Newborns and their families: Newborns receive public health newborn screening so that those born with certain serious health conditions can be identified and referred for treatment, which can extend their lives and improve quality of life. Families interact with the NBS system when a blood spot is taken and when the results are communicated during follow-up.

NBS programs: NBS programs run by U.S. states and territories implement newborn screening for babies born in that state or territory. Not every state program has its own laboratory; some will contract services from other states' laboratories or private laboratories, but every program performs their own follow-up activities. Programs may receive guidance and other forms of support from federal, state, territorial, and other sources, but they operate independently under state or territorial authority.

Federal partners: Federal agencies and advisory bodies provide guidance regarding conditions recommended for screening; issue grants; support research; provide quality assurance and control support; and perform some oversight and regulatory functions relevant to newborn screening, including reviewing test devices and laboratory protocols. There is no formal federal oversight mechanism for newborn screening as a whole and no direct federal source for routine programmatic funding of NBS programs.

State and territorial legislators and policy makers: State and territorial legislators and policy makers contribute to NBS programs through various levers. State and territorial legislatures have the authority to establish and regulate the programs themselves, direct how programs will be administered, make determinations about NBS fees, and allocate federal funding and resources to these programs. State and territorial legislatures may influence which conditions are added to the screening panels directly via legislation or indirectly by authorizing state health departments to do so.

Patient advocates: Advocates play an important role in raising awareness of serious, often rare, disorders, which are often included within the umbrella of rare disease; encouraging their inclusion among the disorders selected for newborn screening; educating families about newborn screening and rare diseases; and helping to facilitate access to care among families of children born with serious disorders. Advocates also contribute to evidence collection to support condition nomination; financially support research initiatives related to newborn screening and advocacy efforts to expand NBS programs; and advocate for federal- and state-level programmatic funding for NBS programs.

Health care providers and health care systems: Health care providers communicate with families about newborn screening, collect blood spots for testing, and convey the results back to families. Providers and health care systems carry out clinical and administrative processes as required by NBS programs in both hospital birth settings, birthing centers, and midwife-facilitated home births. Primary care providers and specialty clinicians facilitate diagnostic testing and clinical care for infants identified as at risk via newborn screening.

BOX 2-2 Continued

As the process moves from screening to diagnosis to treatment and long-term follow-up, the responsibility for follow-up transitions from the NBS program to health care systems.

Payors: Health insurers and programs such as Medicaid and the Children's Health Insurance Program determine and comply with policies regarding coverage of fees for care related to newborn screening, which may include fees related to blood collection, follow-up diagnostic testing, and clinical care.

Researchers and research organizations: Researchers and research organizations produce the scientific evidence that advisory bodies and NBS programs use to inform decisions about which conditions to screen, which testing methods to use, and best practices for providing clinical care. Researchers also investigate ethical, legal, and social issues related to newborn screening to inform policy and practice.

Industry: Private companies provide for purchase laboratory equipment and supplies necessary to conduct newborn screening. Some state- and territorial-run programs use private laboratories to screen their dried blood spots. Private companies also develop new screening and diagnostic tools as well as drugs or other treatments for disorders. Industry often provides financial support for selected research initiatives related to newborn screening and advocacy efforts to expand screening programs.

SOURCE: Andrews et al., 2022; APHL, 2015; HRSA, 2023b; Severin and Jones, 2023; Watson et al., 2022.

BOX 2-3
Federal Partners Involved in Newborn Screening

The primary federal partners involved in newborn screening include the Health Resources and Services Administration (HRSA), the Centers for Disease Control and Prevention (CDC), the National Institutes of Health (NIH), Food and Drug Administration (FDA), and the Agency for Healthcare Research and Quality (AHRQ) (HHS, 2015). Each agency works with its partners to support newborn screening, including through ex officio membership on the Advisory Committee on Heritable Disorders in Newborns and Children, described below.

HRSA: HRSA provides grants and programmatic support for state and territorial NBS programs in their efforts to implement screening for new conditions and provide appropriate follow-up care for children with serious conditions identified via newborn screening. HRSA also administers processes related to the Federal Advisory Committee on Heritable Disorders in Newborns and Children (ACHDNC).

BOX 2-3 Continued

ACHDNC advises the secretary of the U.S. Department of Health and Human Services on newborn and childhood screening, including the appropriate application of tests, technologies, policies, guidelines, and standards to effectively reduce morbidity and mortality in newborns with serious disorders. ACHDNC makes recommendations to the secretary on which conditions should be added to the Recommended Uniform Screening Panel (HRSA, 2022a, 2024a).

FDA: FDA regulates in vitro diagnostics, a category of medical devices that includes the tests used for newborn screening. FDA does not perform any direct testing of devices but reviews data and protocols from tests conducted by device manufacturers and determines whether the device has substantial equivalence (if there is a similar existing device) or a reasonable assurance of safety and effectiveness (if it is a new type of device) (Caposino, 2024; Watson et al., 2022). FDA also regulates drugs and biological products used to treat disorders, including overseeing approval processes for new products (Watson et al., 2022).

CDC: CDC's Newborn Screening and Molecular Biology Branch supports quality assurance for laboratories and screening tools involved in newborn screening through the Newborn Screen Quality Assurance Program (CDC, 2024d). It also assists NBS programs in their efforts to implement screening for new conditions, works to improve screening test performance and interpretation, facilitates training and technology transfer, and provides a national data platform to improve quality and interpretation of NBS results – Enhancing Data-Driven Disease Detection in Newborns (CDC, 2024a,c). CDC's National Center on Birth Defects and Developmental Disabilities also contributes to the broader NBS ecosystem through many avenues, including supporting other forms of screening relevant to infants, developing surveillance systems and registries, and creating resources for primary providers, patients, and their families (Boyle et al., 2012; CDC, 2024f).

NIH: NIH and its institutes fund research projects, infrastructure, and collaborations that provide evidence used for decision making around newborn screening. This includes research to understand diseases that are or may be selected for newborn screening; develop and improve screening and diagnostic tests; develop treatment and management strategies; investigate ethical, legal, and social implications associated with newborn screening; and facilitate translational research (Parisi, 2024; Watson et al., 2022).

AHRQ: AHRQ awards research grants and supports the dissemination of findings related to improving the safety and quality of public health systems and care delivery. It does not have a program specific to newborn screening but has supported research focused on assessing and improving NBS programs (Mistry, 2024).

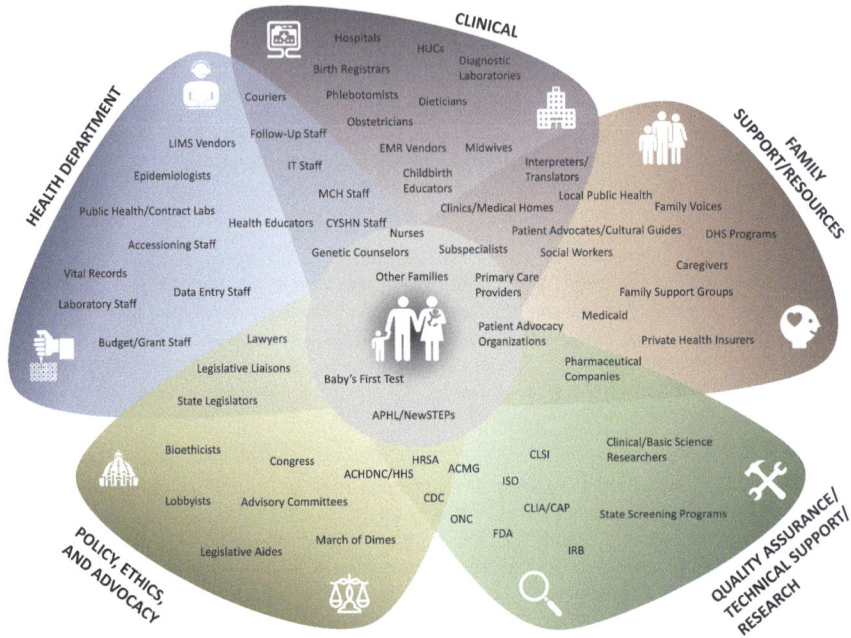

FIGURE 2-2 Players in the NBS ecosystem.
NOTES: ACHDNC = Advisory Committee on Heritable Disorders in Newborns and Children; ACMG = American College of Medical Genetics and Genomics; APHL = Association of Public Health Laboratories; CAP = College of American Pathologists; CLIA = Clinical Laboratory Improvement Amendments; CLSI = Clinical and Laboratory Standards Institute; CYSHN = Children and Youth with Special Health Care Needs; DHS = Department of Human Services; EMR = electronic medical record; FDA = Food and Drug Administration; HHS = Department of Health and Human Services; HRSA = Health Resources and Services Administration; HUC = health unit coordinator; IRB = institutional review board; ISO = International Organization for Standardization; IT = information technology; LIMS = laboratory information management system; MCH = Maternal and Child Health; NBS = newborn screening; NewSTEPs = Newborn Screening Technical assistance and Evaluation Program; ONC = Office of the National Coordinator for Health IT.
SOURCE: Amy Gaviglio, Connetics Consulting. Used with permission.

DISORDERS INCLUDED IN PUBLIC HEALTH NEWBORN SCREENING

Phenylketonuria (PKU) was the first condition for which newborns were routinely screened in the United States (NICHD, 2017a). An inherited disorder affecting the body's ability to metabolize the amino acid phenylalanine, PKU causes phenylalanine to accumulate in the body and interfere with brain development. If left untreated, it can lead to intellectual disability and seizures. Starting a low-protein diet in the first days of life can prevent these issues; as such, identifying infants with PKU shortly after birth can dramatically improve quality of life for these infants and their families (NHGRI, 2014). The development of an inexpensive blood test for PKU in 1961 made it possible to screen for the disorder shortly after birth and begin treatment for those identified to have the disease (Levy, 2021). Routine PKU screening of newborns was enacted into Massachusetts law in 1963 and adopted by most other states within the decade that followed. The implementation of this routine screening is credited with virtually eliminating PKU as a cause of intellectual disability in the United States (NICHD, 2017a).

As a disorder that (1) affects health, (2) is detectable in newborns, and (3) has improved health outcomes when treatment is delivered presymptomatically, PKU is emblematic of the types of conditions that have historically been the focus of newborn screening (NHGRI, 2014; Schnabel-Besson et al., 2024). To achieve the public health goals of screening, it is important for screening to result in better outcomes than would have occurred in the absence of screening (Wilson and Jungner, 1968). This determination involves weighing multiple potential benefits and harms related to early detection and treatment for a given health condition. As science and technology have advanced and it has become feasible to detect and treat a variety of other medical conditions manifesting in newborns, an increasingly broad array of conditions has been deemed suitable for public health newborn screening (Currier, 2022).

While various federal advisory groups, research, and programs have supported and informed state NBS programs over the decades, the determination of how many and which disorders to screen has always rested with the individual state and territorial NBS programs (Fabie et al., 2019). This has led to substantial variation in the disorders included in public health newborn screening from state to state. By the early 2000s, some states screened for as few as 3 conditions while others screened for as many as 43 (ACMG Newborn Screening Expert Group, 2005). In 2003, the Department of Health and Human Services (HHS) established the Advisory Committee on Heritable Disorders in Newborns and Children (ACHDNC) to advise the secretary of Health and Human Services about newborn and childhood screening, and in 2010 the secretary established the Recommended Uniform Screening Panel (RUSP), a list of disorders programs are encouraged to screen (HRSA, 2021).

Federal Processes for Selecting Disorders

The RUSP is the primary mechanism through which the federal government helps to guide state and territorial decisions about the selection of disorders for public health newborn screening. Informed by an expert analysis by the American College of Medical Genetics (ACMG) released in 2005, the RUSP was established in 2010 with an initial list of 29 core

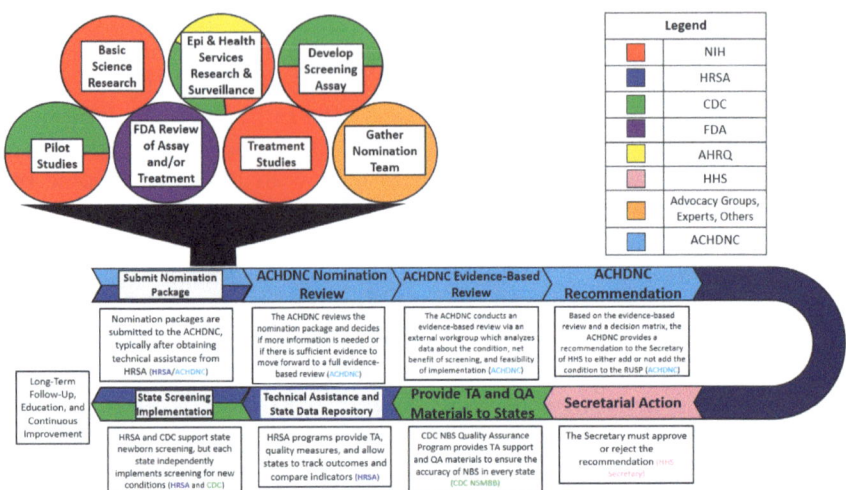

FIGURE 2-3 The process for adding a condition to the Recommended Uniform Screening Panel (RUSP) and the roles of various players involved.
NOTES: ACHDNC = Advisory Committee on Heritable Disorders in Newborns and Children; AHRQ = Agency for Healthcare Research and Quality; CDC = Centers for Disease Control and Prevention; Epi = epidemiological; FDA = Food and Drug Administration; HHS = Department of Health and Human Services; HRSA = Health Resources and Services Administration; NIH = National Institutes of Health; NBS = newborn screening; NSMBB = CDC's Newborn Screening and Molecular Biology Branch; RUSP = Recommended Uniform Screening Panel; TA = technical assistance.
SOURCE: Presented by Jeffrey Brosco, HRSA, January 26, 2024. Minear et al., 2022. CC PDM 1.0.

conditions identified as primary targets for screening and 25 secondary conditions (disorders that are detected in the differential diagnosis of a core disorder, but lack an effective treatment or are poorly understood) (ACMG Newborn Screening Expert Group, 2006).[6] As of August 2024, the RUSP includes 38 core conditions and 26 secondary conditions (HRSA, 2024d). Only 2 of 56 programs currently screen for all 38 RUSP core conditions.[7] Once added to the RUSP, there is not a formal mechanism for removing a condition if population screening reveals that the condition does not meets selection criteria (e.g., net benefit) (Kemper et al., 2014).

The process for adding conditions to the RUSP involves the collective efforts of hundreds of people across the NBS ecosystem (Figure 2-3).

---

[6] ACMG released its report in 2005, and an executive summary was published in *Genetics in Medicine* in 2006.

[7] See https://www.newsteps.org/resources/data-visualizations/newborn-screening-status-all-disorders (accessed January 28, 2025) for up-to-date information on the number of RUSP conditions screened by each program.

The submission of a preliminary nomination form to ACHDNC marks the beginning of the official process to add a condition to the core RUSP panel, but the process actually begins much earlier (Armstrong, 2024; HRSA, 2024c). Prior to submitting a full nomination package, nominators first submit a preliminary nomination form, which is considered by the Nomination and Prioritization workgroup of ACHDNC. The nominators can complete a full nomination package once the working group verifies that the following requirements are met for the condition: an NBS test is available; there is an agreed-upon case definition; a prospective population-based study has been conducted that has identified at least one infant with the condition; and identification before clinical onset allows provision of an effective, approved therapy.[8] To generate a nomination package requires conducting and reviewing research on the health condition, its causes, and its effects; strategies for detecting the condition in newborns, including a population-based pilot study; and approved treatments for the condition (HRSA, 2022b).

Multiple federal and other partners play a role in funding, carrying out, and evaluating studies and technologies relevant to the condition to be nominated. This includes National Institutes of Health (NIH) and Agency for Healthcare Research and Quality (AHRQ) support for basic and translational research; Food and Drug Administration (FDA) reviews of the screening assay and/or treatment; and Centers for Disease Control and Prevention (CDC) contributions to disease surveillance, screening tool validation, and pilot studies for newborn screening using the proposed assay (Brosco, 2024). Critically, this process also relies on the establishment of a nomination team that typically includes patient advocates, scientific and medical experts, and other partners who gather and evaluate the evidence and assemble the nomination package, a process that typically takes several years (HRSA, 2022b).

After an initial review, the ACHDNC decides if sufficient evidence is available, and votes to assign, or not assign, the nominated condition to the external Evidence-Based Review Group (ERG). The ERG systematically reviews the evidence, models the expected effect on health outcomes if the condition were to be added to the RUSP, and assesses the feasibility of implementation by NBS programs. The goal of this review is to not only assess the potential benefits and harms of screening newborns for the disorder but also to identify gaps and anticipate challenges to implementation if screening were to be recommended (HRSA, 2024c).

ACHDNC uses the evidence review group's report along with a decision matrix (Figure 2-4) to make a recommendation to the secretary of HHS regarding whether the condition should be added to the RUSP. The decision matrix, updated in August 2024, prompts each committee

---

[8] The nomination process was updated to include a preliminary nomination form in May 2024 in response to feedback from families, clinicians, and other affected individuals. See https://www.hrsa.gov/advisory-committees/heritable-disorders/rusp/nominate (accessed March 24, 2025).

Recommended Uniform Screening Panel Decision Matrix

ACHDNC — Advisory Committee on Heritable Disorders in Newborns and Children

Certainty of Net Benefit	Magnitude of Net Benefit		
	Substantial	Moderate	Zero, Small or Negative
High	A	B	C
Moderate	B	B	C
Low	I (Insufficient)		

Letter Grade	Description	Action
A	High certainty of substantial net benefit	Recommend addition to the RUSP
B	At least moderate certainty of at least moderate net benefit	Discuss and vote on recommending addition to the RUSP
C	At least moderate certainty of less than moderate net benefit	Do not recommend addition to the RUSP; Identify evidence gaps
I	Low certainty of net benefit	Do not recommended addition to the RUSP; Identify evidence gaps

Public Health Impact Assessment for implementation in 2 years	
% of states reporting effort required as high (# of states reporting high / # states reporting)	
% of states reporting effort required as moderate (# of states reporting moderate / # of states reporting)	
% of states reporting effort required as low (# of states reporting low / # of states reporting)	

FIGURE 2-4 Recommended Uniform Screening Panel decision matrix.
SOURCE: HRSA, 2024e.

member to assess the net benefit of screening all newborns and the certainty of the evidence regarding the net benefit. Designations for net benefit were adapted from the U.S. Preventative Services Task Force with an *A* designation indicates a high certainty of net benefit and leads to recommendation for addition to the RUSP (Calonge, 2023). Using the decision matrix, members also assess the feasibility of implementing screening, and the readiness of programs to implement expanded screening (HRSA, 2024c), although cost-effectiveness of screening, diagnosis, and treatment is not usually considered in this process (Grosse et al., 2016). The decision matrix is a tool to support the committee's decision making, but members ultimately make the decision that is then passed along to the secretary. The secretary then accepts or rejects the recommendation. If a condition is recommended for inclusion and that recommendation is accepted, the condition is added to the RUSP (HRSA, 2024c).

While ACHDNC and the RUSP are mechanisms for providing evidence-based guidance to state and territorial NBS programs, the process of adding conditions to the RUSP also poses challenges. One challenge is the length of time the process takes. According to Health Resources and Services Administration (HRSA) documentation, the shortest time elapsed from the submission of a nomination package to secretarial action was 21 months and the longest was 10 years, with most taking 3–4 years

(HRSA, 2022b). Several stages of review and decision making coupled with the frequency of ACHDNC meetings (only a few times a year) can contribute to the length of the RUSP process. The duration can be further prolonged by necessary resubmissions of nomination packages with additional information that required further research (HRSA, 2022b). Such information is often essential to inform how to screen for the targeted condition safely and effectively (see Box 2-4). While acknowledging the reasons behind the duration of the process, the RUSP process also faces scrutiny for its ability to keep up with medical advances and for the burden it places on the rare disease advocacy community (Andrews et al., 2022; Armstrong, 2024; Kennedy, 2024). These frustrations can drive some advocates to bypass the evidence-based RUSP review process, turning instead to state legislatures to expedite the addition of conditions to NBS panels (APHL, 2015; Susanna Haas Lyons Consulting, 2024).

A related challenge is the sheer amount of effort and time required to assemble the necessary evidence and clear the required reviews at each stage. Generating the evidence used as part of this process reflects an enormous undertaking across the NBS ecosystem—spanning basic science, translational and clinical research, technology development, and population-based pilot studies. These studies must be proposed, funded, conducted, and interpreted. Maintaining the attention and funding necessary to drive this evidence-generation process can also require significant effort on the part of advocacy groups (Armstrong, 2024).

Population-based pilot studies are a particularly onerous component of the nomination package that pose a "chicken or the egg" dilemma: to be considered for nomination to the RUSP for screening, a condition must have already been screened as part of a population-based study. These studies are important to demonstrate feasibility and public health impact (ACHDNC Pilot Studies Workgroup, 2016). However, they require significant funding and effort or may be initiated after a condition is added by a state following political advocacy, thus circumventing other evidence-based mechanisms for addition to newborn screening (APHL, 2015).

A final challenge, and one which could further compound the first two, is that emerging knowledge and technologies present a more complicated array of options—and a more complicated array of potential benefits and harms—for public health newborn screening (Currier, 2022). New technologies pose resource and expertise demands on state- and territorial-run programs, including purchasing new equipment, validating new testing processes, training personnel, storing data, handling sensitive genetic information, and more (Currier, 2022; Watson et al., 2022). Beyond the practical demands and challenges to programs, ethical, legal, and social questions are raised by employing new technologies in newborn screening (Grant, 2022; Ram, 2022; Ross and Clayton, 2019). As it becomes possible to test for an ever broader range of conditions, including

BOX 2-4
Case Study: SCID

The process by which severe combined immunodeficiency (SCID) was incorporated into routine newborn screening provides an illustrative example of the complexity of the review, recommendation, and implementation processes for adding new conditions to screening panels; the many stakeholders and rights holders involved; and challenges related to assessing and implementing new screening technology.

SCID is a rare disorder in which a person's immune system is compromised, leaving them extremely vulnerable to infection. There are several forms of the condition, most of which have a genetic cause. Because babies born with SCID do not have a normally functioning immune system, they can become seriously ill or die from infections. SCID can be effectively treated with a bone marrow transplant, gene therapy, and other established therapies (NIAID, 2019).

The addition of SCID to the Recommended Uniform Screening Panel (RUSP) marked the culmination of many years of effort on the part of physicians and researchers, individuals and families, state newborn screening (NBS) laboratories, SCID experts and advisors, patient advocacy groups, and other partners (Ballard, 2024). Advocacy for adding SCID to the RUSP started well before the RUSP existed, at the first meeting of the Advisory Committee on Heritable Disorders in Newborns and Children (ACHDNC) in 2004 (Ballard, 2024). In the years that followed, the development of an assay to measure a marker known as a T-cell receptor excision circle (TREC), which is absent or low in infants with SCID, made it more feasible to screen for SCID using dried blood spots (Chan and Puck, 2005). The first pilot study for TREC-based newborn screening for SCID began in Wisconsin in 2008 (Baker et al., 2010). ACHDNC initially voted against recommending SCID for the RUSP in 2009, citing five key evidence gaps including the lack of identification of a confirmed case through population-based screening, but in 2010 voted in favor of recommending SCID for the RUSP after receiving additional information to address these gaps (Geleske, 2010; HRSA, 2021).

SCID was officially added to the RUSP as a core condition shortly after the RUSP was established in 2010, and by the end of that year several states had begun routine screening (HRSA, 2021). However, the road to implementation was only just beginning; it was not until 2018—a full 8 years after SCID was added to the RUSP—that SCID newborn screening was adopted across all state and territorial NBS programs (Currier and Puck, 2021).

The implementation of universal newborn screening for SCID was associated with significant improvements in survival for babies born with SCID in the United States (Thakar et al., 2023). However, SCID's path to the RUSP—and the long road to universal implementation—also highlights challenges. One challenge cited by those involved is that generating the evidence necessary for approval and urging the actions necessary for implementation required considerable time and effort on the part of advocates at every step (Ballard, 2024). Another challenge stems from the fact that the TREC test was the first DNA-based test to be proposed for newborn screening, creating a learning curve requiring decision makers, NBS laboratories, and other players to establish new frameworks and processes for reviewing the evidence for the test, supporting quality assurance and validation, and conducting pilot studies (HRSA, 2010). Lastly, unbiased

BOX 2-4 Continued

population screening for SCID using the TREC test presents the challenge of uncovering secondary findings of non-SCID T-cell lymphocyte deficiencies (Kwan et al., 2014). Best practices for follow-up of infants at risk for non-SCID T-cell lymphopenias remain unclear (Kubala et al. 2022). Non-SCID T-cell lymphocyte deficiencies are included as secondary RUSP conditions as secondary findings when screening for SCID (HRSA, 2024d).

As technology continues to advance and additional test modalities are proposed for newborn screening, similar issues may emerge for future disorders. In addition, even many years after the TREC test was developed and SCID was recommended for newborn screening, questions remain regarding best practices for screening, follow-up diagnostic testing, and treatment for babies born with SCID, as well as gaps in communication, data collection and reporting, and uneven access to specialized care (Currier and Puck, 2021, Gaviglio et al., 2023; Sheller et al., 2020). These challenges demonstrate that for many disorders selected for newborn screening, the job is not finished when a condition is added to the RUSP; there remains a need for continued investment in scientific research and program evaluation to elucidate best practices, improve public health systems, and ensure the best possible outcomes for people born with serious disorders.

---

adult-onset conditions, carrier status, and others, there is not always a clear action associated with the test results, a clear benefit to screening in the newborn period, or a complete understanding of the potential psychosocial harms (Currier, 2022). Such considerations can make it more difficult to assess the evidence and guide decision making.

A case study describing how severe combined immunodeficiency (SCID) was added to the RUSP (Box 2-4) illustrates how the process works and some of the challenges involved.

State Processes for Selecting Disorders

Although the RUSP exists to help inform and harmonize newborn screening across the country, there is no federal law or regulation requiring state NBS programs to align with the RUSP (HRSA, 2024d). Each NBS program establishes its own processes for selecting disorders and implementing screening according to state and territorial laws and regulations. The responsibility for carrying out decision-making processes around NBS panels (and overseeing screening programs) typically rests with state or territorial public health departments, the state board of health, or a combination of such bodies (HRSA, 2024b). Some states have laws or proposed legislation requiring public health departments to align their NBS panels with the RUSP, while other states have no requirements regarding RUSP alignment (EveryLife Foundation for Rare Diseases, n.d.).

Most states have expert committees (akin to a state-level ACHDNC) that consider conditions nominated for screening, review the evidence, and make a formal recommendation to approve or reject the nomination (APHL, 2015).[9] This process often involves receiving public comments and assessing projected costs and logistical considerations in addition to considering the scientific evidence about the disorder, its detection, and its treatment. States often use criteria similar to those used by ACHDNC to guide decisions at a national level, but they do so in a state context, gauging the expected benefits, harms, and feasibility of implementation in the context of the particular state or territory and its population (Montana DPHHS, n.d.). Moving through such state-level processes involved in reviewing, recommending, and implementing newborn screening for a new condition often takes several years (Singh et al., 2023).

Cost can be an important issue at the state and territorial level, with some states performing cost-benefit analyses comparing the status quo to adding the nominated condition to the updated screening panel (Thompson, 2024). Adding a condition to a state or territory's NBS panel typically increases the cost of screening, and while some federal grants may be available to offset this (see Chapter 4), most states usually raise NBS fees to accommodate adding new conditions (Dorley, 2024).

IMPLEMENTATION OF NBS PROGRAMS

Newborn screening in the United States is carried out by state and territorial NBS programs. These programs receive guidance and support from federal entities but operate independently under the authority of their state or territory. As a result, programs vary substantially.

Program Oversight and Operations

NBS programs are generally run by state or territorial health departments with oversight and support from state legislatures and other officials, boards of health, or other entities (GAO, 2003).[10] Coordinating a state NBS program is a complex endeavor. In addition to determining which conditions to screen, states must address countless details about how screening is performed, including policies and practices for blood spot collection and parental consent, qualifications and training for personnel, the laboratory equipment and test protocols to be used, how results are

---

[9] See https://www.newsteps.org/resources/data-visualizations/newborn-screening-advisory-committees (accessed September 26, 2024) for up-to-date information on whether programs currently have an advisory committee, if the advisory committee is mandatory or voluntary, meeting frequency, and other details.

[10] See https://www.newsteps.org/data-center/state-profiles?q=data-resources/state-profiles (accessed January 30, 2025) for additional details about how each state and territorial program is run.

communicated and clinically assessed, and how all these activities will be financed (Dubay and Zach, 2023; Lewis et al., 2011). These factors can also change as laws, technologies, and funding structures evolve over time, necessitating careful management and frequent adjustments.

The addition of a new condition to a state's screening panel sets off a cascade of additional tasks and decisions on top of the program's continuing operations. When a new condition is approved for the state panel, the NBS program must do the following:

- coordinate with hospitals, laboratories, health care providers, payors, and others to identify, validate, and establish standard operating procedures for the testing methods to be used;
- establish expected ranges for interpreting the results;
- identify equipment needs and secure the necessary funding, facility space, and infrastructure to perform the new tests;
- incorporate the new condition into electronic data management and tracking systems;
- establish follow-up protocols;
- identify health care providers and specialists as needed; and
- educate and train personnel.

All of this happens within systems that often require complex processes for establishing contracts, procuring materials, hiring staff, obtaining approvals, and communicating with stakeholders. In addition, all of these decisions have financial implications. When adding a new condition for screening, states must identify a funding mechanism to cover the initial implementation and continued ongoing operations (Dorley, 2024; Thompson, 2024).

The complexity of operating NBS programs and onboarding new conditions contributes to a significant lag time between when a new condition is added to the RUSP and/or state screening panel and when screening is universally implemented. According to one analysis, implementation for disorders added to the RUSP between 2010 and 2018 took as few as 2.1 years on average for spinal muscular atrophy and as many as 4 years on average for Pompe disease among states and territories that incorporated those conditions into their screening panels (Singh et al., 2023).

Variation Across Programs

Since the inception of newborn screening in the 1960s, there has been substantial variation in how NBS programs operate (Watson, 2006). As discussed above, programs have long varied regarding the number and types of conditions they screen. Program implementation also differs widely (see Box 2-5).

BOX 2-5
Variability Across State and Territorial NBS Programs

Considerable variability exists across state- and territorial-run newborn screening (NBS) programs. Each program must comply with the legislative requirements of their jurisdiction and implement the program using the funding, workforce, and other resources available to them. As such, programs vary in terms of the number of core Recommended Uniform Screening Panel (RUSP) conditions screened, the timeliness with which results are returned, and the fee charged to hospitals for screening each newborn, among other factors. NBS programs also have variable health information technology (IT) infrastructure at hand to ensure rapid, accurate, and effective communication between laboratories, follow-up programs, and clinical care. Health IT infrastructure can also allow for greater interoperability and comprehensive data capture as greater emphasis is placed on longitudinal follow-up for infants identified through newborn screening (Abhyanker et al., 2015). Below provides a snapshot of the variability of state-run programs across the United States.

Core RUSP conditions screened: State and territorial programs screen from 31 to 38 of the 38 conditions on the RUSP.

Timeliness: In 2022, 18 programs reported from 3 percent to 100 percent of time-critical results within 5 days birth, with a median of 57 percent of results reported (NewSTEPs, 2023).

Fees: For programs that charge fees (typically billed to hospitals), fees for each baby screened range from $30 to $258 with a median cost of $185. Five programs do not charge a fee.

Electronic messaging: There are 15 programs that can both send and receive Health Level Seven (HL7) electronic messaging, 3 programs can only receive HL7 electronic messaging, 3 programs can only send electronic messaging, and 25 programs can neither send nor receive electronic messaging; 10 programs did not provide data.

Information systems:
- Laboratory information management system (LIMS): 23 programs use Revvity, 14 use Neometrics/Natus, 6 use internally developed programs, 3 use StarLims, 9 use other LIMS, and 1 program did not provide data.
- Follow-up information management system: 16 programs use Revvity, 10 use Neometrics/Natus, 17 use internally developed programs, 2 use StarLims, 9 use other information systems including Excel, and 1 program did not provide data.
- Only 25 programs use the same information systems for both laboratory and follow-up.

NOTE: See https://www.newsteps.org/data-center/dashboards-and-reports (accessed January 30, 2025) for up-to-date information on each state or territory's NBS program, including their responsible laboratory.

Although the procedure for collecting a blood spot is consistent across states and collection contexts, the processes surrounding collection vary, and are not always well documented. For example, there are few data about how and when parents are informed about newborn screening. Most state programs have no formal opt-in process but allow parents to opt out of newborn screening for religious or other reasons (President's Council on Bioethics, 2008). The information that is collected on the sample card (including details about the infant such as race or ethnicity, home address, and other features) also varies from state to state. In addition, some states perform only a single screen in the first days of life, while others perform an additional screen 12 weeks later with a new dried blood spot sample.

These second screens are typically collected by the primary care provider and sent for testing with the goal of increasing identification of children for certain conditions (e.g., congenital hypothyroidism) (HRSA, 2023b; Shapira et al., 2015). This second screen is different from second-tier or reflex testing which is performed for only a subset of infants who have an out-of-range result on their initial screen; second-tier screening is performed using the same blood spot, whereas second screen uses a newly collected blood spot (Caggana et al., 2013).

Testing of blood spots may be done in state laboratories, university centers, private laboratories, or even be outsourced to laboratories in other states (GAO, 2003; NewSTEPs, 2021). Laboratories may use different tests or methodologies to detect risk for the same condition with variable accuracy, specificity, and sensitivity (Dubay and Zach, 2023; McGarry et al., 2023; Rehani et al., 2023). Most NBS programs operate their laboratories 6 days per week and their follow-up offices 5 days per week, although operational hours can range between 5 and 7 days per week for both.[11] Programs that operate for more days per week are more likely to achieve compliance with timeliness goals (Sontag et al., 2020).

The funding mechanisms for supporting NBS programs also vary from state to state (Johnson et al., 2006). While many programs receive state funding and federal grants, most funding for NBS program operations comes from fees that NBS programs charge to birthing facilities. These fees are often bundled with other charges for newborn care that are billed to insurance companies (Costich and Durst, 2016). Newborn screening is required coverage for most health plans under the Affordable Care Act.[12] Therefore, insurance will cover the cost of newborn screening

---

[11] See https://www.newsteps.org/resources/data-visualizations/operating-days-and-hours (accessed September 26, 2024) for up-to-date information on each program's operating days and hours for both laboratory and follow-up.

[12] Patient Protection and Affordable Care Act of 2010, Pub. L. No. 111-148, 124 Stat. 119.

for most newborns, either through Medicaid—which covers the cost of approximately 40 percent of births in the United States annually (CMS, 2024)—or private insurance. Hospitals are required to perform screening even for families who cannot pay (NICHD, 2017b). However, uninsured individuals may be asked to pay the NBS fee depending on the program.[13] For those delivering outside of hospital settings, these fees can be a challenge as home births and birth center births are much less likely to be covered by insurance (AABC, 2024; Coupal et al., 2021; MacDorman and Declerq, 2019). Birthing centers and birth workers report that they often assume the cost of NBS tests or pass the cost onto families (AABC, 2024). The fees NBS programs charge range from $0 to over $200 per blood collection card purchased or processed, with most programs' fees falling between $51 and $150 per card.[14] An analysis revealed no correlation between the fees charged and the number of conditions screened, laboratory operating hours, or follow-up activities (Ojodu, 2024).

Finally, programs differ in their processes for following up on screening results. Each NBS program develops its own protocols for testing blood samples, with many using a tiered system to analyze secondary parameters and increase the specificity of results for screens that fall outside of expected ranges in first-tier testing (Furnier et al., 2020; Rehani et al., 2023). Programs may vary in their processes for handling repeat screening or additional diagnostic testing for presumptive positive, borderline, or unsatisfactory results, as well as the involvement of NBS program personnel and laboratories versus primary care providers or specialty clinicians in these processes (HRSA, 2023b). As infants with serious health conditions transition from screening to diagnosis and care—thus transitioning from a public health program to the health care system—the extent of NBS program involvement in facilitating clinical care or ongoing surveillance can also vary.

Timely identification of infants with serious disorders is at the core of the value proposition for newborn screening; as such, compliance with timeliness goals is a key quality indicator for NBS programs. According to timeliness goals articulated by ACHDNC in 2015, blood samples should be collected within 48 hours after birth and received at the laboratory within 24 hours of collection, presumptive positive results for time-critical conditions should be communicated to the baby's health care provider no later than 5 days of life, and presumptive positive results for all other conditions should be communicated to the baby's health care

---

[13] For example, see https://doh.wa.gov/you-and-your-family/infants-and-children/newborn-screening/screening-cost (accessed February 19, 2025).

[14] See https://www.newsteps.org/data-resources/reports/nbs-fees-report (accessed September 26, 2024) for up-to-date information on fees associated with each program.

provider no later than 7 days of life (HRSA, 2017). Data for 2012–2015 showed that most states were not meeting these goals for 95 percent of specimens (GAO, 2016). Recent data collected from 25 state-run programs indicated an improvement in timeliness metrics especially for programs open 7 days per week; however, timeliness goals are still not being fully met (NewSTEPs, 2023; Sontag et al., 2020). Other quality indicators that have been used to assess NBS programs include percentage of infants lost to follow-up (i.e., infants that did not receive a confirmed diagnosis or diagnosis ruled out), percentage of newborns not screened, percentage of unsatisfactory specimens, and more.[15]

Many factors may influence states' ability to meet timeliness goals and other quality indicators. For example, the task of transporting samples from isolated communities in Alaska to a testing laboratory in Iowa is drastically different from transporting samples from a major university hospital to a laboratory on the same campus.[16] The vulnerability of systems to events such as power outages, blizzards, and hurricanes can also affect NBS program performance (National Center on Birth Defects and Developmental Disabilities, 2017). The complexity of the conditions being screened can also challenge timeliness. As with any program administered by state and territorial governments, NBS programs are also vulnerable to evolving legislative priorities and variability in state budget allocations. In addition, disease prevalence, population demographics, and clinical capacity for specialized management and treatment can be different between states, all of which affect newborn screening. While variation in the practice of public health newborn screening may be understandable and even inevitable given these circumstances, to fulfill the value proposition of newborn screening requires that such variability does not extend to the outcomes experienced by newborns and their families.

Support for Public Health NBS Programs

State and territorial NBS programs receive both programmatic and monetary support from federal sources. This support can take a variety of forms, from crosscutting resources intended to benefit all NBS programs to grants issued for specific NBS programs or activities. Organizations outside the federal government, such as professional organizations and advocacy groups, also provide support and resources to NBS programs and the NBS system as a whole.

---

[15] See https://www.newsteps.org/data-center/quality-indicators?q=data-resources/quality-indicators (accessed September 26, 2024).
[16] See https://www.newsteps.org/data-resources/reports/courier-system-report (accessed September 26, 2024).

Several laws have played an important role in federal activities relevant to public health newborn screening. Examples include the Children's Health Act of 2000,[17] which led to the establishment of ACHDNC; the Newborn Screening Saves Lives Act of 2007,[18] which provided funding for various NBS activities and led to the establishment of the RUSP; and the Newborn Screening Saves Lives Reauthorization Act of 2014, which extended and expanded upon the 2008 legislation but expired in 2019 when it was not reauthorized a second time (HRSA, 2021).[19] Although there is no direct federal source for routine programming support of NBS programs, programs can receive federal funding through Title V block grants and grants from the Heritable Disorders Program under the Children's Health Act of 2000 (Johnson et al., 2006).

HRSA leads several efforts aimed at facilitating effective public health newborn screening across the country. In addition to its direct involvement administering ACHDNC and the RUSP, HRSA provides support to state and territorial NBS programs through state grant mechanisms known as NBS Propel and Co-Propel, a national coordinating center known as NBS Excel, and family engagement and leadership projects. These efforts began in 2023 and the period of performance for these grant programs will end in 2028. These efforts are intended to help NBS programs address state- or territory-specific challenges, support screening implementation for core RUSP conditions, and improve follow-up (HRSA, 2024a,e). Where particular gaps in access to follow-up and treatment have been identified (for example, in access to high-quality treatment and follow-up for sickle cell disease), HRSA also funds condition-specific programs to address these gaps (HRSA, 2023c).

A variety of federal, state, and nonprofit partners play critical roles in carrying out activities supported by HRSA. For example, the Association of Public Health Laboratories receives HRSA funding to develop and maintain the Newborn Screening Technical assistance and Evaluation Program (NewSTEPs),[20] a program that provides data, technical assistance, and training to support some NBS programs. Another example is Baby's First Test, an educational resource for families and health professionals (Baby's First Test, 2024b). Baby's First Test was initially funded through a cooperative agreement between HRSA and the nonprofit organization Genetic Alliance; it is now maintained through partnership agreements, licensing, and sponsorship (Baby's First Test, 2024b).

---

[17] Children's Health Act of 2000, Public Law 106-310, 106th Cong., 2nd sess. (October 17, 2000).

[18] Newborn Screening Saves Lives Act of 2008, S1858, 110th Cong., 1st sess., Congressional Record 153, No. 191, daily ed. (December 13, 2007).

[19] Newborn Screening Saves Lives Reauthorization Act of 2014, HR1281, 113th Congress., 2nd sess., Congressional Record 160, No. 158, daily ed. (December 8, 2014).

[20] See https://www.newsteps.org/ (accessed September 26, 2024). Although there are 56 newborn screening programs, only 53 are actively providing data to NewSTEPS.

CDC also provides substantial support to state NBS programs. Its efforts focus on building capacity directly within state NBS programs as well as through CDC's Newborn Screening and Molecular Biology Branch, which provides a variety of services to support NBS laboratories. CDC activities have included issuing grants to support state implementation of screening for conditions added to the RUSP; developing a national contingency plan for ensuring continued NBS program operation during crises; providing reference materials and improving test performance for biochemical and DNA-based screening through its national Newborn Screening Quality Assurance Program; and providing technical assistance, training, and site visits to inform and enhance laboratory practices (CDC, 2024a,e).

In addition, CDC's Enhancing Data-Driven Disease Detection in Newborns (ED3N) project is under way to establish a national data platform to improve the quality and interpretation of NBS results (CDC, 2024c). A new funding program starting in 2024 will establish a Center of Excellence to Enhance Disease Detection in Newborns with a goal of positioning NBS programs to adapt in response to new technological developments and meet increasing demands (CDC, 2024b).

These and other sources of support can play a vital role in facilitating quality assurance, operational improvements, and education and outreach to support high-quality NBS programs across the country. However, the availability of grants and other mechanisms of support does not automatically mean that all NBS programs will benefit from them. Lower-resourced states and programs may face greater challenges allocating staff resources toward applying for grants and taking advantage of various opportunities for programmatic support and improvement. Unchecked, this dynamic could lead to a situation where well-resourced NBS programs get stronger while federal channels of support do not always effectively reach the programs that could use them most.

COLLECTION AND USE OF BLOOD SPOTS

Blood samples are central to newborn screening. An examination of the practices and processes for the collection and use of samples—from obtaining consent for the initial heel stick all the way through to the eventual destruction of samples and data—highlights important facets of the current NBS system and some of the challenges it raises.

Consent and Sample Collection

Questions about parental consent have been raised throughout the history of newborn screening (Annas, 1982; Faden et al., 1982). When should parental consent be required, and when should parents be able to opt out of screening? Can a parent's right to refuse screening be outweighed by the potential harm that occurs if a child with a serious and treatable condition is not identified in time to fully benefit from treatment? When parents opt out of newborn screening, does it undermine not only their own child's right to access screening but also the public health benefits of newborn screening more broadly?

Consent requires that a participant must be informed, demonstrate understanding, and voluntarily agree to participate. NBS programs take a variety of approaches to consent (King and Smith, 2016). Since newborns cannot speak for themselves, consent for newborn screening applies to the infant's parent(s) or guardian(s). The vast majority of NBS programs take an opt-out approach, which assumes the baby will be screened unless a parent opts out, rather than requiring parents to affirmatively opt in. Most states allow parents to opt out for reasons of religious belief, and some allow parents to opt out for religious or personal reasons. A few programs include stipulations that parents should provide informed consent, be informed of their right to object, and/or be given a reasonable opportunity to opt out (President's Council on Bioethics, 2008). Bioethical foundations underpinning newborn screening are explored further in Chapter 3.

Although NBS programs in general have thus far been allowed to set their own processes for obtaining consent or allowing parents to opt out of universal screening, these are not settled questions. Debates related to these matters have surfaced repeatedly during the history of NBS programs and are likely to continue to arise in the future (Annas, 1982; Currier, 2022; Faden et al., 1982; Ross, 2010). The factors that influence the outcomes of these debates may also change as technologies and social contexts evolve (Goldenberg and Sharp, 2012). For example, if new screening technologies raise concerns about the risks of screening (e.g., psychosocial effects; data privacy; false positives and misinterpretation; ethical, legal, and social issues), it could tip the balance in favor of more parental control over participation in screening. The public's level of trust in science, medicine, and government could also influence how people view opt-out screening and the restrictions that should be placed upon these activities. Questions about who reaps the benefits and who incurs harms from newborn screening can also raise important considerations relevant to the conditions included on screening panels and the use of opt-out versus consented screening.

Testing Methods

Tests with the appropriate specificity and sensitivity are critical to the effectiveness of newborn screening as a public health intervention (Wilson and Jungner, 1968). A test with too many false positives burdens families and health care systems with unnecessary stress and expense, whereas a test with too many false negatives undermines the value of universal screening and leads to missed or delayed diagnoses (Goldenberg et al., 2016). In addition, to be viable for newborn screening at a population level it is important for tests to be cost-effective and feasible to implement rapidly at scale using dried blood spots (Wilson and Jungner, 1968). Achieving and demonstrating all of these parameters requires substantial investments in basic research, test development and refinement, and pilot testing within NBS programs (Watson et al., 2022).

The tests used for newborn screening have evolved over time (Watson et al., 2022). Most tests used or proposed for newborn screening fall into two main categories: biochemical tests and molecular (or DNA-based) tests (Almannai et al., 2016; CDC, 2024c). Biochemical tests measure biomarkers contained in blood that are associated with specific health conditions. For example, the test for PKU measures the amount of the amino acid phenylalanine in a baby's blood since children with PKU have elevated phenylalanine. Similarly, the test for cystic fibrosis measures the amount of the protein immunoreactive trypsinogen, which is typically elevated in babies with this condition (Minnesota Department of Health, 2022). Biochemical methods are used in both first-tier and second-tier testing (see Box 2-1 for definitions) (Almannai et al., 2016; CDC, 2024c).

Technology improvements in the 1990s enabled scientists to develop tests that measure multiple biomarkers with a single test, an approach called multiplexing. Tandem mass spectrometry (MS/MS) is the main platform used for multiplex testing (Chace et al., 2003). The availability of MS/MS made it feasible for NBS programs to efficiently screen for more disorders, which ultimately led many states to substantially expand their screening panels between 1990 and 2008 (ACMG Newborn Screening Expert Group, 2005; Tarini, 2007). Other biochemical testing methods include high-performance liquid chromatography, liquid chromatography tandem mass spectrometry, fluorometry, and isoelectric focusing (Minnesota Department of Health, 2022).

Molecular or nucleic acid-based tests identify genetic markers that are associated with health conditions. These genetic markers can be found in the DNA that each of us has within our cells (the genome), or they can be produced from various biological processes. The adoption of molecular tests for newborn screening is in its early stages. SCID was the first condition recommended for the RUSP that required the use of a molecular screening test, the TREC test (Van Der Spek et al., 2015). This test detects small DNA segments that are produced by certain immune cells, which are absent or low in infants with SCID, using a technique known as quantitative real-time polymerase chain reaction (PCR) (Chan and Puck, 2005). Other molecular testing methods include various other forms of PCR, next-generation sequencing, and whole genome sequencing (Friedman et al., 2017).

Currently, NBS programs use nucleic acid-based methods to detect specific diseases with single gene or targeted genotyping, most often as a second-tier screen to achieve greater specificity when a first-tier biochemical test shows results outside of the expected range (Smith et al., 2020). These methods can also be used to provide just-in-time information to help clinicians prepare for their initial communication with families regarding NBS-positive results (Furnier et al., 2020). However, the potential capabilities represented by methods such as next-generation sequencing and whole genome sequencing extend far beyond this targeted use. If used as a first-tier strategy, genetic sequencing could theoretically be used to identify a much broader array of conditions than is currently included in newborn screening (Goldenberg and Sharp, 2012). For example, genome-based screens could enable easier identification of not only the types of conditions that have historically been included in NBS programs—serious, identifiable in newborns, and treatable if identified early—but also health conditions that may emerge later in life, conditions for which no treatments are available, and even other genetic information not directly related to health. This possibility raises questions about what types of information parents and the state should be able to obtain about newborns, how this information should be used and how it should be protected, and what additional benefits and harms may result (King and Smith, 2016).

Limited representation of different ancestral groups in genomic databases further complicates opportunities to expand the use of nucleic acid-based methods in newborn screening. Underrepresented ancestral backgrounds have higher rates of variants of uncertain significance,[21] which could lead to misclassification of benign variants as pathogenic or missed diagnoses owing to an inability to recognize pathogenic variants (Rosamilia et al., 2024). Current second-tier testing for cystic fibrosis reveals these vulnerabilities as babies from underrepresented ancestral backgrounds are at a higher risk of receiving false-negative results and delays in intervention (McGarry et al., 2023). There are ongoing efforts to increase representation of different ancestral groups in genomic databases to ensure that all individuals receive access to the benefits of nucleic acid-based screening (All of Us Research Program Investigators, 2019; Fatumo et al., 2022; Wonkam

---

[21] Variants, or genetic differences, are categorized as either pathogenic, likely pathogenic, uncertain significance, likely benign, and benign based on the ACMG guidelines. A variant is categorized as uncertain significance if there is insufficient or conflicting evidence to determine its clinical significance (Richards et al., 2015).

et al., 2022). See Chapter 5 for further discussion of the applications for nucleic acid-based methods in newborn screening with a focus on genomic sequencing.

Storage and Secondary Use of Blood Spots

The blood spots collected for newborn screening can be useful for various purposes after the initial screening tests are completed (Baby's First Test, 2024a). Some of these potential uses are essential to the operation of NBS programs, others may benefit the infant or their family, while others may benefit society more broadly. Issues around the storage and subsequent use of blood spots after newborn screening raise important ethical, legal, and practical questions.

For families, blood spots from newborn screening can potentially be used to carry out subsequent testing (for example, to clarify an uncertain result or test for additional conditions) without requiring another blood draw (Baby's First Test, 2024a).

Further, the use of leftover blood spots is instrumental for improving and ensuring the quality of NBS programs. These residual blood spots, which match the composition of the state's population, are used by the NBS program for quality assurance and quality control purposes to continuously validate that the test methods used are accurate and reliable for each baby born (De Jesús et al., 2015; Texas Health and Human Services, 2024a,b).

Blood spots can also help advance biomedical research. Since a vast majority of infants participate in newborn screening, blood spot cards represent a large collection of biological samples that is broadly representative of the population. Blood spots can be used for environmental pollutant tracking and detection, genetic and epigenetic studies, biomarker detection, and drug monitoring (McClendon-Weary et al., 2020). Studying these samples can also lead to new insights about health and disease, including opportunities to identify, treat, and even prevent certain health conditions (Rothwell et al., 2019).

Like other aspects of newborn screening, there is no standard or universal practice for the storage and secondary use of blood spots across NBS programs; each state or territory establishes its own policies and practices (Lewis et al., 2011). Blood spots may be retained for a month or indefinitely; most states retain them for at least 6 months. They are typically stored in facilities managed by the laboratories that carry out NBS tests.[22]

---

[22] See https://www.newsteps.org/data-resources/reports/dbs-retention-report (accessed September 26, 2024) for up-to-date information on the length of time programs retain dried blood spots associated with each program.

Privacy and security are important concerns with storage and secondary use of blood spots and associated data. Since blood spots can potentially be used to identify individuals or their family members and uncover details about their health, people have raised concerns about the harms that could result if law enforcement personnel, health insurers, or others gained access to them (Grant, 2022; NASEM, 2010; Ram, 2022). A recent incident in New Jersey of law enforcement subpoenaing a newborn blood spot to investigate a 1996 cold case has exacerbated worries and distrust (Grant, 2022; Hughes et al., 2022). To safeguard privacy and reduce the risk of a security breach, states may use a variety of practices including separating biological samples from the details about the infant that are contained on the collection card, securing samples within locked facilities, employing best practices for securing electronic data, training personnel and restricting access to samples and data, and establishing oversight bodies that determine when and how samples may be accessed for research or other purposes (Baby's First Test, 2024a).

Consent to secondary reuse of blood spots is another important issue. In many cases, little or no information is provided to parents about what will happen to the blood spot after newborn screening is complete (Botkin et al., 2014). Even in states where parents are asked to consent to their infant's blood sample being used for research or other purposes, there may be questions about whether parents truly understand or whether the days following birth are an appropriate time to request consent (Kaeser, 2023; Rothwell et al., 2016). The storage and subsequent use of blood spots has sparked lawsuits in several states and resulted in judgments and settlements that have required states to destroy millions of stored blood spots (Hughes et al., 2022). See Chapter 4 for an exploration of policies and case law concerning storage and use of residual dried blood spots.

FOLLOW-UP CARE

To fulfill the public health promise of newborn screening and benefit people born with serious conditions, it is critical that individuals identified to have health conditions via screening receive follow-up care, not only when they are infants but throughout life (Howell and Engelson, 2007). In some cases, treatment must begin during an infant's first days of life to prevent death or severe disability. In other cases, monitoring the infant's health is the appropriate response and treatment decisions can wait until there is a clearer understanding of the person's condition and how their disease is progressing (Berry et al., 2016). In practice, ensuring appropriate follow-up care after newborn screening is a complex endeavor involving multiple sectors and partners, and it may not always result in access to and delivery of high-quality care for all (Houtrow et al., 2022).

The responsibility for short-term follow-up initially rests with the NBS program. When screening generates a result that is outside of the expected range, NBS programs may repeat the initial screening test or conduct second-tier testing of blood spots to provide further clarity on the result. The NBS program then communicates the results to the baby's primary care provider or a specialty clinician, who shares the results with the newborn's family. NBS program personnel, the primary care provider, or the specialty clinician may then recommend further testing or other steps to confirm a diagnosis and take medical action as appropriate (HRSA, 2023b).

As the process moves from screening to diagnosis to treatment and long-term follow-up, the responsibility for follow-up transitions from the NBS program to the health care system. The question of who pays for testing and follow-up at each stage is complex and varies from state to state. Although the Affordable Care Act requires most health plans to cover screening for RUSP conditions with no cost sharing, this does not address costs associated with confirmatory testing, counseling, medical food and formula, or future health care for infants with positive diagnoses—many of whom require special foods, medicines, or other interventions throughout their lifespan (Costich and Durst, 2016). Other costs incurred as part of newborn screening play out in different ways depending on the funding structures of state NBS programs, how NBS fees are bundled with other care costs associated with childbirth, and other factors. Some states cover or mandate insurance coverage for some of these costs, whereas others do not; for example, some states require health insurers cover medical formulas and food for children born with inborn errors of metabolism (Johnson Policy Consulting, 2008; Schuett, 2022). Coverage for services also may vary among Medicaid programs, Medicare,[23] and commercial insurance plans.

Like other aspects of the U.S. health care system, the task of ensuring access and delivery of high-quality care for all has raised challenges in the context of newborn screening. Infants with special health care needs who are born to families with fewer economic or social resources, language barriers, and difficulty accessing transportation can face challenges receiving the care they need. Infants born in areas that lack specialty clinics or equipment required for the diagnosis and treatment of their condition can also face limitations (Houtrow et al., 2022). Since so much about the

---

[23] The first individuals identified with PKU by newborn screening over 60 years ago will soon become Medicare eligible. Medicare has a non-coverage determination for enteral medical food and formula. Therefore, these individuals could lose coverage for these necessary medical foods and formulas. See https://www.cms.gov/medicare-coverage-database/view/ncd.aspx?ncdid=242&ncdver=3& (accessed January 30, 2025).

implementation and funding of NBS programs varies from state to state, the families of children born in one state can experience significantly different challenges than those born just over the state border.

Questions and challenges related to follow-up care also become increasingly complex if screening panels expand to include a broader array of conditions, including more conditions with expensive and medically complex treatments such as gene therapy (Brown and Koenig, 2021). To raise awareness and help address these issues, public health researchers and patient advocates have created programs and policy initiatives aimed at improving care access and delivery, recognizing and addressing disparities, and empowering families to support the needs of their loved ones living with serious disorders.

RESEARCH PROGRAMS

Achieving the goals of public health newborn screening and ensuring its quality and cost-effectiveness requires ongoing research, both to keep existing tests and systems running well and to adopt new screening tests that can improve the lives of more people with serious disorders. Practitioners, researchers, and funding agencies play a critical role in advancing this work at the local, state, and federal levels.

Research studies across the country assess applications for emerging technologies in newborn screening and pilot test screens for new conditions (Early Check, 2024; GUARDIAN Study, 2021; Montefiore Einstein, 2024). Most of these studies are primarily funded by NIH and many also receive support from industry or advocacy organizations. They are typically conducted as partnerships involving academic research institutions, state departments of health, and state or private laboratories.

Many state NBS programs also conduct research to develop screening tests for conditions that are on or being considered for their state screening panel and implement those assays and others as part of population-based pilot studies (New England Newborn Screening Program, 2024; Rothwell et al., 2019). This work helps states to ensure that the methods used in their screening program are achieving the appropriate level of specificity and sensitivity in the specific context of the population they serve and with the equipment and protocols they use (ACHDNC Pilot Studies Workgroup, 2016). This work is also vital for developing a nomination package to the RUSP, adopting new conditions that are added to a state screening panel, and helping state programs identify opportunities to increase efficiency and cost-effectiveness in their operations.

Federal agencies including NIH, CDC, and AHRQ provide critical funding, infrastructure, and programmatic support to propel research programs relevant to newborn screening. NIH and its institutes have been instrumental in generating fundamental knowledge about rare diseases and their detection and treatment, as well as in spurring technology development and facilitating translational research. The *Eunice Kennedy Shriver* National Institute on Child Health and Human Development (NICHD) and the National Human Genetics Research Institute (NHGRI) have led many of the NIH activities that are most directly relevant to newborn screening.

NIH supports research through both grants and contracts. NICHD awards grants for investigator-initiated research projects related to developing new screening approaches and therapies for disorders that can be screened in newborns, as well as research into the natural history of such disorders (HHS, 2021a,b; NICHD, 2024). Studies funded through these mechanisms span the spectrum from fundamental research to translational research that benefits patients, health systems, and communities. NICHD also contracts with state and private research organizations to conduct NBS pilot studies for conditions that are nominated for or recently added to the RUSP (Parisi, 2024). NICHD and NHGRI also support investigator-initiated research projects in ethical, legal, and social issues related to newborn screening or newborn sequencing (NHGRI, 2023).

NIH also has spearheaded several crosscutting initiatives aimed at facilitating collaboration and guiding research directions related to emerging developments in newborn screening and rare diseases. From 2008 to 2024 NICHD supported the Newborn Screening Translational Research Network through a contract with the ACMG, which developed research infrastructure to facilitate data sharing and information exchange to support collaboration across the NBS research community (NICHD, 2023). In addition, NICHD and NHGRI jointly established the Newborn Sequencing in Genomic Medicine and Public Health (NSIGHT) program, which ran from 2013 to 2019. Informed by research needs identified at a 2010 workshop, NSIGHT funded four studies examining exome sequencing and genome sequencing approaches in newborn screening and rare disease diagnostics (NHGRI, 2022). These still-ongoing studies and others (e.g., Early Check, BabySeq, Screen Plus, GUARDIAN, BeginNGS) are investigating the feasibility of using dried blood spots for genomic sequencing, defining panels of genes that could be useful for newborn screening, comparing sequencing and biochemical methods in different screening contexts, and assessing parent perspectives on newborn sequencing (NASEM, 2023; NICHD, 2010).

In addition to its programs supporting NBS program implementation, CDC advances NBS research with a primary focus on developing and improving reference materials and assays that screening laboratories can use to validate and refine their testing methods (CDC, 2024d).

CDC's current efforts in this space aim to modernize and automate the production of the dried blood spot reference materials laboratories use for quality assurance and enhance interpretation of screening test results (Cuthbert, 2024). To provide risk assessment and clinical decision support across the NBS system, CDC's ED3N initiative focuses on developing a national data solution that would make advanced data processing, analytics, and visualization capabilities available to all NBS programs (CDC, 2024c).

CONCLUSIONS

Conclusion 2-1: Newborn screening programs perform an essential public health service by screening almost every baby born in the United States and connecting the thousands of newborns annually identified as at risk for a condition with diagnosis and clinical care.

Conclusion 2-2: The goals of screening and diagnostic testing are often conflated, but each serves a different purpose. In the context of newborn screening, screening tests determine whether a baby is at risk of a certain condition, whereas diagnostic testing confirms whether a baby that had an out-of-range screening result in fact has a certain condition. Newborn screening occurs as part of public health, and diagnostic testing of at-risk infants occurs in clinical care.

Conclusion 2-3: The process for incorporating new conditions into public health newborn screening is long and burdensome. Identifying opportunities to systematize, streamline, and support evidence generation and assessment and harmonize the onboarding of screening new conditions could increase efficiency and reduce times to adding appropriate conditions. While the addition of new conditions to screening panels necessitates a rigorous evidence review to verify that the individual and public health benefits outweigh the costs and potential harms, it is also important to avoid unnecessary delays to ensure the U.S. population reaps the benefits in a timely manner.

Conclusion 2-4: The implementation of public health newborn screening is variable across the country. Variation across state- and territorial-run programs is inevitable and may enable programs to address their specific circumstances and populations. When this variability arises from insufficient resources or support and negatively affects health outcomes, it weakens the value proposition of newborn screening.

Conclusion 2-5: The landscape of U.S. public health newborn screening (NBS) is disjointed and not systematic in its implementation. An informal NBS ecosystem supports and informs the work of public health NBS programs, research into conditions, and diagnosis and provision of subsequent clinical care. Thus, this ecosystem extends beyond what public health programs can accomplish both to collect evidence through research and as infants identified as at risk make the transition to clinical care. An aligned vision and greater coordination would be more robust, efficient, and better prepare public health newborn screening for the future.

REFERENCES

AABC (American Association of Birth Centers). 2024 (unpublished). *AABC survey on funding of newborn screening.* Perkiomenville, PA: AABC.

Abhyanker, S., R. M. Goodwin, M. K. Sontag, C. Yusuf, J. Ojodu, and C. J. McDonald. 2015. An update on the use of health information technology in newborn screening. *Seminars in Perinatology* 39(3):188-193.

ACHDNC (Advisory Committee on Heritable Disordes in Newborns and Chilren) Pilot Studies Workgroup. 2016. *Report and recommendations of the pilot studies workgroup.* https://www.hrsa.gov/sites/default/files/hrsa/advisory-committees/heritable-disorders/achdnc-pilot-studies-report.pdf (accessed December 30, 2024).

ACMG (American College of Medical Genetics) Newborn Screening Expert Group. 2005. *Newborn screening: Toward a uniform screening panel and system.* https://www.hrsa.gov/sites/default/files/hrsa/advisory-committees/heritable-disorders/newborn-uniform-screening-panel.pdf (accessed September 26, 2024).

ACMG Newborn Screening Expert Group. 2006. Newborn screening: Toward a uniform screening panel and system. *Genetics in Medicine* 8(Suppl 1):1S-252S.

All of Us Research Program Investigators. 2019. The "all of us" research program. *New England Journal of Medicine* 381(7):668-676.

Almannai, M., R. Marom, and V. R. Sutton. 2016. Newborn screening: A review of history, recent advancements, and future perspectives in the era of next generation sequencing. *Current Opinion in Pediatrics* 28(6):694-699.

Andrews, S. M., K. A. Porter, D. B. Bailey, and H. L. Peay. 2022. Preparing newborn screening for the future: A collaborative stakeholder engagement exploring challenges and opportunities to modernizing the newborn screening system. *BMC Pediatrics* 22(1):90.

Annas, G. J. 1982. Mandatory PKU screening: The other side of the looking glass. *American Journal of Public Health* 72(12):1401-1403.

APHL (Association of Public Health Laboratories). 2015. *Adding conditions to state newborn screening panels.* https://www.aphl.org/aboutAPHL/publications/Documents/NBS_NBSPanelConditions_FactSheet_updated102015.pdf (accessed September 26, 2024).

Armstrong, N. 2024. *Advocacy perspectives on adding new diseases: Experiences with developing a nomination package.* PowerPoint Presentation, National Academies Committee on Newborn Screening: Current Landscape and Future Directions Meeting 2, Washington, DC, March 26, 2024. https://www.nationalacademies.org/event/42052_03-2024_newborn-screening-current-landscape-and-future-directions-meeting-2 (accessed January 17, 2025).

Baby's First Test. 2024a. *What happens to the blood sample.* https://www.babysfirsttest.org/newborn-screening/what-happens-to-the-blood-sample (accessed September 18, 2024).

Baby's First Test. 2024b. *What is newborn screening?* https://www.babysfirsttest.org/ (accessed September 18, 2024).

Baker, M. W., R. H. Laessig, M. L. Katcher, J. M. Routes, W. J. Grossman, J. Verbsky, D. F. Kurtycz, and C. D. Brokopp. 2010. Implementing routine testing for severe combined immunodeficiency within Wisconsin's newborn screening program. *Public Health Reports* 125(Suppl 2):88-95.

Ballard, B. 2024. *Perspectives on the process of adding SCID newborn screening to the RUSP and all 50 states: A retrospective review.* PowerPoint Presentation, National Academies Committee on Newborn Screening: Current Landscape and Future Directions Meeting 2, Washington, DC, March 26, 2024.

Berry, S. A., N. D. Leslie, M. J. Edick, S. Hiner, K. Justice, and C. Cameron. 2016. Inborn errors of metabolism collaborative: Large-scale collection of data on long-term follow-up for newborn-screened conditions. *Genetics in Medicine* 18(12):1276-1281.

Botkin, J. R., E. Rothwell, R. A. Anderson, A. Goldenberg, M. Kuppermann, S. M. Dolan, N. C. Rose, and L. Stark. 2014. What parents want to know about the storage and use of residual newborn bloodspots. *American Journal of Medical Genetics Part A* 164(11):2739-2744.

Botkin, J. R., E. Rothwell, R. A. Anderson, N. C. Rose, S. M. Dolan, M. Kuppermann, L. A. Stark, A. Goldenberg, and B. Wong. 2016. Prenatal education of parents about newborn screening and residual dried blood spots. *JAMA Pediatrics* 170(6):543-549.

Boyle, C. A., J. F. Cordero, and E. Trevathan. 2012. The national center on birth defects and developmental disabilities: Past, present, and future. *American Journal of Preventive Medicine* 43(6):655-658.

Brosco, J. P. 2024. *Perspectives from federal NBS partners: HRSA.* PowerPoint Presentation, Webinar on Perspectives from Federal NBS Partners, Washington, DC, March 8, 2024. https://www.nationalacademies.org/event/42199_03-2024_newborn-screening-current-landscape-and-future-directions-webinar-on-perspectives-from-federal-nbs-partners (accessed September 27, 2024).

Brosco, J. P., S. D. Grosse, and L. F. Ross. 2015. Universal state newborn screening programs can reduce health disparities. *JAMA Pediatrics* 169(1):7-8.

Brown, J. E. H., and B. Koenig. 2021. Ethical, legal, and social implications of fetal gene therapy. *Clinical Obstetrics and Gynecology* 64(4):933-940.

Caggana, M., E. A. Jones, S. I. Shahied, S. Tanksley, C. A. Hermerath, and I. M. Lubin. 2013. Newborn screening: From Guthrie to whole genome sequencing. *Public Health Reports* 128(Suppl 2):14-19.

Calonge, N. 2023. *ACHDNC decision matrix.* PowerPoint Presentation, ACHDNC Meeting, Washington, DC, November 2, 2023. https://www.hrsa.gov/sites/default/files/hrsa/advisory-committees/heritable-disorders/meetings/achdnc-decision-matrix-tool.pdf (accessed September 27, 2024).

Caposino, P. 2024. *Aims, efforts and opportunities in newborn screening - FDA perspective.* PowerPoint Presentation, Webinar on Perspectives from Federal NBS Partners, Washington, DC, March 8, 2024. https://www.nationalacademies.org/event/42199_03-2024_newborn-screening-current-landscape-and-future-directions-webinar-on-perspectives-from-federal-nbs-partners (accessed September 26, 2024).

CDC (Centers for Disease Control and Prevention). 2024a. *About newborn screening laboratories.* https://www.cdc.gov/newborn-screening/php/about/index.html (accessed September 18, 2024).

CDC. 2024b. *Centers of excellence to enhance disease detection in newborns.* https://www.grants.gov/search-results-detail/349850 (accessed September 27, 2024).

CDC. 2024c. *Enhancing data-driven disease detection in newborns.* https://www.cdc.gov/newborn-screening/php/about/ed3n-project.html (accessed September 20, 2024).

CDC. 2024d. *Newborn screening quality assurance program.* https://www.cdc.gov/laboratory-quality-assurance/php/newborn-screening/index.html (accessed July 31, 2024).

CDC. 2024e. *Supporting state newborn screening laboratories.* https://www.cdc.gov/newborn-screening/php/about/state-newborn-screening-laboratories.html (accessed September 20, 2024).

CDC. 2024f. *National Center on Birth Defects and Developmental Disabilities (NCBDDD).* https://www.cdc.gov/ncbddd/index.html (accessed February 24, 2025).

Chace, D. H., T. A. Kalas, and E. W. Naylor. 2003. Use of tandem mass spectrometry for multianalyte screening of dried blood specimens from newborns. *Clinical Chemistry* 49(11):1797-1817.

Chan, K., and J. M. Puck. 2005. Development of population-based newborn screening for severe combined immunodeficiency. *Journal of Allergy and Clinical Immunology* 115(2):391-398.

CLSI (Clinical and Laboratory Standards Institute). 2023. *Newborn screening glossary.* https://htd.clsi.org/listalltermsNewborn.asp (accessed September 26, 2024).

CMS (Centers for Medicare & Medicaid Services). 2024. *2024 Medicaid & CHIP beneficiaries at a glance: Maternal health.* https://www.medicaid.gov/medicaid/benefits/downloads/2024-maternal-health-at-a-glance.pdf (accessed February 19, 2025).

Costich, J. F., and A. L. Durst. 2016. The impact of the Affordable Care Act on funding for newborn screening services. *Public Health Reports* 131(1):160-166.

Coupal, E., K. Hart, B. Wong, and E. Rothwell. 2021. Newborn screening knowledge and attitudes among midwives and out-of-hospital-birth parents. *Journal of Perinatal and Neonatal Nursing* 34(4): 357-364.

Currier, R., and J. M. Puck. 2021. SCID newborn screening: What we've learned. *Journal of Allergy and Clinical Immunology* 147(2):417-426.

Currier, R. J. 2022. Newborn screening is on a collision course with public health ethics. *International Journal of Neonatal Screening* 8(4):51.

Cuthbert, C. 2024. *CDC's role in supporting newborn screening laboratory quality and enhancing disease detection in newborns: Current activities and programmatic vision.* PowerPoint Presentation, Webinar on Perspectives from Federal NBS Partners, Washington, DC, March 8, 2024. https://www.nationalacademies.org/event/42199_03-2024_newborn-screening-current-landscape-and-future-directions-webinar-on-perspectives-from-federal-nbs-partners (accessed September 2024).

De Jesús, V., J. Mei, S. Cordovado, and C. Cuthbert. 2015. The newborn screening quality assurance program at the Centers for Disease Control and Prevention: Thirty-five year experience assuring newborn screening laboratory quality. *International Journal of Neonatal Screening* 1(1):13-26.

Dorley, M. C. 2024. *Adding disorders to the Tennessee NBS panel: Public health perspective.* PowerPoint Presentation, National Academies Committee on Newborn Screening: Current Landscape and Future Directions Meeting 2, Washington, DC, March 26, 2024. https://www.nationalacademies.org/event/42052_03-2024_newborn-screening-current-landscape-and-future-directions-meeting-2 (accessed September 27, 2024).

Dubay, K., and T. L. Zach. 2023. *Newborn screening.* StatPearls Publishing. https://www.ncbi.nlm.nih.gov/books/NBK558983/ (accessed September 24, 2024).

Early Check. 2024. *What is Early Check?* https://earlycheck.org/ (accessed September 19, 2024).

EveryLife Foundation for Rare Diseases. n.d. *RUSP alignment legislation.* https://everylifefoundation.org/newborn-screening-take-action/support-legislation/ (accessed February 21, 2024).

Fabie, N. A. V., K. B. Pappas, and G. L. Feldman. 2019. The current state of newborn screening in the United States. *Pediatric Clinics of North America* 66(2):369-386.

Faden, R. R., N. A. Holtzman, and A. J. Chwalow. 1982. Parental rights, child welfare, and public health: The case of PKU screening. *American Journal of Public Health* 72(12):1396-1400.

Fatumo, S., T. Chikowore, A. Choudhury, M. Ayub, A. R. Martin, and K. Kuchenbacker. 2022. Diversity in genomic studies: A roadmap to address the imbalance. *Nature Medicine* 28(2):243-250.

Friedman, J. M., M. C. Cornel, A. J. Goldenberg, K. J. Lister, K. Sénécal, and D. F. Vears. 2017. Genomic newborn screening: Public health policy considerations and recommendations. *BMC Medical Genomics* 10(1):9.

Furnier, S. M., M. S. Durkin, and M. W. Baker. 2020. Translating molecular technologies into routine newborn screening practice. *International Journal of Neonatal Screening* 6(4):80.

GAO (Government Accountability Office). 2003. *Newborn screening: Characteristics of state programs.* GAO-03-449. Washington, DC: GAO.

GAO. 2016. *Newborn screening timeliness: Most states had not met screening goals, but some are developing strategies to address barriers.* GAO-17-196. Washington, DC: GAO.

Gaviglio, A., M. Lasarev, R. Sheller, S. Singh, and M. Baker. 2023. Newborn screening for severe combined immunodeficiency: Lessons learned from screening and follow-up of the preterm newborn population. *International Journal of Neonatal Screening* 9(4):68.

Geleske, T. A. 2010. Weighing the evidence: Recommendation made to add SCID to uniform newborn screening panel. *AAP News* 31(6):22.

Goldenberg, A. J., and R. R. Sharp. 2012. The ethical hazards and programmatic challenges of genomic newborn screening. *Journal of the American Medical Association* 307(5):461-462.

Goldenberg, A. J., A. M. Comeau, S. D. Grosse, S. Tanksley, L. A. Prosser, J. Ojodu, J. R. Botkin, A. R. Kemper, and N. S. Green. 2016. Evaluating harms in the assessment of net benefit: A framework for newborn screening condition review. *Maternal and Child Health Journal* 20(3):693-700.

Grant, C. 2022. *Police are using newborn genetic screening to search for suspects, threatening privacy and public health.* https://www.aclu-nj.org/en/news/police-are-using-newborn-genetic-screening-search-suspects-threatening-privacy-and-public (accessed July 23, 2024).

Grosse, S. D., J. D. Thompson, Y. Ding, and M. Glass. 2016. The use of economic evaluation to inform newborn screening policy decisions: The Washington state experience. *Milbank Quarterly* 94(2):366-391.

GUARDIAN Study. 2021. *The GUARDIAN study is a free newborn screening study to help all babies have healthier lives.* https://guardian-study.org/ (accessed September 2024).

HHS (U.S. Department of Health and Human Services). 2015. *Report to Congress: Newborn screening activities.* https://mchb.hrsa.gov/sites/default/files/mchb/programs-impact/nbs-report.pdf (accessed February 21, 2025).

HHS. 2021a. *Innovative screening approaches and therapies for screenable disorders in newborns (R01 - clinical trial optional): R01 research project grant.* https://grants.nih.gov/grants/guide/pa-files/PAR-21-353.html (accessed September 18, 2024).

HHS. 2021b. *Innovative screening approaches and therapies for screenable disorders in newborns (R03 - clinical trial optional): R03 small grant program.* https://grants.nih.gov/grants/guide/pa-files/PAR-21-354.html (accessed September 18, 2024).

Houtrow, A., A. J. Martin, D. Harris, D. Cejas, R. Hutson, Y. Mazloomdoost, and R. K. Agrawal. 2022. Health equity for children and youth with special health care needs: A vision for the future. *Pediatrics* 149(Suppl 7):e2021056150F.

Howell, R. R., and G. Engelson. 2007. Structures for clinical follow-up: Newborn screening. *Journal of Inherited Metabolic Disease* 30(4):600-605.

HRSA (Health Resources and Services Administration). 2010. *Report: Newborn screening for severe combined immunodeficiency disorder.* https://www.hrsa.gov/sites/default/files/hrsa/advisory-committees/heritable-disorders/reports-recommendations/newborn-screening-scid-report.pdf (accessed January 8, 2025).

HRSA. 2017. *Newborn screening timeliness goals.* https://www.hrsa.gov/advisory-committees/heritable-disorders/newborn-screening-timeliness (accessed September 18, 2024).

HRSA. 2021. *History of the ACHDNC.* https://www.hrsa.gov/advisory-committees/heritable-disorders/timeline (accessed July 31, 2024).

HRSA. 2022a. *Advisory committee on heritable disorders in newborns and children charter.* https://www.hrsa.gov/sites/default/files/hrsa/advisory-committees/heritable-disorders/achdnc-charter.pdf (accessed January 8, 2025).

HRSA. 2022b. *Nominating a condition for the Recommended Uniform Screening Panel for newborn screening: Frequently asked questions and other guidance.* https://www.hrsa.gov/advisory-committees/heritable-disorders/frequently-asked-questions (accessed July 31, 2024).

HRSA. 2023a. *About newborn screening.* https://newbornscreening.hrsa.gov/about-newborn-screening (accessed July 29, 2024).

HRSA. 2023b. *Newborn screening process.* https://newbornscreening.hrsa.gov/newborn-screening-process (accessed July 29, 2024).

HRSA. 2023c. *Sickle cell disease programs.* https://mchb.hrsa.gov/programs-impact/programs/sickle-cell (accessed September 26, 2024).

HRSA. 2024a. *Cooperative newborn screening system priorities (NBS Co-Propel) program.* https://mchb.hrsa.gov/programs/cooperative-newborn-screening-system-priorities (accessed September 26, 2024).

HRSA. 2024b. *Newborn screening in your state.* https://newbornscreening.hrsa.gov/your-state (accessed September 27, 2024).

HRSA. 2024c. *Nominate a condition.* https://www.hrsa.gov/advisory-committees/heritable-disorders/rusp/nominate (accessed September 18, 2024).

HRSA. 2024d. *Recommended Uniform Screening Panel.* https://www.hrsa.gov/advisory-committees/heritable-disorders/rusp (accessed July 31, 2024).

HRSA. 2024e. *Commitee approach to evaluating the condition review report (decision matrix).* https://www.hrsa.gov/advisory-committees/heritable-disorders/decision-matrix (accessed December 17, 2024).

Hughes, R., IV, S. Choudhury, and A. Shah. 2022. Newborn screening blood spot retention and reuse: A clash of public health and privacy interests. *Health Affairs Forefront.* https://www.healthaffairs.org/content/forefront/newborn-screening-blood-spot-retention-and-reuse-clash-public-health-and-privacy (accessed January 17, 2025).

Johnson, K., M. A. Lloyd-Puryear, M. Y. Mann, L. R. Ramos, and B. L. Therrell. 2006. Financing state newborn screening programs: Sources and uses of funds. *Pediatrics* 117(Suppl 3):S270-S279.

Johnson Policy Consulting. 2008. *State statutes and regulations on dietary treatment of disorders identified through newborn screening.* https://www.hrsa.gov/sites/default/files/hrsa/advisory-committees/heritable-disorders/reports-recommendations/state-laws-medical-foods-tab.pdf (accessed January 8, 2025).

Kaeser, E. 2023. *Legal challenges to dried blood spot use in Michigan highlight the role of informed consent in valuable public health activities.* Network for Public Health Law. https://www.networkforphl.org/news-insights/legal-challenges-to-dried-blood-spot-use-in-michigan-highlight-the-role-of-informed-consent-in-valuable-public-health-activities/ (accessed September 23, 2024).

Kanungo, S., D. R. Patel, M. Neelakantan, and B. Ryali. 2018. Newborn screening and changing face of inborn errors of metabolism in the United States. *Annals of Translational Medicine* 6(24):468.

Kemper, A. R., N. S. Green, N. Calonge, W. K. K. Lam, A. M. Comeau, A. J. Goldenberg, J. Ojodu, L. A. Prosser, S. Tanksley, and J. A. Bocchini. 2014. Decision-making process for conditiosn nominated to the Recommended Uniform Screening Panel: Statement of the US Department of Health and Human Services Secretary's Advisory Committee on Heritable Disorders in Newborns and Children. *Genetics in Medicine* 16:183-187.

Kennedy, A. 2024. *Child health and rare disease organizations – Perspectives on the study task.* PowerPoint Presentation, National Academies Committee on Newborn Screening: Current Landscape and Future Directions Meeting 1, Washington, DC, January 26, 2024. https://www.nationalacademies.org/event/41786_01-2024_newborn-screening-current-landscape-and-future-directions-meeting-1b (accessed January 17, 2025).

King, J. S., and M. E. Smith. 2016. Whole-genome screening of newborns? The constitutional boundaries of state newborn screening programs. *Pediatrics* 137(Suppl 1):S8-S15.

Kubala, S. A., A. Sandhu, T. Palacios-Kibler, B. Ward, G. Harmon, M. L. DeFelice, V. Bundy, M. E. M. Younger, H. Lederman, H. Liang, M. Anzabi, M. K. Ford, J. Heimall, M. D. Keller, and M. G. Lawrence. 2022. Natural history of infants with non-SCID T cell lymphopenia identified on newborn screen. *Clinical Immunology* 245:109182.

Kwan, A., R. S. Abraham, R. Currier, A. Brower, K. Andruszewski, J. K. Abbott, M. Baker, M. Ballow, L. E. Bartoshesky, V. R. Bonagura, F. A. Bonilla, C. Brokopp, E. Brooks, M. Caggana, J. Celestin, J. A. Church, A. M. Comeau, J. A. Connelly, M. J. Cowan, C. Cunningham-Rundles, T. Dasu, N. Dave, M. T. De La Morena, U. Duffner, C.-T. Fong, L. Forbes, D. Freedenberg, E. W. Gelfand, J. E. Hale, I. C. Hanson, B. N. Hay, D. Hu, A. Infante, D. Johnson, N. Kapoor, D. M. Kay, D. B. Kohn, R. Lee, H. Lehman, Z. Lin, F. Lorey, A. Abdel-Mageed, A. Manning, S. McGhee, T. B. Moore, S. J. Naides, L. D. Notarangelo, J. S. Orange, S.-Y. Pai, M. Porteus, R. Rodriguez, N. Romberg, J. Routes, M. Ruehle, A. Rubenstein, C. A. Saavedra-Matiz, G. Scott, P. M. Scott, E. Secord, C. Seroogy, W. T. Shearer, S. Siegel, S. K. Silvers, E. R. Stiehm, R. W. Sugerman, J. L. Sullivan, S. Tanksley, M. L. Tierce, IV, J. Verbsky, B. Vogel, R. Walker, K. Walkovich, J. E. Walter, R. L. Wasserman, M. S. Watson, G. A. Weinberg, L. B. Weiner, H. Wood, A. B. Yates, and J. M. Puck. 2014. Newborn screening for severe combined immunodeficiency in 11 screening programs in the United States. *JAMA* 312(7):729-738.

Levy, H. L. 2021. Robert Guthrie and the trials and tribulations of newborn screening. *International Journal of Neonatal Screening* 7(1):5.

Lewis, M. H., A. Goldenberg, R. Anderson, E. Rothwell, and J. Botkin. 2011. State laws regarding the retention and use of residual newborn screening blood samples. *Pediatrics* 127(4):703-712.

MacDorman, M., and E. Declercq. 2019. Trends and state variations in out-of-hospital births in the United States, 2004-2017. *Birth* 46(2):279-288.

McClendon-Weary, B., D. L. Putnick, S. Robinson, and E. Yeung. 2020. Little to give, much to gain - what can you do with a dried blood spot? *Current Environmental Health Reports* 7(3):211-221.

McGarry, M. E., C. L. Ren, R. Wu, P. M. Farrell, and S. A. McColley. 2023. Detection of disease-causing CFTR variants in state newborn screening programs. *Pediatric Pulmonology* 58(2):465-474.

Minear, M. A., M. N. Phillips, A. Kau, and M. A. Parisi. 2022. Newborn screening research sponsored by the NIH: From diagnostic paradigms to precision therapeutics. *American Journal of Medical Genetics Part C: Seminars in Medical Genetics* 190(2):138-152.

Minnesota Department of Health. 2022. *Newborn screening infomation for families: Laboratory testing overview.* https://www.web.health.state.mn.us/people/newbornscreening/families/testing.html (accessed September 23, 2024).

Mistry, K. 2024. *Agency for Healthcare Research and Quality (AHRQ) overview.* PowerPoint Presentation, Webinar on Perspectives from Federal NBS Partners, Washington, DC, March 8, 2024. https://www.nationalacademies.org/event/42199_03-2024_newborn-screening-current-landscape-and-future-directions-webinar-on-perspectives-from-federal-nbs-partners (accessed September 24, 2024).

Montana DPHHS (Montana Department of Public Health and Human Services). n.d. *Newborn screening advisory committee.* https://dphhs.mt.gov/boardscouncils/NBS/index (accessed September 26, 2024).

Montefiore Einstein. 2024. *ScreenPlus.* https://einsteinmed.edu/research/screenplus/ (accessed September 23, 2024).

NASEM (National Academies of Sciences, Engineering, and Medicine). 2010. Concerns about the use of residual newborn screening samples. In *Institute of Medicine (US) Challenges and opportunities in using residual newborn screening samples for translational research: Workshop summary.* Washington, DC: The National Academies Press.

NASEM. 2023. *The promise and perils of next-generation DNA sequencing at birth.* Washington, DC: The National Academies Press.

National Center on Birth Defects and Developmental Disabilities. 2017. *Newborn screening contingency plan.* Version II. Atlanta, GA: Centers for Disease Control and Prevention.

New England Newborn Screening Program. 2024. *Voluntary newborn screening.* https://nensp.umassmed.edu/screening-programs/massachusetts/voluntary-newborn-screening (accessed September 23, 2024).

NewSTEPs (Newborn Screening Technical assistance and Evaluation Program). 2021. *NewSTEPs annual report 2020*. Association of Public Health Laboratories. https://www.newsteps.org/sites/default/files/resources/download/NewSTEPs%20Annual%20Report%209%2022%2021.pdf (accessed December 30, 2024).

NewSTEPs. 2023. *NewSTEPs 2022 annual report*. Association of Public Health Laboratories. https://www.newsteps.org/sites/default/files/resources/download/NewSTEPS-2022-Annual-Report.pdf (accessed December 30, 2024).

NHGRI (National Human Genome Research Institute). 2014. *About phenylketonuria*. https://www.genome.gov/Genetic-Disorders/Phenylketonuria (accessed July 25, 2024).

NHGRI. 2022. *Newborn sequencing in genomic medicine and public health (NSIGHT)*. https://www.cdc.gov/newborn-screening/php/about/state-newborn-screening-laboratories.html (accessed September 23, 2024).

NHGRI. 2023. *ELSI: Participating NIH ICs*. https://www.genome.gov/Funded-Programs-Projects/ELSI-Research-Program-ethical-legal-social-implications/domains/participating-ICs (accessed September 26, 2024).

NIAID (National Institute of Allergy and Infectious Diseaes). 2019. *Severe combined immunodeficiency (SCID)*. https://www.niaid.nih.gov/diseases-conditions/severe-combined-immunodeficiency-scid (accessed September 26, 2024).

NICHD (National Institue of Child Health and Human Development). 2010. *Newborn screening in the genomic era: Setting a research agenda: Meeting summary*. https://www.genome.gov/Pages/PolicyEthics/StaffArticles/Newborn_Screening_Meeting_Summary.pdf (accessed December 30, 2024).

NICHD. 2017a. *Phenylketonuria (PKU) and newborn screening*. https://www.nichd.nih.gov/about/accomplishments/contributions/pku (accessed September 23, 2024).

NICHD. 2017b. *Who pays for newborn screening?* https://www.nichd.nih.gov/health/topics/newborn/conditioninfo/how-used/pays (accessed September 23, 2024).

NICHD. 2023. *Notice of information regarding close-out and transition planning for the newborn screening translational research network*. https://grants.nih.gov/grants/guide/notice-files/NOT-HD-23-012.html (accessed September 27, 2024).

NICHD. 2024. *Newborn screening research activities and advances*. https://www.nichd.nih.gov/health/topics/newborn/researchinfo/activities (accessed September 23, 2024).

NICHD. n.d. *Newborn screening*. https://www.nichd.nih.gov/health/topics/factsheets/newborn (accessed September 26, 2024).

Ojodu, J. 2024. *The state of the newborn screening system in the United States*. PowerPoint Presentation, National Academies Committee on Newborn Screening: Current Landscape and Future Directions Meeting 2, Washington, DC, March 26, 2024. https://www.nationalacademies.org/event/42052_03-2024_newborn-screening-current-landscape-and-future-directions-meeting-2 (accessed October 2, 2024).

Parisi, M. A. 2024. *Perspectives from federal NBS partners: National Institutes of Health*. PowerPoint Presentation, Webinar on Perspectives from Federal NBS Partners, Washington, DC, March 8, 2024. https://www.nationalacademies.org/event/42199_03-2024_newborn-screening-current-landscape-and-future-directions-webinar-on-perspectives-from-federal-nbs-partners (accessed September 24, 2024).

President's Council on Bioethics. 2008. *The changing moral focus of newborn screening: An ethical analysis by the President's Council on Bioethics*. Washington, DC: President's Council on Bioethics.

Ram, N. 2022. America's hidden national DNA database. *Texas Law Review* 100(7):1253-1325.

Rehani, M. R., M. S. Marcus, A. B. Harris, P. M. Farrell, and C. L. Ren. 2023. Variation in cystic fibrosis newborn screening algorithms in the United States. *Pediatric Pulmonology* 58(3):927-933.

Richards, S., N. Aziz, S. Bale, D. Bick, S. Das, J. Gastier-Foster, W. W. Grody, M. Hegde, E. Lyon, E. Spector, K. Voelkerding, and H. L. Rehm. 2015. Standards and guidelines for the interpretation of sequence variants: A joint consensus recommendation of the

American College of Medical Genetics and Genomics and the Association for Molecular Pathology. *Genetics in Medicine* 17(5):405-424.

Rosamilia, M. B., A. M. Markunas, P. S. Kishnani, and A. P. Landstrom. 2024. Underrepresentation of diverse ancestries drives uncertainty in genetic variants found in cardiomyopathy-associated genes. *JACC: Advances* 3(2):100767.

Ross, L. F. 2010. Mandatory versus voluntary consent for newborn screening? *Kennedy Institute of Ethics* 20(4):299-328.

Ross, L. F., and E. W. Clayton. 2019. Ethical issues in newborn sequencing research: The case study of BabySeq. *Pediatrics* 144(6):e20191031.

Rothwell, E., B. Wong, R. A. Anderson, and J. R. Botkin. 2016. The influence of education on public trust and consent preferences with residual newborn screening dried blood spots. *Journal of Empirical Research on Human Research Ethics* 11(3):231-236.

Rothwell, E., E. Johnson, N. Riches, and J. R. Botkin. 2019. Secondary research uses of residual newborn screening dried bloodspots: A scoping review. *Genetics in Medicine* 21(7):1469-1475.

Schnabel-Besson, E., U. Mütze, N. Dikow, F. Hörster, M. A. Morath, K. Alex, H. Brennenstuhl, S. Settegast, J. G. Okun, C. P. Schaaf, E. C. Winkler, and S. Kölker. 2024. Wilson and Jungner revisited: Are screening criteria fit for the 21st century? *International Journal of Neonatal Screening* 10(3):62.

Schuett, V. 2022. *State laws and policies for the coverage of metabolic food and formula*. https://nucdf.org/file_download/a176f34f-8813-4ae5-a33a-baea9fd2850e (accessed September 24, 2024).

Severin, C., and L. Jones. 2023. Handle with care: State newborn screening policies. https://www.astho.org/communications/blog/handle-with-care-state-newborn-screening-policies/ (accessed February 4, 2024).

Shapira, S. K., C. F. Hinton, P. K. Held, E. Jones, W. Harry Hannon, and J. Ojodu. 2015. Single newborn screen or routine second screening for primary congenital hypothyroidism. *Molecular Genetics and Metabolism* 116(3):125-132.

Sheller, R., J. Ojodu, E. Griffin, S. Edelman, C. Yusuf, T. Pigg, A. Huston, B. Fitzek, J. G. Boyle, and S. Singh. 2020. The landscape of severe combined immunodeficiency newborn screening in the United States in 2020: A review of screening methodologies and targets, communication pathways, and long-term follow-up practices. *Frontiers in Immunology* 11:577853.

Singh, S., J. Ojodu, A. R. Kemper, W. K. K. Lam, and S. D. Grosse. 2023. Implementation of newborn screening for conditions in the United States first recommended during 2010-2018. *International Journal of Neonatal Screening* 9(2):20.

Smith, L. D., M. N. Bainbridge, R. B. Parad, and A. Bhattacharjee. 2020. Second tier molecular genetic testing in newborn screening for Pompe disease: Landscape and challenges. *International Journal of Neonatal Screening* 6(2):32.

Sontag, M. K., J. I. Miller, S. McKasson, R. Sheller, S. Edelman, C. Yusuf, S. Singh, D. Sarkar, J. Bocchini, J. Scott, J. Ojodu, and Y. Kellar-Guenther. 2020. Newborn screening timeliness quality improvement initiative: Impact of national recommendations and data repository. *PLoS One* 15(4):e0231050.

Susanna Haas Lyons Engagement Consulting. 2024. *What we heard: Newborn screening in the United States*. Presented to the Committee on Newborn Screening: Current Landscape and Future Directions at the National Academies of Sciences, Engineering, and Medicine. https://www.nationalacademies.org/documents/embed/link/LF2255DA3DD1C41C0A42D3BEF0989ACAECE3053A6A9B/file/D35FB72C883DD3F3496A747004FB20B434E54764D1D0?noSaveAs=1 (accessed December 18, 2024).

Tarini, B. A. 2007. The current revolution in newborn screening. *Archives of Pediatrics & Adolescent Medicine* 161(8):767-772.

Texas Health and Human Services. 2024a. *Newborn screening - use and storage of dried blood spots after NBS*. https://www.dshs.texas.gov/laboratory-services/programs-laboratories/newborn-screening-laboratory/newborn-screening-use-storage (accessed September 24, 2024).

Texas Health and Human Services. 2024b. *Newborn screening - use of NBS blood spots after completion of newborn screening*. https://www.dshs.texas.gov/laboratory-services/programs-laboratories/newborn-screening-laboratory/newborn-screening-use-nbs (accessed September 24, 2024).

Thakar, M. S., B. R. Logan, J. M. Puck, E. A. Dunn, R. H Buckley, M. J. Cowan, R. J. O'Reilly, N. Kapoor, L. Forbes Satter, S.-Y. Pai, J. Heimall, S. Chandra, C. L. Ebens, D. Chellapandian, O. Williams, L. M. Burroughs, B. D. Saldana, A. Rayes, L. M. Madden, S. Chandrakasan, J. J. Bednarski II, K. B. DeSantes, G. D. E. Cuvelier, P. Teira, A. P. Gillio, H. Eissa, A. P. Knutsen, F. D. Goldman, V. M. Aquino, E. B. Shereck, T. B. Moore, E. H. Caywood, M. T. V. Lugt, J. Rozmus, L. Broglie, L. C. Yu, A. J. Shah, J. R. Andolina, X. Liu, R. E. Parrott, J. Dara, S. Prockop, C. A. Martinez, M. Kapadia, S. C. Jyonouchi, K. E. Sullivan, J. J. Bleesing, S. Chaudhury, A. Petrovic, M. D. Keller, T. C. Quigg, S. Parikh, S. Shenoy, C. Seroogy, T. Rubin, H. Decaluwe, J. M. Routes, T. R. Torgerson, J. W. Leiding, M. A. Pulsipher, D. B. Kohn, L. M. Griffith, E. Haddad, C. C. Dvorak, and L. D. Notarangelo. 2023. Measuring the effect of newborn screening on survival after haematopoietic cell transplantation for severe combined immunodeficiency: A 36-year longitudinal study from the primary immune deficiency treatment consortium. *Lancet* 402(10396):129-140.

Thompson, J. D. 2024. *Perspective on the process of adding new conditions*. PowerPoint Presentation, National Academies Committee on Newborn Screening: Current Landscape and Future Directions Meeting 2, Washington, DC, March 26, 2024. https://www.nationalacademies.org/event/42052_03-2024_newborn-screening-current-landscape-and-future-directions-meeting-2 (accessed September 27, 2024).

Van Der Spek, J., R. H. H. Groenwold, M. Van Der Burg, and J. M. Van Montfrans. 2015. TREC based newborn screening for severe combined immunodeficiency disease: A systematic review. *Journal of Clinical Immunology* 35(4):416-430.

Watson, M. S. 2006. Current status of newborn screening: Decision-making about the conditions to include in screening programs. *Mental Retardation and Developmental Disabilities Research Reviews* 12(4):230-235.

Watson, M. S., M. A. Lloyd-Puryear, and R. R. Howell. 2022. The progress and future of US newborn screening. *International Journal of Neonatal Screening* 8(3):41.

Wilson, J. M. G., and G. Jungner. 1968. Principles and practice of screening for disease. *Public Health Papers* 34. Geneva: World Health Organization.

Wonkam, A., N. S. Munung, C. Dandara, K. K. Esoh, N. A. Hanchard, and G. Landoure. (2022). Five priorities of African genomics research: The next frontier. *Annual Review of Genomics and Human Genetics* 23(1):499-521.

3

Grounding NBS Decision Making in Ethical Principles and Values

"Nothing is perfect. It's subjective to every parent. Some people want to have the peace of mind [by knowing all the likelihoods] and some people just want to have a clear answer. It just depends on the parent . . . do they want to live in the gray?" – Parent

Newborn screening (NBS) in the United States continues to evolve in response to discussions over inclusion of additional conditions, incorporation of new screening technologies, increased understanding of diseases and treatments, and ongoing efforts to connect screening with clinical follow-up and care. It also contends with overarching considerations around family choice and autonomy, and issues that raise technical, ethical, legal/policy, and implementation questions. As a result, a foundation to inform decision making for NBS programs, funding processes, insurance coverage, informed consent, and related research remains timely and necessary. This chapter explores principles, values, and considerations that help guide ethical decision making in the context of public health programs. It discusses this report's application of such principles and values to newborn screening to inform the analyses presented in the remainder of the report.

EXAMINING NEWBORN SCREENING AS A PUBLIC HEALTH SERVICE

Newborn screening as a public health service and the role of government in its implementation emerged as an "accident of history" and a practical necessity as this service took shape in its early years

(Clayton, 2024; Levy, 2021) (see Chapter 1 for a brief history of public health newborn screening). When looking to the future of newborn screening in the United States, it is worth stepping back to reexamine whether this premise still holds true.

Newborn screening as a universally provided service can draw on philosophical concepts around the value of enabling a just or fair society, equality of opportunity, and investment of resources where they can create the greatest opportunity (Rawls, 2001). Equality of opportunity draws on the idea that every individual—regardless of their background or circumstances—should have a chance to succeed. Public health newborn screening contributes to this chance for the approximately 7,000 infants identified each year as at risk for conditions that affect their morbidity or mortality (Gaviglio et al., 2023a). Newborn screening as a public health intervention also represents an investment of resources toward ensuring that no child dies from a preventable or treatable condition. Two examples help illustrate the positive health impacts of newborn screening:

- Eleven NBS programs identified severe combined immunodeficiency (SCID) in 1 in 58,000 infants. Infants identified through screening had a high rate of survival (87 percent) for SCID, which is an otherwise fatal diagnosis (Kwan et al., 2014).
- Public health newborn screening in Utah identified spinal muscular atrophy (SMA) in 1 in 20,000 infants. All infants identified met important developmental milestones through up to 5 years of age—inconsistent with the natural history of SMA (Wong et al., 2024).

The field of public health is sometimes perceived as focusing on preventing infectious disease, with vaccination programs being one of the most visible examples. However, its role is much broader, encompassing many facets that impact the health of populations. The 10 Essential Public Health Services,[1] originally released in 1994 and revised in 2020, has stood for three decades as a key framework outlining core public health functions. Newborn screening programs align with the public health services embedded in this framework, including monitoring and addressing the causes of health risks. Providing a universal means to identify infants born with serious, urgent, and treatable health conditions supports the underlying goal of promoting the health of all people in the United States. To be successful in this mission, newborn screening involves other public health functions and services, including effective communication, evaluation and quality improvement, workforce development, and organizational infrastructure.

It is also worth considering the potential implications were newborn screening provided in alternative ways, rather than as a service

---

[1] https://www.cdc.gov/public-health-gateway/php/about/index.html (accessed March 24, 2025).

implemented through public health programs. The primary alternative to the current public health approach to newborn screening would likely be to carry out all newborn screening through health care systems, as part of birth and clinical care services. Indeed, care providers and health care systems already fulfill important roles in implementing public health newborn screening and delivering care to babies identified through screening (see Chapter 2 and elsewhere in the report). However, variation in resources, priorities, and practices between and even within health care systems suggests that newborn screening communications, blood spot collection and screening, reporting of results, follow-up, and other performance aspects would likely vary not only state to state, as in the current system, but from hospital or birth setting to hospital. Health care settings are not designed to fulfill the same obligations to all babies or to operate with the same resources and authorities as state/territorial and federal governments. Leaving the implementation of newborn screening programs to private or nonprofit sectors (through health care systems or others) appears likely to reduce consistency, could limit or negatively affect the near-universal provision of newborn screening to all babies born in the United States, and could amplify existing differences around diseases and variants included on screening panels and other program features.

A role for newborn screening as a public health service in the United States remains relevant, and for public entities to be involved in overseeing and implementing it fairly, effectively, and sustainably. Subsequent sections of this chapter describe how the committee approached the mission and scope of newborn screening as a public health endeavor upholding public health principles, and the relationship of public health newborn screening to other parts of the ecosystem, such as clinical care and research. This analysis also informed the vision described throughout this report for the next chapter of public health newborn screening.

ESTABLISHING A FOUNDATION FOR ALIGNED AND CONSISTENT DECISION MAKING

As public health newborn screening moves into its next era, competing needs and tensions persist. Those who benefit from public health newborn screening through detection and connection to care are often a different group than experiences harms related to screening (e.g., false positives, unclear results, psychosocial stress)—each of these groups may have different priorities and concerns related to the future of newborn screening. Patient advocacy groups have expressed deep concerns with barriers to adding conditions to NBS panels. Ethicists and policy makers have raised concerns regarding the opportunity costs of expanding newborn screening, as well as continued differences among programs arising from variation in screening panels and follow-up within and across states. As technology has evolved, scientists, advocates, and others have suggested an expanded role for genomic sequencing in NBS programs, raising technical, ethical, legal, and implementation questions. The introduction of new classes of therapies with high price tags raises concerns about access to treatment for diagnosed patients. Lawsuits brought by privacy advocates over storage and secondary uses of newborn dried blood spots have led to the destruction of millions of specimens in Minnesota, Texas, and Michigan (Hughes et al., 2022). Legal scholars and others have strongly criticized the use of blood spots by law enforcement (Grant, 2022; Ram, 2022). If unaddressed, these and other tensions, challenges, and pressures may imperil the effectiveness of this essential public health service (Currier, 2022; McCandless and Wright, 2020).

One approach to making choices when faced with tensions and competing priorities is to look to the process of ethical decision making. In addition to complying with legal obligations, a process of ethically informed analysis aims to ground decisions guiding newborn screening around shared commitments, principles, and values that can be explained and justified to those involved with and affected by these programs. Such a process can promote clarity of reasoning and support greater consistency and efficiency.

The process of ethical decision making provides philosophical and methodological tools to examine the goals and values of screening, help weigh trade-offs among options when making decisions, understand tensions that may arise between or among these alternatives, and, when appropriate, identify the path chosen based on principles and priorities. As highlighted by the American Public Health Association, "Resolving ethical tensions does not mean finding the right answer; rather, it means searching for a morally appropriate way forward, all things considered" (APHA, 2019, p. 7). As drawn from Mattison (2000) and APHA (2019), features of this process include attention to

- Determining the public health goals, gathering information, and understanding the circumstances affecting the decision.
- Identifying ethical principles and values, including where such principles and values are in tension, and look to guidance from relevant ethical and theoretical frameworks, codes of conduct, or other guidance.
- Considering possible courses of action, and assessing their implications for affected individuals and communities, including the consequences of different choices on anticipated benefits, harms, and outcomes.
- Analyzing how a course of action aligns with core values, and making a choice that can be explained and justified.

Attention to these concepts helps to ensure more intentional, transparent decisions to preserve and improve newborn screening.

UNDERSTANDING COMMUNITY VIEWS TO INFORM ETHICALLY GROUNDED DECISION MAKING

Grounding decisions in an ethical manner involves assessing the best available factual evidence, understanding the lived experience of those involved, providing opportunities for direct or indirect participation of those communities and stakeholders toward finding solutions and informing the decision-making process, and explicitly thinking through how the proposed public health action or program can be publicly justified and explained. As stated in the American Public Health Association (APHA) Code of Ethics, "Empirical studies and anecdotal evidence show that when done well, public deliberation can yield more informed, considered, civic-minded, egalitarian discussions and mutually supported decisions" (APHA, 2019, p. 10).

Eliciting information on views, concerns, and priorities of a wide array from individuals and groups who compose the NBS community is key. A number of prior publications have assessed such views, particularly from parents and providers, in areas that include the focus of newborn screening, role of new genomic technologies, preferences around decision making and consent, and experiences in the context of specific diseases (see, for example, Andrews et al., 2022 Bailey et al., 2006; Crossnohere et al., 2022; Goldenberg et al., 2014; Hiraki et al., 2006; Lisi and McCandless, 2016; Miller et al., 2015; Tarini et al., 2018). As additional input to this study and to better understand the wide-ranging perspectives of individuals or groups interested in or affected by newborn screening—including laboratory and follow-up professionals, patients, families, advocacy organizations, care providers, administrators, and technology and therapeutics developers—input was sought through virtual listening sessions and an online questionnaire.[2] Selected issues and quotes below reflect the challenges and opportunities facing the NBS system and participants' views on charting an ethical and equitable course forward.

Scaling Condition-by-Condition Review in an Era of Rapid Discovery

Each state determines which conditions to include on its routine, public health NBS panel. As described in Chapter 2, states draw on federal guidance provided through the Recommended Uniform Screening Panel (RUSP). Adding a condition to the RUSP is a lengthy and multistep process that typically takes several years (HRSA, 2022). The slow nature of this process is inherent in the comprehensiveness of the required nomination package, the rigor of the evidence review, and the need to provide national guidance (Bailey et al., 2021; Kemper et al., 2014). As of 2024,

---

[2] See Appendix A for details on this component of information gathering; input received is summarized in Susanna Haas Lyons Engagement Consulting, 2024.

only nine conditions have been added to the RUSP since its creation in 2010 (HRSA, 2024a). The sustainability of this process has come under scrutiny for its limited capacity to keep pace with the development of new disease therapies and for the burden it places on the rare disease advocacy community and others to support the development of the evidence base needed for RUSP nomination (Andrews et al., 2022; Armstrong, 2024; Kennedy, 2024).

> A valid NBS test and valid treatment may exist for a disease, [but] it takes the better part of a decade to get it [added to the RUSP], and taxes the advocacy organizations who can least afford to spend their valuable time and resources on this.
>
> —Parent of a child with a rare disease

> New conditions are added to the RUSP regularly and are expected to be added to each NBS program in a timely manner. Tremendous resources and expertise including laboratory technology, clinical care, informatics, data analytics, and project management are required to add new conditions to programs that have limited resources and daily responsibilities of screening and following thousands of newborns.
>
> —NBS lab professional

> The process of adding conditions to NBS programs is way too slow and reliant on old criteria that are no longer valid [in] our era of increasingly precise and cost-effective genomic screening tools. That's why federal guidance through the RUSP is, in my view, excessively conservative. This conservatism trickles down to state labs, which often follow the guidance and don't have the resources to add much else through pilot programs.
>
> —Parent of a child with a rare disease

Embedding Equity Within the NBS System

Universal access to newborn screening is a deeply valued feature of current NBS programs that can reduce health disparities (Brosco et al., 2015). Although every baby has access to newborn screening, an infant will receive screening for different conditions depending on the state or territory in which they are born, meaning a baby born in one state may receive screening for a condition while a baby born in another state may not (NewSTEPs, 2023a). The quality and timeliness of screening vary from state to state as well, furthering geographic inequities (GAO, 2016; McGarry et al., 2023; NewSTEPs, 2023b). Molecular screening tests may not be designed inclusively for babies of different ancestral origins, leading to false positives and negatives for children of non-European descent (Bosfield et al., 2021; McGarry et al., 2023).

Babies identified via newborn screening will have different access to the provision of evidence-based care based on where they live as well as their socioeconomic status and race (McColley et al., 2022; Sohn and Timmermans, 2019). There are noteworthy gaps in care for certain conditions, including sickle cell disease; fewer than half of Medicaid-enrolled children with sickle cell anemia receive annual transcranial doppler screening—a standard of care—and only half receive disease-modifying treatment (Schieve et al., 2022). Different conditions attract different levels of financial research investment from industry and advocacy groups, which may ultimately lead to gaps in evidence generation (Bailey, 2022). The NBS system wrestles with how to embed equity throughout the system, beyond initial screening access, and across geographic, socioeconomic, ancestral, and racial/ethnic dimensions.

> There isn't uniformity from state to state, meaning sometimes families find out about their child's condition based on luck of residence alone. Even federally recommended disease[s] don't have to be added in every state. Luck or happenstance shouldn't be a factor in determining if a child has a rare disease not immediately apparent at birth.
>
> —Parent of a child with a rare disease

> While infants are generally screened universally, the system for follow-up and treatment for screen-positive infants mirrors our health care system. [Some] Infants are lost to follow-up or don't receive treatment in a timely manner.
>
> —Health care provider

> Although I appreciate the desire to press forward and help more children, we absolutely need to make sure that the current system is equitably working for everyone. Otherwise, we will continue to leave children behind. Progress rarely appreciates thoughtful reassessments, so we need to prioritize ensuring that public health interventions work for the entire population before moving forward and continuing to drive health disparities.
>
> —Health researcher

Considering New Screening Technologies in an Underresourced System

Echoing debates around incorporating tandem mass spectrometry into newborn screening in the 1990s, the NBS system currently wrestles with whether and, if so, how to apply emerging screening technologies, such as next-generation DNA sequencing. DNA sequencing as a platform technology for newborn screening could exponentially expand the number of conditions screened (Brunelli et al., 2023; Tarini, 2007). It could also create a deluge of complex and/or uncertain results for families and providers who may not have the expertise to interpret such information (Ross and Clayton, 2019; Tarini and Goldenberg, 2012). Furthermore, the collection and reuse of personal genetic information raises evolving social, ethical, and legal implications (Grant, 2022; Ram, 2022; Ross and Clayton, 2019). What factors should guide decision making on the role of this technology for newborn screening, while maintaining turnaround deadlines and the quality of service delivery required for the programs, remain open questions.

> Expanding a system that is underresourced and therefore inefficient and underperforming, fails more people while continuing to fall short of current goals. Improvements to the current system, achieving better efficiency would free up resources for new efforts.
>
> —Public health professional

> As technology advances, it's easy to want to advance newborn screening as well. However, it requires thoughtful consideration about whether these advances truly advance newborn screening. Are we doing things for research purposes or to actually help babies and their families?
>
> —NBS follow-up professional

> The next evolution in newborn screening is going to be sequencing . . . using sequencing technology. We've been bound or limited by tandem mass spectrometry, which is limited [to] inborn errors of metabolism . . . Most conditions are not inborn errors of metabolism that affect infants and children. . . . There are therapies for these conditions now. And there's a way to identify [infants] before they become symptomatic . . . I can give you numerous examples of children, where their lives were saved by newborn screening, the new newborn screening of sequencing.
>
> —Health industry representative

Balancing the Universality of Screening and Parental Choice

The near universality of newborn screening in the United States is seen as one of the program's greatest strengths, and many argue that this would not last if screening involved a parental informed consent process (APHL, 2016). The current nonconsented (opt-out) screening approach is generally based on the benefits to the child and society of screening for conditions that are serious, urgent, and treatable, and the potential for harm if a parent refuses such screening (APHL, 2016; Faden et al., 1982). As conditions that stray from the criteria of urgent, severe, and treatable are considered for inclusion, there are calls to (1) reassess the consented or nonconsented approach to screening, (2) consider risks—both known and unknown, and (3) explore other potential models (Bailey and Gehtland, 2015; Currier, 2022; Ross, 2010; Tarini, 2007).

> As we move forward, maybe the question that needs to be asked is, "Is identification and treatment of this condition urgent enough that parental consent should be waived?" And if that answer is "No," then the condition may not belong with NBS but could [be] offered to parents at a later date outside of the NBS program.
>
> —NBS laboratory professional

> The current system provides not enough information and agency to parents. Informed consent should be required, and it should not be an opt-out system.
>
> —Parent

Addressing the Unmet Needs of the Rare Disease Community

Rare disease patients and their families contend with gaps in research, treatment options, and access to care, along with significant obstacles to obtain diagnoses (EveryLife Foundation, 2023; Halley et al., 2022; Stoller, 2018; Von Der Lippe et al., 2022). Many within the rare disease community see the NBS system as a critical tool to avert a protracted diagnostic odyssey and jumpstart research into treatments (EveryLife Foundation, 2023). What information should guide evidence review and decision making for inclusion of conditions in newborn screening and whether conditions without current medical treatments or interventions should be included on screening panels are of interest to many involved with or affected by rare diseases. Whether public health newborn screening should be the mechanism to meet many unmet needs affecting the rare disease community and how to address strains on the current NBS system remain unanswered questions.

> The most important need of the rare disease community is more effective treatments for more diseases. . . . Development of new treatment or more effective treatment of any rare disease depends on identifying patients early enough, ideally presymptomatic, so the treatment benefits can be better demonstrated. Newborn screening can be the spark of treatment development that in turn fuels the further expansion of newborn screening. . . . It's a chicken-and-egg dilemma that constrains both newborn screening and treatment development. We can only break out of it if we find a way to tackle both at the same time.
>
> —Parent of a child with a rare disease

> Every day that a test is not made available is a day that a child entering this world can be missed and forced to endure unnecessary hardship. Knowledge doesn't take away the condition, it is always there. Knowledge allows informed decision making. Knowledge helps to avoid unnecessary burdens on exploratory pipelines. Knowledge allows for quality-of-life improvements. Knowledge allows for future family planning decision making. Knowledge allows for memories to me made, for the precious lives of our children to not be wasted searching for answers. Knowledge is everything.
>
> —Parent of a child with a rare disease

Colliding Interests over Storage and Secondary Use of Blood Spots

Potential conflicts between public health and privacy concerns over storage and secondary use of blood spots pose a threat to public health newborn screening and have erupted into several court cases in recent years. Although the landscape of policies regulating this issue vary, states typically retain the dried blood spots collected from babies for quality assurance and control, and often for secondary research that can advance public health or other goals. Legal challenges have disputed various retention and consent policies and specific uses of these dried blood spots, including access to specimens by law enforcement in New Jersey and storage and secondary research use in Michigan (Hughes et al., 2022). Concerns around retention and reuse of blood spots without informed consent have also contributed, at least in part, to reauthorization failures for the NBS Saves Lives Act (Sterman and Molina, 2023). Privacy and civil rights concerns about storage and secondary use of blood spots must be considered to preserve trust and build trustworthiness in the NBS system.

> Although these bloodspots have amazing potential for equitable public health research, the failure to protect bloodspots from misuse in criminal investigations and the lack of transparency in storing and using these bloodspots severely damages public trust.
>
> —Health researcher

> A nonconsented/mandated public health program has a big responsibility to promote trust and to not inadvertently cause harm by being distracted by special interests outside of the scope of newborn screening.
>
> —Health care provider

Wavering Public Trust amid Limited Awareness

The effectiveness of public health actions and policies is rooted in public trust gained through basing decisions on ethical, scientific, and professional standards. Trust is a key component for acceptance of public health guidance, and the COVID-19 pandemic brought to light the consequence of weak or absent trust and the importance of building institutional accountability and trustworthiness (Best et al., 2021; Taylor et al., 2023 Warren et al., 2020). Trust in public health broadly has eroded among several constituencies, and the growing number of lawsuits concerning residual dried blood spots threaten to undermine trust in the NBS system specifically (Hughes et al., 2022; RWJF, 2021). For many parents whose child does not receive an at-risk screening result, newborn screening is a barely recalled experience, contributing to lack of awareness of the program and its goals (DeLuca, 2018; Hasegawa et al., 2011). Ensuring that newborn screening is a trustworthy system will be important to the ability of programs to meet their mandate to screen all infants born in the United States.

> In a post-COVID America, it appears that the more parents hear about newborn screening, the more they may distrust and seek to opt out of it, despite its demonstrated benefits for newborns as a whole. Better, more nuanced, and earlier parent education may help to enhance parental and community trust—as would more robust privacy protections for NBS samples/data on the back end.
>
> —Privacy advocate

> I think I do remember them taking blood from my second baby, but that was it. They never came back and never reported the results.
>
> —Parent

> The general public has poor understanding of [newborn screening]. There's a lack of trust by many about any government programs—add to this the apprehension about genetic information being shared. Lack of education about newborn screening leaves state and federal programs vulnerable to funding loss or worse. At a minimum, there should be more education for expectant parents (grandparents) to prepare them for potentially receiv[ing] out-of-range results.
>
> —Health care provider

Improving NBS Delivery Without Systems for Data Collection and Integration

"Evidence is also an ethical issue" in policy and programmatic decisions on the future of newborn screening (Baily, 2023). Which information on potential benefits, harms, and suitability of screening for a condition through public health newborn screening should guide assessment, and the extent and types of evidence required remain areas of debate.

Data collection through state and territorial NBS programs is also currently siloed and typically ends when a tested infant transitions to the health care system. Recently, there has been a push to collect and connect screening, short-term, and longitudinal data to improve NBS delivery, assess and address disparities, and better understand how newborn screening affects longer-term health outcomes. The current system is limited by information technology and data capacity and lack of interoperability, hindering achievement of these aims (Watson et al., 2022).

> We focus a lot on screening, but there's no data or national system to count the number of kids who are screened positive.
>
> —Medical geneticist

A PATH FORWARD FOR PUBLIC HEALTH NEWBORN SCREENING GROUNDED IN BIOETHICAL FOUNDATIONS

These and other areas identified raise questions about the path forward for public health newborn screening. One of the reasons decision making for newborn screening is complex is because it involves an interplay not only of multiple viewpoints, but also of multiple bioethical contexts. Dried blood spot screening, in which every baby's blood is collected and tested at birth, is designed as a public health program. As such, its fundamental purpose is rooted in improving the collective health of the U.S. population (Currier, 2022; Kass, 2001). However, the implementation of newborn screening is experienced by individual families as part of clinical care, with samples typically collected in the hospital, birth center, or at home after birth, results follow-up communicated by their primary care provider, and the health effects ultimately experienced by individual patients (HRSA, 2023). Public health infrastructure involved in newborn screening can also be used as part of research efforts, such as to conduct consented pilot studies that evaluate the risks and benefits of screening for new conditions, advances that can be difficult (or arguably impossible) to gather through other means (see Chapter 6).

Public health ethics, clinical ethics, and research ethics address ethical issues in these different health and research contexts. While these three areas draw on shared principles such as autonomy, beneficence, nonmaleficence, and justice (Beauchamp and Childress, 1979, 2019), they can approach or weigh such principles differently depending on the populations and fundamental goals being served, with implications for decision making in these domains. The following sections briefly explore how ethical principles are applied in these three contexts.

Public Health Ethics

Public health as a discipline focuses on health challenges at the population level and particularly on programs designed to prevent disease or to promote or sustain health (Kass, 2001).[3] The Centers for Disease Control and Prevention defines public health ethics as the following:

> Because public health actions are often undertaken by governments and are directed at the population level, the principles and values which guide public health can differ from those which guide actions in biology and clinical medicine (bioethics and medical ethics) which are more patient or individual-centered.[4]

The ethics of public health interventions are generally judged based on the balance of harms and benefits across the population as a whole. In prioritizing the health of a population, most or all individuals in that population take on some degree of burden for a clear health benefit that can only be achieved through population-level interventions, although individuals may or may not directly benefit from the intervention. Population-level public health interventions are justified based on a shared understanding of benefit and minimal risk. As wide participation in screening is necessary for the desired benefits, and as risks are minimal, NBS programs may involve minimal procedures for obtaining individual consent. State and territorial public health newborn screening, for example, is generally opt-out, meaning the baby's blood is automatically collected and screened unless the parent or caregiver refuses (King and Smith, 2016).

Because of the focus of public health programs on *population* health, the types of interventions employed align with criteria that include the following:

- The risks are low, and there is clear and convincing evidence of significant benefit.
- The risks and benefits are such that the majority of the community would reasonably be expected to agree that the balance of risks and benefits is appropriate (with some important considerations for equity, discussed below).
- No subset of the population systematically receives a greater share of the benefits and burdens.
- There is no alternative approach that can achieve the same goal as well as the proposed public health program (Kass, 2001).

---

[3] See https://www.cdc.gov/public-health-gateway/php/about/index.html (accessed March 20, 2024).
[4] See https://www.cdc.gov/scientific-integrity/php/public-health-ethics/index.html (accessed December 12, 2024).

Contemporary public health ethics frameworks also emphasize values such as transparent and trustworthy governance and decision making and equity as critical elements (APHA, 2019; Lee et al., 2020; Parasidis and Fairchild, 2022).

Clinical Ethics

The study of clinical ethics is generally focused on guiding the care of individual patients by their clinicians. Clinical ethics centers the best interests of the individual person, prioritizing the capacitated patient's right to autonomous decision making and evaluating risks and benefits of alternatives in terms of the individual patient's or family's goals, values, and preferences (Varkey, 2021). The range of potential interventions that can be offered in the context of clinical care are broader than those that can be ethically justified in the context of public health because they are specifically targeted for the betterment of an individual and can incorporate a wider range of benefits and risks that reflect patients' diverse preferences (Kass, 2001; Swain et al., 2008; Thomas et al., 2002). In clinical care, an individual is in a position to weigh these risks and benefits and make decisions according to their own values and preferences (Varkey, 2021).

Being able to respect a patient's autonomy via informed consent requires three elements: the capacity to make a decision that reflects one's own values; adequate information about the risks, benefits, and alternatives of a choice to inform that decision; and freedom from coercion that could otherwise limit that choice (Faden and Beauchamp, 1986). If an otherwise fully capacitated adult lacks capacity temporarily (e.g., due to unconsciousness) or has become incapacitated indefinitely (e.g., a patient affected by Alzheimer's disease), a surrogate decision maker who is often the next of kin is generally asked to make a substituted judgment on the patient's behalf. This allows a trusted associate of the patient to apply known values to a clinical decision (Varkey, 2021).

As a further specification of clinical ethics, pediatric ethics helps assess how to respect autonomy, ensure beneficence, and protect against nonmaleficence in the context of a primary patient who does not have practical (i.e., a younger child or infant) or at least legal (i.e., an older adolescent) capacity to make medical decisions on behalf of themselves. The American Academy of Pediatrics recognizes multiple standards that may be employed when surrogates (usually parents) make decisions on behalf of children and conversations around the issues involved in pediatric clinical decision making continue (Katz et al., 2016; Salter et al., 2023). Historically, medical decision making in children has centered on a "best-interest" standard, meaning adhering to a decision that would be in the best interests of an average patient in the same situation (Kopelman, 1997; Varkey, 2021). However, parental decisions about their child's medical care are generally respected, understanding that parents must balance the needs of the minor patient with those of the entire family and are rarely overridden unless such decisions cross a threshold of abuse or neglect (Diekema, 2004; Ross, 2019). Newborn screening and subsequent care, by definition, involve infants without capacity to consent and are thus informed by the frameworks employed for surrogate decision making in pediatric contexts.

Research Ethics

Research ethics generally guides the study and generation of new medical and scientific knowledge. A primary goal of such research is often not to benefit the individual participant, but rather future patients like them. The ethical protection of human research participants (human subjects) has been the focus of landmark reports such as the Belmont Report (National Commission for the Protection of Human Subjects of Biomedical and Behavioral Research, 1979) and is subject to regularity requirements that include attention to whether risks to the individual participant are likely to outweigh potential benefits to the participant, or to the patient community of which they are a part (see 45 CFR Part 46). An adult patient may reasonably decide to enroll in a clinical trial for a novel treatment with a higher risk profile if they assess that the risk is outweighed by the potential benefit to their own health, for example if they have terminal cancer that has been resistant to all authorized and widely used treatments.

Additional research protections exist for certain groups of people, including fetuses, neonates, and children. As described in a Presidential Commission report, a "key impetus for a separate regulatory subpart addressing additional protections for child participants in research was the recognition that, while adults can consent to assume research risks, children cannot" (Presidential Commission for the Study of Bioethical Issues, 2013, p. 37). Under 45 CFR 46, along with conducting the research in accordance with sound ethical principles and making adequate provision for soliciting assent of the children and permission of their parents or guardians, children are allowed to be enrolled in clinical trials that are of minimal risk to themselves; greater than minimal risk if there is the prospect of direct benefit to the child or "the research is likely to yield generalizable knowledge about the [child]'s disorder or condition" (§46.406), or with authorization from the secretary of the Department of Health and Human Services when "the research presents an opportunity to understand, prevent, or alleviate a serious problem affecting the health or welfare of children" (§46.407). Contemporary and responsive research ethics models also emphasize engaging individuals and communities to inform ethically grounded approaches to conducting research and mitigating potential research-related harms. Such models emphasize public engagement by funding agencies, research institutions, institutional review boards, and investigators to understand the needs, values, and preferences across the research continuum. As part of this process, it is important to include the voices of persons traditionally underrepresented in research and those who face vulnerabilities in the research process (Dawson et al., 2020; Fisher 2014; Schott et al., 2023; Solomon, 2013).

EXAMPLES OF PRIOR APPROACHES TO ETHICAL DECISION MAKING IN NEWBORN SCREENING

The current approach to newborn screening in the United States draws on a history of literature and analyses that have guided program choices, including on diseases that are appropriate to include in screening. The current criteria for conditions included on NBS panels, which focus on conditions that significantly affect health, are detectable in newborns, and for which effective treatment is available, hearken back to an influential set of criteria proposed by Wilson and Jungner in 1968 to guide public health screening programs (see Box 3-1). Wilson and Jungner's criteria were developed largely to inform a different public health context—screening adults for chronic diseases. However, two inborn errors

---

BOX 3-1
Criteria Proposed by Wilson and Jungner for Public Health Disease Screening Programs

1. The condition sought should be an important health problem.
2. There should be an accepted treatment for patients with recognized disease.
3. Facilities for diagnosis and treatment should be available.
4. There should be a recognizable latent or early symptomatic stage.
5. There should be a suitable test or examination.
6. The test should be acceptable to the population.
7. The natural history of the condition, including development from latent to declared disease, should be adequately understood.
8. There should be an agreed policy on whom to treat as patients.
9. The cost of case-finding (including diagnosis and treatment of patients diagnosed) should be economically balanced in relation to possible expenditure on medical care as a whole.
10. Case-finding should be a continuing process and not a "once and for all" project.

SOURCE: Wilson and Junger, 1968.

of metabolism—phenylketonuria and galactosemia—were mentioned in the paper, suggesting this guidance was not solely meant for application toward adult public health (Wilson and Jungner, 1968). As such, these criteria have both utility and limitations when applied to the context of screening newborns. Nevertheless, they have provided an important foundation for subsequent analyses and critiques.

In the 2000s, in response to the highly variable landscape of conditions screened across state-run NBS programs since their inception in the 1960s, developments in screening technologies, and advancing understanding of medical genetics, the Health Resources and Services Administration's Maternal and Child Health Bureau commissioned the American College of Medical Genetics and Genomics (ACMG) to develop recommendations to inform newborn screening (ACMG Newborn Screening Expert Group, 2006). Guiding principles identified in the 2006 ACMG report included newborn screening as a public health responsibility; benefit to affected newborns as the primary driver of policy decisions with secondary consideration to the interests of unaffected newborns, families, health professionals, and the public; the importance of evidence in making decisions about newborn screening; and public and professional education and awareness as essential to NBS success. The ACMG report identified 29 primary conditions it recommended be part of public health newborn screening.

Others expressed reservations with aspects of the evaluation process used to generate the ACMG report and its recommendations (Botkin et al., 2006; Moyer et al., 2008; Natowicz, 2005). Concerns were raised about the report's emphasis on professional opinion, which is considered the weakest form of evidence for policy decisions by the U.S. Preventative Services Task Force and others. The rigor with which these opinions were ascertained was also questioned, both in terms of the survey design as well as in the composition and balance of expertise surveyed. Literature reviews supporting the ACMG recommendations were criticized for potential lack of independence and lack of appropriate methodology. Nevertheless, the ACMG's recommendations and ensuing critiques, along with subsequent refinements to the process for evaluating and considering diseases for inclusion, have elevated the importance of rigorous evidence review as a foundation for the program (ACMG Newborn Screening Expert Group, 2006; Botkin et al., 2006; Kemper et al., 2014; Moyer et al., 2008; Natowicz, 2005). A 2008 ethical analysis undertaken by the President's Council on Bioethics reflected on how benefits and harms from newborn screening are conceived, including the potential social or research benefits beyond those to an identified child's well-being. The resulting report sought a framework to balance benefits and harms of screening, respect for parental decision making, concerns about the implications of unclear results, the role of research in understanding currently untreatable conditions, the promise of further technical advances, the scale of resources required by population-level health programs, ultimately distinguishing between conditions ethically appropriate to include in mandatory screening (having an effective treatment and direct benefit to child welfare), and conditions that could be part of voluntary screening panels and would require parental consent (President's Council on Bioethics, 2008).

The approaches articulated in these reports and others have informed NBS decision making. These developments collectively focused on creating a more equitable screening system for all Americans and ultimately led to the creation of the RUSP, greater uniformity across state and territorial NBS programs, and incorporation of a framework for reviewing conditions considered for addition to the RUSP (CDC, 2012). Since these analyses, decision making and criteria for inclusion on the RUSP have continued to evolve (HRSA, 2024b; Kemper et al., 2014). Notably, the original conditions named in the ACMG report—which formed the basis for the RUSP—have never been reassessed.

The past two decades have seen additional calls to expand newborn screening beyond conditions that meet criteria articulated in these reports, such as including conditions with less severe effects, that emerge later in childhood, or that lack available treatments (Currier, 2022). There have been calls to expand research associated with state and territorial NBS public health programs to facilitate addition of new conditions to NBS panels, better understand and treat heritable disease, or study other health issues.[5] There have been ongoing debates about the appropriate roles for newer, genomic-based screening technologies (see Chapter 5). Ethical decision-making frameworks for the next era of newborn screening remain necessary and timely in light of these ongoing debates on the scope and aims of newborn screening and the range of needs and tensions described earlier in this chapter.

PRINCIPLES AND VALUES CENTRAL TO EXCELLENCE IN PUBLIC HEALTH NEWBORN SCREENING

Contemporary public health codes of ethics elevate additional principles and values as part of identifying appropriate paths forward around public health actions, particularly when faced with multiple goals and competing viewpoints (APHA, 2019). These considerations include not only the ethical permissibility of a course of action, but also its inter-

---

[5] See Chapter 5 for a discussion of research needs relevant to newborn screening and an explanation of the legal landscape guiding storage and reuse of newborn screening blood spots for research.

sections with respect for individuals and communities, reciprocity and proportionality around anticipated benefits and harms, effectiveness and responsible use of scare resources, accountability and transparency, and consultation with affected parties through public participation (APHA, 2019). While additional values and broader system-level considerations can be incorporated in multiple ways, this report highlights the role of three closely intertwined concepts that are critical for maintaining and strengthening an excellent NBS system now and into the future: effectiveness, trustworthiness, and equity.

Achieving and Maintaining the Effectiveness of NBS Programs

Effectiveness is central to achieving the value proposition of public health newborn screening (Berberich, 2024; Holtzman and Watson, 1998). Ensuring that public health newborn screening is effectively meeting its goals is supported by the provision of validated, timely, and accurate newborn screening, coupled with timely linkage from screening to confirmatory or follow-up testing, and to genetic counseling and care when necessary. NBS effectiveness enables infants and their families to benefit from treatments for screened conditions in time to make a difference in reducing morbidity and mortality.

Maintaining NBS effectiveness is a necessary part of preserving broad support for the mission and implementation of newborn screening as a public health endeavor, not only among the millions of parents and caregivers whose babies are screened each year, but also among the range of federal, state, and local policy makers who put in place the policies, programs, and resources guiding and sustaining this effort; the networks of public health and clinical professionals essential to carrying out screening, diagnosis, and care; and the U.S. public willing to support the role and purpose of newborn screening.

Sustaining Trustworthiness in the Mission and Implementation of Public Health Newborn Screening

"The most important asset that public health can have is the public's trust that work is being done on its own behalf" (Kass, 2001, p. 1782). An ethical and high-quality NBS system must be one that is trustworthy; it must deserve to be trusted by the many constituencies participating in and using this system. Strengthening the NBS system to address ethical complexities, mitigate harms, and maximize benefits requires trustworthiness, which in turn entails features such as transparency and engagement (Beans, 2024; Clayton, 2024; Goldenberg, 2024; Hassan, 2024; Ram, 2024; Tanksley, 2024; Wallis, 2024).

As the committee heard during the study, building trust takes time. Legal and ethical thinking has moved toward the position that people are entitled to know their health information and be part of the process (NASEM, 2018).[6] Public health newborn screening often operates in the background as an essentially mandated program, but ongoing and expanding calls seek to bring greater systematic awareness and understanding of newborn screening to families and providers (ACOG Committee on Genetics, 2019; Botkin et al., 2016; Davis et al., 2006; Therrell et al., 2011). Greater family awareness and education about public health newborn screening are particularly important given the tension between building trustworthiness and the nonconsented nature of screening in many jurisdictions. Educating about public health newborn screening—particularly its purpose and benefits, when and how it will happen, and parental options concerning both screening and the retention and reuse of the residual dried blood spots—provides families the agency to act as partners in the NBS system, and in turn build trust. Understanding who is best equipped to deliver this information to families and communities in a way that builds trustworthiness is important, and newborn screening decision makers may be able to learn from other health interventions that engage pregnant patients in the community, where they live. See Chapter 4 for the importance of viewing families as partners in the NBS system.

Building trust will also require engaging with community views to continue to ground decision making about the future of newborn screening in an ethical manner. Many ethical and social concerns about the practice of public health newborn screening can be better understood through research on community views. Such research could be designed to understand views on consent for public health newborn screening, storage and reuse of dried blood spots, or a broader range of screening-related benefits (see Chapter 6). Building public trust without losing communities that have little earned trust in public health and health care programs and understanding and mitigating issues that may lead people to opt out of public health newborn screening will all be important.

Understanding and operationalizing the concept of trustworthiness involves multiple dimensions and has been the subject of a body of prior research (Nong, 2023; Taylor et al., 2023). For example, features that feed into and support trustworthiness include acting in accordance with ethical principles, prioritizing the public's best interests and needs, and maintaining excellence in the performance of major program functions. These include ensuring the timeliness, validity, and accuracy of screening test results; safely, securely, and ethically managing storage and use of dried blood spots and any derived data; and demonstrating high performance

---

[6] 21st Century Cures Act, Pub. L. No. 114-255.

through quality assurance and improvement measures. Operating with transparency and proactively addressing sources of mistrust, engaging stakeholders to understand values and needs and participate as partners, and creating and using clear and effective communication materials also build trustworthiness. Examples of areas highlighted during the study's information gathering that affect public perceptions of trustworthiness include earlier, more effective, and more nuanced education about newborn screening and the importance of data privacy protections (see Chapter 4).

Paying Attention to Equity Dimensions that Affect How Well Public Health Newborn Screening Serves All Babies

As a population-level investment in the well-being of infants born in U.S. states and territories, equity is a foundational aspect of newborn screening. NBS programs, subsequent diagnosis and care for identified babies, and the surrounding research enterprise need to serve the needs of all infants born in the United States and their families.

The nature of newborn screening, designed to reach every baby born in the United States, has the potential to serve as a powerful tool to reduce disparities in time to diagnosis for communities underserved by the health care system (Brosco et al., 2015). Just because babies may be screened *equally*, in the sense that their blood is collected and sent to a laboratory for testing, does not necessarily mean that all aspects of NBS programs, or the larger system, are *equitable*. Paying careful attention to equity in newborn screening involves multiple dimensions (see Table 3-1). When screening tests are not designed inclusively, infants of non-European descent tend to have higher rates of false positives and negatives (Bosfield et al., 2021; Gaviglio, 2021; McGarry et al., 2023; Peng et al., 2020). Studies suggest that infants from underserved communities experience longer times to confirmatory diagnosis and treatment initiation after identification through newborn screening (Gaviglio, 2021; McColley et al., 2023; Singh, 2022). In addition, care for diagnosed babies can depend on family circumstances, which may be affected by geographic and socioeconomic factors such as uneven distribution of specialists, ability to travel to appointments or specialized facilities, and the nature of the family's health insurance coverage.

Expanding public health screening without recognizing or addressing major inequities in other parts of the NBS system will never be more than partially successful and could even exacerbate disparities, particularly in the context of limited resources and new high-priced therapies such as gene therapies (Gaviglio et al., 2023b; Sobotka and Ross, 2023). Although not every dimension of equity described in Table 3-1 is in the purview

TABLE 3-1 Several Dimensions of Equity and Their Relevance to Newborn Screening

Conceptual Dimension	Illustrative Example in the Context of Newborn Screening
Policy and Input (Nature and inclusiveness of decision making) Prioritization, investment, and other decision-making processes need to elevate a range of voices. Attention needs to be paid to how newborn screening can avoid perpetuating past injustices and/or correct past injustices when possible.	Current focus and composition of voting members of the federal Advisory Committee on Heritable Disorders in Newborns and Children (ACHDNC) is not representative of the breadth of issues and full range of interested and affected parties involved in public health newborn screening.
Geography Not all states screen for the same diseases, the screening assays used by different states vary in their performance, and not all states have the same access to specialists for identified conditions.	Genetic counselors and clinical geneticists are geographically concentrated in metropolitan areas, and some states have few to no practitioners (Jenkins et al., 2021; NSGC, 2020).
Screening Deployment All babies need fair and equal opportunities to receive newborn screening.	Newborn screening generally reaches all babies and families; it is carried out on an estimated 98% of babies born in U.S. states and territories (Sohn and Timmermans, 2019).
Assay Performance and Evaluation Screening assays and confirmatory diagnostic tests need to perform accurately for all members of the population; performance should be evaluated in representative populations to ensure accuracy and reduce the likelihood of disparate effectiveness.	Infants of African descent are at a higher risk of receiving false positives from commonly used molecular NBS assays for mucopolysaccharidosis type I (Bosfield et al., 2021).
Diagnosis All babies identified through screening need an equitable opportunity to receive timely confirmatory diagnostic testing and be handed off to the clinical care system where needed.	Infants from minoritized racial/ethnic groups who screen positive for cystic fibrosis receive diagnostic follow-up later than recommended and later than their White peers (McColley et al., 2023).
Care/Treatment All identified babies need longer-term connection and access to care, but disparities reflect features of the U.S. health care system.	Fewer Medicaid-enrolled children with congenital hypothyroidism receive recommended, evidence-based care (i.e., follow-up thyroid stimulating hormone testing) than their privately insured peers (Kemper et al., 2020).

TABLE 3-1 Continued

Conceptual Dimension	Illustrative Example in the Context of Newborn Screening
Research/Attention The research portfolio informing newborn screening (and heritable disorders more broadly) needs to include topics relevant to diverse communities, including those that have been historically underserved.	Different conditions attract different levels of financial research investment from industry and advocacy groups, which may ultimately lead to gaps in evidence generation (Bailey, 2022).

NOTE: NBS = newborn screening.

of public health newborn screening to address, the ramifications of each must be considered when making decisions about the policy and practice of newborn screening.

PUBLIC HEALTH NEWBORN SCREENING FOR THE ERA AHEAD: THIS REPORT'S APPROACH

Drawing on these frameworks and values, the approach taken by this report emphasizes how public health newborn screening aligns with ethical foundations informing public health and focuses on supporting and strengthening the excellence of the NBS through effectiveness, trustworthiness, and equity where opportunities exist. It is essential to emphasize that some elements intertwined with newborn screening or that help fully address needs of the many parties who participate in this system remain critically important, but they are not well suited to public health programs or do not fall within the ability of public health to address in isolation. Intersecting needs in clinical care and research settings require taking a system-level approach, with active and ongoing engagement among the diversity of stakeholders and rightsholders involved. This is necessary to align values as issues continue to emerge and evolve, and to support effective decision making for both NBS programs and for the broader NBS and disease treatment system.

The report emphasizes the following features in guiding decision making about newborn screening as a public health endeavor.

Align Decisions for Newborn Screening Conducted as a Universal, Public Health Service with Public Health Ethics

Universal newborn screening, implemented through state and territorial public health departments to screen all babies at birth, falls within the purview of public health ethics. Newborn screening as a public health program uses a population-level screening paradigm that considers balancing risks, benefits, and decision making through a population-level lens rather than an individual, person-level lens. Such a mandated public health program is generally only justifiable if risks are minimal, benefits are viewed as significant and important by a majority of the population, and alternative approaches (such as relying on detection and diagnosis of a condition later as part of clinical care) are unlikely to achieve the same benefit.

Focus Public Health Newborn Screening on Reducing Morbidity and Mortality

To align with public health values and principles, universal, at-birth newborn screening conducted as a population-level screening program needs to focus on conditions that are serious, urgent, and have a therapeutic intervention rigorously shown to reduce babies' morbidity and mortality. These criteria align with the public health mission of newborn screening to reduce morbidity and mortality and advance child welfare.

Focus Public Health Newborn Screening on Certain Types of Conditions

Deploying universal, population-level screening requires there to be widely shared views that anticipated benefits are significant, that these outweigh anticipated harms, and that alternative approaches (such as diagnosis later through the care system) are unlikely to achieve these benefits. The public health aim that justifies universal newborn screening focuses on child welfare through the identification of conditions that affect screened infants' morbidity and mortality because they are serious, urgent, and treatable. Practically and ethically, it is also important to ensure that the current foundation of public health newborn screening works effectively and equitably for everyone before pressing forward with large expansions.

Rare diseases, though individually rare, collectively affect an estimated 10 percent of the U.S. population.[7] Screening for a greater number of rare diseases that meet the criteria for public health newborn screening would mean that a greater number of infants with disease will be identified as at risk, diagnosed, and treated. As such, expanding the *number* of conditions included in public health newborn screening could be one potential way to increase the net population benefit of the NBS program; however, expanding the *scope* of newborn screening to include conditions that are, for example, later onset or have no available treatment, would not align with the public health paradigm of the program. Other

---

[7] See https://rarediseases.info.nih.gov (accessed March 24, 2025).

approaches, including through clinical care or research, may need to be explored to screen for conditions that do not meet the high bar necessary for inclusion in public health newborn screening.

Subsections below describe how the terms *serious*, *urgent*, and *treatable* can be conceptualized in the context of public health newborn screening and how the committee considered them for the purposes of this report.

Screening for Conditions Having Serious Health Effects

In alignment with public health criteria and prior reports from ACMG and others, the approach to public health at-birth newborn screening primarily focuses on identifying serious genetic conditions prior to the onset of symptoms (Andermann et al., 2008). It is difficult to define terms such as *serious*. Many definitions have been used, often focusing on morbidity and mortality. Such concepts are always viewed through the lens of an individual's or their family's subjective experience and priorities regarding their quality of life; what is serious for one individual may be deemed relatively unimportant for another (Boardman and Clark, 2022; FDA, 2022; Kleiderman et al., 2024; Roy et al., 2021; Wertz and Knoppers, 2002). In addition, context matters, as living with certain diseases or disabilities can be facilitated or greatly impeded by a person's surrounding environment. Lack of agreement on the meaning of *serious* is particularly relevant when considering whether or not to expand newborn screening to include conditions that less clearly meet current inclusion criteria, those with a less clear knowledge base on the range of disease variants and their manifestations, or where there is less agreement on the nature, severity, and timing of the effects. Although the term *serious* cannot be easily defined, the committee generally considered it to mean diseases that have significant negative health effects on an affected baby's morbidity and/or mortality.

Screening for Conditions That Are Urgent to Address

Although the term *urgent* can be interpreted in variable ways, the committee generally viewed it as indicating a need to act presymptomatically early in a baby's life—or to be primed to act quickly during early life—to prevent negative effects on morbidity and mortality (e.g., dietary management for medium-chain acyl-coenzyme A dehydrogenase deficiency to prevent death) (Marsden et al., 2021).

Perspectives differ on whether to expand public health NBS panels to conditions that have later onset of symptoms during childhood or conditions that can be effectively treated later, after symptoms arise. Some have argued for the value of reducing the diagnostic odyssey and ensuring timely treatment, while others have argued that to screen for these in the newborn period introduces potential burdens or harms of providing information that creates undue stress associated with being "patients in waiting" (Kelly et al., 2016; Moyer et al., 2008).

Including such conditions in public health newborn screening is one mechanism to meet diagnostic and treatment aims, but it is not the only one. Later onset conditions and/or those that can be effectively treated when symptoms arise could arguably be addressed through clinical screening or diagnostic testing later in childhood, rather than through public health screening at birth (Sobotka and Ross, 2023). While there are significant barriers associated with clinical diagnosis and care, these barriers can be better addressed by interventions to improve clinical care systems for such patients and families, as opposed to using population-level newborn screening.

Similarly, perspectives differ on reporting information for the purposes of understanding a baby's carrier status for a disease (rather than being affected by the disease itself), informing parental health or lifestyle choices, informing family reproductive choices, or realizing other potential benefits as part of public health newborn screening. In these cases, the balance of potential benefits and harms is less certain in the context of a large-scale public program and individual parents have widely variable preferences in desire for this information (Joseph et al., 2016; Moultrie et al., 2020; Tluczek et al., 2022). A patient's own preferences (i.e., the child's) would guide this decision but their preferences are unknowable as newborns. Although clinical care and research settings have substantial challenges and limitations of their own, it is again difficult to make a clear case for these types of conditions as part of routine, population-wide public health newborn screening.

Screening for Conditions That Are Treatable

Similar logic applies when considering whether universal, at-birth newborn screening as a public health program should expand to include conditions that lack demonstrably efficacious interventions. Arguments for expansion point to the potential benefits to families with rare conditions of avoiding the diagnostic odyssey, accessing clinical trials while the child is still presymptomatic, informing reproductive choices for the family, and others (Alexander and van Dyck, 2006; EveryLife Foundation, 2023; Susanna Haas Lyons Engagement Consulting, 2024). While some families will undoubtedly derive value from this knowledge, surveys suggest that perspectives on having screening for these types of conditions vary widely (Ersig et al., 2023; Timmins et al., 2022). Parents are free to request screening for additional conditions as part of their child's clinical care, if they are able to do so. This is, of course, with the acknowledgment that the cost of clinical testing can be a high, and sometimes insurmountable, burden for some families. But as discussed above, public health decisions are generally targeted toward improving the health of a community, necessarily balancing scarce resource allocation at state and federal levels, rather than on the personalized needs of any given individual child or family to tailor clinical interventions.

It is important to note that the definition of *treatment* can be interpreted narrowly, focusing primarily on interventions such as drugs or dietary changes. However, other kinds of health interventions, including physical, occupational, and speech therapy, may significantly improve functional status and quality of life for affected children. The linchpin of the definition of *treatment* is evidence of significant benefit, such that most people would agree that its potential benefits outweigh the burdens of screening. If a treatment is demonstrated to reduce morbidities and mortality, then the actual mechanism of treatment (e.g., drug versus physical therapy) should not be a barrier to inclusion in public health newborn screening. The concept of medical interventions needs to account for multiple types of evidence-based interventions that reduce morbidity for individuals identified through screening and prioritize research and investment into these varied forms of interventions and services.

Questions about Carrier Status

Questions have been raised about testing for or reporting carrier status as part of public health newborn screening. If carrier status manifests in infancy as a serious, urgent, and treatable condition, then that would align with the mission of public health newborn screening, which focuses on detecting serious, urgent conditions that are treatable if identified in infancy. For example, in rare instances, female carriers of X-linked conditions can be symptomatic (Migeon, 2020), which has been a point of consideration for X-linked conditions previously considered for NBS panels (Condition Review Workgroup, 2017). For autosomal recessive conditions, being a carrier can have health risks or implications that may impact an infant later in life (NASEM, 2020; Shi et al., 2021). However, this information has no immediate clinical usefulness for the newborn (Clayton, 2010). Ultimately, health implications related to carrier status that arise in adulthood and/or cannot be intervened on in infancy do not align with the public health mission of newborn screening to detect infants with serious conditions and connect them to care and intervention.

However, the reality is that carrier status may be detected when screening for a primary condition (e.g., detection of sickle cell trait when screening for sickle cell disease) (APHL, 2015). This issue raises practical, ethical, and legal questions concerning whether to report such information. A core tension lies between the desire for transparency on the one hand and the protection of individual and public health goals on the other (Miller et al., 2009). The rationale for an opt-out (rather than opt-in) consent model for public health newborn screening rests on the premise that the anticipated benefits of identifying babies with serious, treatable conditions outweigh the potential harms of sharing that information, and there is a different set of benefits and harms when it comes to carrier status. For example, disclosing carrier status could result in psychological harms to the family, who may not wish to receive information about their baby's genetic status that is not actionable, and could elicit concerns about the possibility of insurance or reproductive discrimination later in life (Tluczek et al., 2022). However, generating a finding and withholding that information from families could undermine public trust in the newborn screening (Goldenberg et al., 2019). Further conversations and empirical research are needed to understand the balance of benefits and harms, and spectrum of parental perspectives, for reporting such information.

In light of these issues, wherever a newborn screening program is aware that incidental or secondary findings may be generated, it is important to plan for those situations in program policies and practices. If programs elect to notify families or clinicians of such findings, it is vital that this notification be given thoughtfully, making it clear that there is no immediate health concern and providing appropriate information about what the results mean and what additional steps might be considered (NASEM, 1994).

The Role of Consent in Newborn Screening

Routine public health newborn screening is currently undertaken as a universal screening program at birth, generally through an opt-out (rather than opt-in) approach (King and Smith, 2016). Some have proposed that one solution to needs and tensions around newborn screening is to integrate a wider range of conditions into newborn screening in tandem with a more robust consent process that would allow parents to choose the conditions for which they wish to have their child screened. Theoretically, there are two ways this could be approached: by implementing explicit consent for all at-birth screened conditions, or by moving to a two-panel system in which a subset of urgent, severe and treatable conditions is universally screened and other conditions are included on an optional, consented panel (Currier, 2022; Gaviglio, 2024; President's Council on Bioethics, 2008).

In practice, however, the nature and complexity of the many hundreds of diseases that could be included, the burden of making these complex decisions without the support of their personal physician (e.g., the child's pediatrician), and the complex logistics of its implementation at the population level present major challenges. Some have expressed worries that adding a second, optional panel to at-birth screening might result in a greater number of parents opting out of the recommended universal panel. Further, one would need to consider the public resources that would be required to set up, track, and maintain a system to allow individual consent for a range of diseases, given the widely variable public opinion as to its value.

These costs would also need to be weighed against alternative methods of improving public health, which may be particularly difficult to justify if many of the new conditions lack effective treatments. States already vary in how they implement newborn screening or perform consented pilot studies,[8] and several research initiatives present parents with optional panels of screened diseases (e.g., Early Check, BabySeq); lessons may be able to be drawn from these (Peay et al., 2022). However, all such implications for program excellence, trustworthiness, and equity would need to be better understood before recommending changes to universal public health screening at large scale across the full population.

Addressing System Needs Beyond Routine Public Health Newborn Screening

Newborn screening is often charged as the mechanism to serve disparate needs and stakeholders—all of which are important but not all of which are well suited under the model of a public health program. The parameters guiding ethical decision making for routine, universal, at-birth newborn screening as a public health program are necessarily narrow owing to the population-based nature of the screening program itself. Public health newborn screening cannot and should not be the sole, or even the primary, solution to the broader problem of delays in rare disease diagnosis, to longstanding challenges around access and capacity in the clinical care system for patients and families with genetic diseases, and to the need to identify and develop new treatments for diseases. Taking a more strategic view at the system level will be important to addressing these other priorities.

---

[8] For example, the Massachusetts Department of Public Health may authorize pilot studies for conditions. Participation is voluntary and written consent is collected. See https://nensp.umassmed.edu/sites/nensp.umassmed.edu/files/English.pdf (accessed December 18, 2024).

CONCLUSIONS

A decision-making approach grounded in ethical principles and values can help envision a path forward to navigate the mounting tensions, challenges, and pressures facing newborn screening in the United States while preserving and strengthening what is already considered a public health achievement. This leads to the following conclusions:

Conclusion 3-1: As a program guided by public health ethics, focusing public health newborn screening on conditions that are serious, urgent, and have a therapeutic intervention rigorously shown to reduce morbidity and mortality in affected infants aligns with this mission to advance child welfare. Deploying universal, population-level screening requires there to be widely shared views that anticipated benefits outweigh anticipated harms and that alternative approaches are unlikely to achieve the same net benefits.

Conclusion 3-2: Expanding the scope of universal, at-birth newborn screening would no longer align with the public health mission of the program and would require expanded consent procedures (for example, to include conditions with later onset or no available treatment, or potential benefits beyond babies' morbidity and mortality). However, the ramifications that changing the consent paradigm for performing routine public health newborn screening would have on equity and program performance would need to be better understood before implementing at large scale.

Conclusion 3-3: When considering the concept of an available treatment or intervention in assessing whether to add a condition to public health newborn screening, evidence for the magnitude of benefit (improvement in child morbidity and mortality) is most important rather than the specific type of intervention.

Conclusion 3-4: The rare disease community has unmet needs that are valid, important, and in need of public attention and investment, but not all of them can be well addressed by state-run public health NBS programs. Doing so risks compromising the integrity and sustainability of public health NBS programs; investment in other dimensions of research and care remain essential to address these additional needs.

REFERENCES

ACMG (American College of Medical Genetics) Newborn Screening Expert Group. 2006. Newborn screening: Toward a uniform screening panel and system. *Genetics in Medicine* Suppl 1:1S-252S.

ACOG (American College of Obstetricians and Gynecologists) Committee on Genetics. 2019. Newborn screening and the role of the obstetrician-gynecologist. ACOG Committee Opinion Number 778. *Obstetrics and Gynecology* 133(5):e357-e361.

Alexander, D., and P. C. van Dyck. 2006. A vision for the future of newborn screening. *Pediatrics* 117(5): S350-S354.

Andermann, A., I. Blancquaert, S. Beauchamp, and V. Déry. 2008. Revisiting Wilson and Jungner in the genomic age: A review of screening criteria over the past 40 years. *Bulletin of the World Health Organization* 86(4):317-319.

Andrews, S. M., K. A. Porter, D. B. Bailey, and H. L. Peay. 2022. Preparing newborn screening for the future: A collaborative stakeholder engagement exploring challenges and opportunities to modernizing the newborn screening system. *BMC Pediatrics* 22(1):90.

APHA (American Public Health Association). 2019. *Public health code of ethics*. https://www.apha.org/-/media/files/pdf/membergroups/ethics/code_of_ethics.pdf (accessed January 8, 2025).

APHL (Association of Public Health laboratories). 2015. *Hemoglobinopathies: Current practices for screening, confirmation and follow-up*. https://www.cdc.gov/sickle-cell/media/pdfs/nbs_hemoglobinopathy-testing_122015.pdf (accessed March 10, 2025).

APHL. 2016. *APHL position statement: Parental consent for newborn screening*. Silver Spring, MD: APHL.

Armstrong, N. 2024. *Advocacy perspectives on adding new diseases: Experiences with developing a nomination package*. PowerPoint Presentation, National Academies Committee on Newborn Screening: Current Landscape and Future Directions Meeting 2, Washington, DC, March 26, 2024. https://www.nationalacademies.org/event/42052_03-2024_newborn-screening-current-landscape-and-future-directions-meeting-2 (accessed January 17, 2025)

Bailey, D. B., Jr., 2022. A window of opportunity for newborn screening. *Molecular Diagnosis & Therapy* 26(3):253-261.

Bailey, D. B., and L. Gehtland. 2015. Newborn screening. *Journal of the American Medical Association* 313(15):1511-1512.

Bailey, D. B., Jr., L. M. Beskow, A. M. Davis, and D. Skinner. 2006. Changing perspectives on the benefits of newborn screening. *Mental Retardation and Developmental Disabilities Research Reviews* 12(4):270-279.

Bailey, D. B., K. A. Porter, S. M. Andrews, M. Raspa, A. Y. Gwaltney, and H. L. Peay. 2021. Expert evaluation of strategies to modernize newborn screening in the United States. *JAMA Network Open* 4(12):e2140998.

Baily, M. A. 2023. *Newborn screening. Bioethics Briefings*. The Hastings Center. https://www.thehastingscenter.org/briefingbook/newborn-screening/ (accessed January 8, 2025).

Beans, J. 2024. *Considerations for newborn screening among Alaska Native and American Indian peoples*. PowerPoint presentation and discussion, National Academies Committee on Newborn Screening: Current Landscape and Future Directions Meeting 2, Washington, DC, March 26, 2024. https://www.nationalacademies.org/event/42052_03-2024_newborn-screening-current-landscape-and-future-directions-meeting-2 (accessed September 27, 2024).

Beauchamp, T., and J. Childress. 1979. *Principles of biomedical ethics*. New York: Oxford University Press.

Beauchamp, T., and J. Childress. 2019. Principles of biomedical ethics: Marking its fortieth anniversary. *American Journal of Bioethics* 19(11): 9-12.

Berberich, S. 2024. *Reflections on the mission of NBS programs*. Presentation, National Academies Committee on Newborn Screening: Current Landscape and Future Directions Meeting 2, Washington, DC, March 26, 2024. https://www.nationalacademies.org/event/42052_03-2024_newborn-screening-current-landscape-and-future-directions-meeting-2 (accessed September 27, 2024).

Best, A. L., F. E. Fletcher, M. Kadono, and R. C. Warren. 2021. Institutional distrust among African Americans and building trustworthiness in the COVID-19 response: Implications for ethical public health practice. *Journal of Health Care for the Poor and Underserved* 32(1):90-98.

Boardman, F. K., and C. C. Clark. 2022. What is a 'serious' genetic condition? The perceptions of people living with genetic conditions. *European Journal of Human Genetics* 30(2):160-169.

Bosfield, K., D. S. Regier, S. Viall, R. Hicks, N. Shur, and C. L. Grant. 2021. Mucopolysaccharidosis type I newborn screening: Importance of second tier testing for ethnically diverse populations. *American Journal of Medical Genetics Part A* 185(1):134-140.

Botkin, J. R., E. W. Clayton, N. C. Fost, W. Burke, T. H. Murray, M. A. Bailey, B. Wilfond, A. Berg, and L. F. Ross. 2006. Newborn screening technology: Proceed with caution. *Pediatrics* 117(5):1793-1799.

Botkin, J. R., E. W. Rothwell, R. A. Anderson, N. C. Rose, S. M. Dolan, M. Kuppermann, L. A. Stark, A. Goldenberg, and B. Wong. 2016. Prenatal education of parents about newborn screening and residual dried blood spots: A randomized clinical trial. *JAMA Pediatrics* 170(6):543-549.

Brosco, J. P., S. D. Grosse, and L. F. Ross. 2015. Universal state newborn screening programs can reduce health disparities. *JAMA Pediatrics* 169(1):7-8.

Brunelli, L., H. Sohn, and A. Brower. 2023. Newborn sequencing is only part of the solution for better child health. *Lancet Regional Health - Americas* 25:100581.

CDC (Centers for Disease Control and Prevention). 2012. CDC Grand rounds: Newborn screening and improved outcomes. *Morbidity and Mortality Weekly Report* 61(21):390-393.

Clayton, E. W. 2010. Currents in contemporary ethics: State run newborn screening in the genomic era, or how to avoid drowning when drinking from a fire hose. *Journal of Law, Medicine & Ethics* 38(3):697-700.

Clayton, E. W. 2024. *Panel reflections and discussion on public trust, May 16, 2024*. Presentation and discussion to the Committee on Newborn Screening: Current Landscape and Future Directions. https://www.nationalacademies.org/event/42550_05-2024_newborn-screening-current-landscape-and-future-directions-meeting-3 (accessed March 4, 2025).

Condition Review Workgroup. 2017. *Newborn screening for X-linked adrenoleukodystrophy (X-ALD): A systematic review of evidence*. https://www.hrsa.gov/sites/default/files/hrsa/advisory-committees/heritable-disorders/xald-external-evidence-review-report.pdf (accessed March 10, 2025).

Crossnohere, N. L., N. Armstrong, R. Fischer, and J. F. P. Bridges. 2022. Diagnostic experiences of Duchenne families and their preferences for newborn screening: A mixed-methods study. *American Journal of Medical Genetics. Part C, Seminars in Medical Genetics* 190(2):169-177.

Currier, R. J. 2022. Newborn screening is on a collision course with public health ethics. *International Journal of Neonatal Screening* 8(4):51.

Davis, T. C., S. G. Humiston, C. L. Arnold, J. A. Bocchin, Jr., P. F. Bass, 3rd, E. M. Kennen, A. Bocchini, P. Kyler, and M. Lloyd-Puryear. 2006. Recommendations for effective newborn screening communication: Results of focus groups with parents, providers, and experts. *Pediatrics* 117(5 Pt 2):S326-S340.

Dawson, L., N. Benbow, F. E. Fletcher, S. Kassaye, A. Killelea, S. R. Latham, L. M. Lee, T. Leitner, S. J. Little, S. R. Mehta, O. Martinez, B. Minalga, A. Poon, S. Rennie, J. Sugarman, P. Sweeney, L. V. Torian, and J. O. Wertheim. 2020. Addressing ethical challenges in US-based HIV phylogenetic research. *Journal of Infectious Diseases* 222(12):1997-2006.

DeLuca, J. M. 2018. Public attitudes toward expanded newborn screening. *Journal of Pediatric Nursing* 38:e19-323.

Diekema, D. 2004. Parental refusals of medical intervention: The harm principle as threshold for state intervention. *Theoretical Medicine and Bioethics* 25:243-264.

Ersig, A. L., C. Jaja, and A. Tluczek. 2023. Call to action for advancing equitable genomic newborn screening. *Public Health Genomics* 26(1):188-193.

EveryLife Foundation (EveryLife Foundation for Rare Diseases and The Lewin Group). 2023. *The cost of delayed diagnosis in rare disease: A health economic study*. https://everylifefoundation.org/wp-content/uploads/2023/09/EveryLife-Cost-of-Delayed-Diagnosis-in-Rare-Disease_Final-Full-Study-Report_0914223.pdf.

Faden, R. R., and T. L. Beauchamp. 1986. *A history and theory of informed consent* (1st ed.). Oxford, UK: Oxford University Press.

Faden, R. R., N. A. Holtzman, and A. J. Chwalow. 1982. Parental rights, child welfare, and public health: The case of PKU screening. *American Journal of Public Health* 72(12):1396-1400.

FDA (Food and Drug Administration). 2022. *Expanded access – Keywords, definitions, and resources*. https://www.fda.gov/news-events/expanded-access/expanded-access-keywords-definitions-and-resources (accessed March 10, 2025).

Fisher, C. B. 2014. HIV prevention research ethics: An introduction to the special issue. *Journal of Empirical Research on Human Research Ethics* 2014 9(1):1-5.

GAO (Government Accountability Office). 2016. *Newborn screening timeliness: Most states had not met screening goals, but some are developing strategies to address barriers*. GAO-17-196. Washington, DC: GAO.

Gaviglio, A. 2021. *Exploring equity across the newborn screening system: From discourse to action*. In Association of Public Health Laboratories - Newborn Screening Virtual Symposium. https://vimeo.com/669951228 (accessed January 9, 2025).

Gaviglio, A. 2024. *Implementation of consent models for newborn screening: Historical insights and future considerations*. Presented at Newborn Screening: Current Landscape and Future Directions Meeting 2. https://www.nationalacademies.org/event/42052_03-2024_newborn-screening-current-landscape-and-future-directions-meeting-2 (accessed January 24, 2025).

Gaviglio, A., S. McKasson, S. Singh, and J. Ojodu. 2023a. Infants with congenital diseases identified through newborn screening—United States, 2018–2020. *International Journal of Neonatal Screening* 9(2):23.

Gaviglio, A., M. W. Skinner, L. J. Lou, R. S. Finkel., E. F. Augustine, and A. J. Goldenberg. 2023b. Gene-targeted therapies: Towards equitable development, diagnosis, and access. *American Journal of Medical Genetics* 193(1):56-63.

Goldenberg, A. J. 2024. *History of and ethical justification for NBS programs*. PowerPoint Presentation, National Academies Committee on Newborn Screening: Current Landscape and Future Directions Meeting 2, Washington, DC, March 26, 2024. https://www.nationalacademies.org/event/42052_03-2024_newborn-screening-current-landscape-and-future-directions-meeting-2 (accessed March 10, 2025).

Goldenberg, A. J., D. S. Dodson, M. M. Davis, and B. A. Tarini. 2014. Parents' interest in whole-genome sequencing of newborns. *Genetics in Medicine* 16(1):78-84.

Goldenberg, A. J., M. Lloyd-Puryear, J. P. Brosco, B. Therrell, L. Bush, S. Berry, A. Brower, N. Bonhomme, B. Bowdish, D. Chrysler, and A. Clarke. 2019. Including ELSI research questions in newborn screening pilot studies. *Genetics in Medicine* 21(3):525-533.

Grant, C. 2022. *Police are using newborn genetic screening to search for suspects, threatening privacy and public health*. ACLU New Jersey, July 26. https://www.aclu-nj.org/en/news/police-are-using-newborn-genetic-screening-search-suspects-threatening-privacy-and-public (accessed July 23, 2024).

Halley, M. C., H. S. Smith, E. A. Ashley, A. J. Goldenberg, and H. K. Tabor. 2022. A call for an integrated approach to improve efficiency, equity and sustainability in rare disease research in the United States. *Nature* 54(3):219-222.

Hasegawa, L. E., K. A. Fergus, N. Ojeda, and S. M. Au. 2011. Parental attitudes toward ethical and social issues surrounding the expansion of newborn screening using new technologies. *Public Health Genomics* 14(4-5):298-306.

Hassan, S. 2024. *Panel reflections and discussion on public trust, May 16, 2024*. Presentation and discussion to the Committee on Newborn Screening: Current Landscape and Future Directions. https://www.nationalacademies.org/event/42550_05-2024_newborn-screening-current-landscape-and-future-directions-meeting-3 (accessed March 4, 2025).

Hiraki, S., K. E. Ormond, K. Kim, and L. F. Ross. 2006. Attitudes of genetic counselors towards expanding newborn screening and offering predictive genetic testing to children. *American Journal of Medical Genetics. Part A* 140(21):2312-2319.

Holtzman, N. A., and W. S. Watson. 1998. *Promoting safe and effective genetic testing in the United States*. Johns Hopkins University Press.

HRSA (Health Resources and Services Administration). 2022. *Nominating a condition for the Recommended Uniform Screening Panel for newborn screening: Frequently asked questions and other guidance*. https://www.hrsa.gov/advisory-committees/heritable-disorders/frequently-asked-questions (accessed July 31, 2024).

HRSA. 2023. *Newborn screening process*. https://newbornscreening.hrsa.gov/newborn-screening-process (accessed July 29, 2024).

HRSA. 2024a. *Recommended uniform screening panel*. https://www.hrsa.gov/advisory-committees/heritable-disorders/rusp (accessed July 31, 2024).

HRSA. 2024b. *Commitee approach to evaluating the condition review report (decision matrix)*. https://www.hrsa.gov/advisory-committees/heritable-disorders/decision-matrix (accessed December 17, 2024).

Hughes, R., IV, S. Choudhury, and A. Shah. 2022. Newborn screening blood spot retention and reuse: A clash of public health and privacy interests. *Health Affairs Forefront*. https://www.healthaffairs.org/content/forefront/newborn-screening-blood-spot-retention-and-reuse-clash-public-health-and-privacy (accessed December 18, 2024).

Jenkins, B. D., C. G. Fischer, C. A. Polito, D. R. Maiese, A. S. Keehn, M. Lyon, M. J. Edick, M. R. G. Taylor, H. C. Andersson, J. N. Bodurtha, M. G. Blitzer, M. Muenke, and M. S. Watson. 2021. The 2019 US medical genetics workforce: A focus on clinical genetics. *Genetics in Medicine* 23(8):1458-1464.

Joseph, G., F. Chen, J. Harris-Wai, J. M. Puck, C. Young, and B. A. Koenig. 2016. Parental views on expanded newborn screening using whole-genome sequencing. *Pediatrics* 137 (Suppl 1):S36-S46.

Kass, N. E. 2001. An ethics framework for public health. *American Journal of Public Health* 91(11):1776-1782.

Katz, A. V., S. A. Webb, R. C. Macauley, M. R. Mercurio, M. R. Moon, A. L. Okun, D. J. Opel, M. B. Statter, and Committee on Bioethics. 2016. Informed consent in decision-making in pediatric practice. *Pediatrics* 138(2):e20161485.

Kelly, N., D. C. Makarem, and M. P. Wasserstein. 2016. Screening of newborns for disorders with high benefit-risk ratios should be mandatory. *Journal of Law, Medicine & Ethics* 44(2):231-240.

Kemper, A. R., N. S. Green, N. Calonge, W. K. K. Lam, A. M. Comeau, A. J. Goldenberg, J. Ojodu, L. A. Prosser, S. Tanksley, and J. A. Bocchini, Jr. 2014. Decision-making process for conditions nominated to the Recommended Uniform Screening Panel: Statement of the US Department of Health and Human Services Secretary's Advisory Committee on Heritable Disorders in Newborns and Children. *Genetics in Medicine* 16(2):183-187.

Kemper, A. R., S. D. Grosse, M. Baker, A. J. Pollock, C. F. Hinton, and S. K. Shapira. 2020. Treatment discontinuation within 3 years of levothyroxine initiation among children diagnosed with congenital hypothyroidism. *Journal of Pediatrics* 223:136-140.

Kennedy, A. 2024. *Child health and rare disease organizations – Perspectives on the study task*. PowerPoint Presentation, National Academies Committee on Newborn Screening: Current Landscape and Future Directions Meeting 1, Washington, DC, January 26, 2024. https://www.nationalacademies.org/event/41786_01-2024_newborn-screening-current-landscape-and-future-directions-meeting-1b (accessed January 17, 2025).

King, J. S., and M. E. Smith. 2016. Whole-genome screening of newborns? The constitutional boundaries of state newborn screening programs. *Pediatrics* 137(Suppl 1):S8-S15.

Kleiderman, E., F. Boardman, A. J. Newson, A.-M. Laberge, B. M. Knoppers, and V. Ravitsky. 2024. Unpacking the notion of "serious" genetic conditions: Towards implementation in reproductive decision-making? *European Journal of Human Genetics* 33:158-166.

Kopelman, L. M. 1997. The best interest standards as threshold, ideal, and standard of reasonableness. *Journal of Medicine and Philosophy* 22(3):271-289.

Kwan, A., R. S. Abraham, R. Currier, A. Brower, K. Andruszewski, J. K. Abbott, M. Baker, M. Ballow, L. E. Bartoshesky, V. R. Bonagura, F. A. Bonilla, C. Brokopp, E. Brooks, M. Caggana, J. Celestin, J. A. Church, A. M. Comeau, J. A. Connelly, M. J. Cowan, C. Cunningham-Rundles, T. Dasu, N. Dave, M. T. De La Morena, U. Duffner, C.-T. Fong, L. Forbes, D. Freedenberg, E. W. Gelfand, J. E. Hale, I. C. Hanson, B. N. Hay, D. Hu, A. Infante, D. Johnson, N. Kapoor, D. M. Kay, D. B. Kohn, R. Lee, H. Lehman, Z. Lin, F. Lorey, A. Abdel-Mageed, A. Manning, S. McGhee, T. B. Moore, S. J. Naides, L. D. Notarangelo, J. S. Orange, S.-Y. Pai, M. Porteus, R. Rodriguez, N. Romberg, J. Routes, M. Ruehle, A. Rubenstein, C. A. Saavedra-Matiz, G. Scott, P. M. Scott, E. Secord, C. Seroogy, W. T. Shearer, S. Siegel, S. K. Silvers, E. R. Stiehm, R. W. Sugerman, J. L. Sullivan, S. Tanksley, M. L. Tierce, IV, J. Verbsky, B. Vogel, R. Walker, K. Walkovich, J. E. Walter, R. L. Wasserman, M. S. Watson, G. A. Weinberg, L. B. Weiner, H. Wood, A. B. Yates, and J. M. Puck. 2014. Newborn screening for severe combined immunodeficiency in 11 screening programs in the United States. *JAMA* 312(7):729-738.

Lee, L. M., S. E. Ortiz, G. Pavela, and B. Jennings. 2020. Public health code of ethics: Deliberative decision-making and reflective practice. *American Journal of Public Health* 110(4):489-491.

Levy, H. L. 2021. Robert Guthrie and the trials and tribulations of newborn screening. *International Journal of Neonatal Screening* 7(1):5.

Lisi, E. C., and S. E. McCandless. 2016. Newborn screening for lysosomal storage disorders: Views of genetic healthcare providers. *Journal of Genetic Counseling* 25(2):373-384.

Marsden, D., C. L. Bedrosian, and J. Vockley. 2021. Impact of newborn screening on the reported incidence and clinical outcomes associated with medium- and long-chain fatty acid oxidation disorders. *Genetics in Medicine* 23(5):816-829.

Mattison, M. 2000. Ethical decision making: The person in the process. *Social Work* 45(3):201-212.

McCandless, S. E., and E. J. Wright. 2020. Mandatory newborn screening in the United States: History, current status, and existential challenges. *Birth Defects Research* 112(4):350-366.

McColley, S. A., S. L. Martiniano, C. L. Ren, M. K. Sontag, K. Rychlik, L. Balmert, A. Elbert, R. Wu, and P. M. Farrell. 2022. Disparities in first evaluation of infants with cystic fibrosis since implementation of newborn screening. *Journal of Cystic Fibrosis* 22(1):89-97.

McGarry, M. E., C. L. Ren, R. Wu, P. M. Farrell, and S. A. McColley. 2023. Detection of disease-causing CFTR variants in state newborn screening programs. *Pediatric Pulmonology* 58(2):465-474.

Migeon, B. R. 2020. X-linked diseases: susceptible females. *Genetics in Medicine* 22(7):1156-1174.

Miller, F. A., J. S. Robert, and R. Z. Hayeems. 2009. Questioning the consensus: Managing carrier status results generated by newborn screening. *American Journal of Public Health* 99(2):210-215.

Miller, F. A., R. Z. Hayeems, Y. Bombard, C. Cressman, C. J. Barg, J. C. Carroll, B. J. Wilson, J. Little, J. Allanson, P. Chakraborty, Y. Giguère, and D. A. Regier. 2015. Public perceptions of the benefits and risks of newborn screening. *Pediatrics* 136(2):e413-e423.

Moultrie, R. R., R. Paquin, C. Rini, M. I. Roche, J. S. Berg, C. M. Powell, and M. A. Lewis. 2020. Parental views on newborn next generation sequencing: Implications for decision support. *Maternal and Child Health Journal* 24(7):856-864.

Moyer, V. A., N. Calonge, S. M. Teutsch, and J. R. Botkin. 2008. Expanding newborn screening: Process, policy, and priorities. *Hastings Center Report* 38(3):32-39.

NASEM (National Academies of Sciences, Engineering, and Medicine). 1994. *Assessing genetic risks: Implications for health and social policy.* Washington, DC: The National Academies Press.

NASEM. 2018. *Returning individual research results to participants: Guidance for a new research paradigm.* Washington, DC: The National Academies Press.

NASEM. 2020. *Addressing sickle cell disease: A strategic plan and blueprint for action.* Washington, DC: The National Academies Press.

National Commission for the Protection of Human Subjects of Biomedical and Behavioral Research. 1979. *The Belmont Report: Ethical principles and guidelines for the protection of human subjects of research.* U.S. Department of Health and Human Services. https://www.hhs.gov/ohrp/regulations-and-policy/belmont-report/read-the-belmont-report/index.html (accessed December 19, 2024).

Natowicz, M. 2005. Newborn screening – Setting evidence-based policy for protection. *New England Journal of Medicine* 353:867-870.

NewSTEPs. 2023a. *Newborn screening status for all disorders.* https://www.newsteps.org/resources/data-visualizations/newborn-screening-status-all-disorders (accessed August 12, 2024).

NewSTEPs. 2023b. *NewSTEPs 2022 annual report.* https://www.newsteps.org/sites/default/files/resources/download/NewSTEPS-2022-Annual-Report.pdf (accessed January 9, 2025).

Nong, P. 2023. Demonstrating trustworthiness to patients in data-driven health care. *Hastings Center Report* 53(Suppl 2):S69-S75.

NSGC (National Society of Genetic Counselors). 2020. *Professional status survey 2020: Executive summary.* https://www.nsgc.org/Portals/0/Docs/Policy/PSS%20Executive%20Summary%202020%20FINAL%2005-03-20.pdf (accessed January 9, 2025).

Parasidis, E., and A. L. Fairchild. 2022. Closing the public health ethics gap. *New England Journal of Medicine* 387(11):961-963.

Peay, H. L., A. Y. Gwaltney, R. Moultrie, H. Cope, B. L. Boyea, K. A. Porter, M. Duparc, A. A. Alexander, B. B. Biesecker, A. Isiaq, and J. Check. 2022. Education and consent for population-based DNA screening: A mixed-methods evaluation of the early check newborn screening pilot study. *Frontiers in Genetics* 13:891592.

Peng, G., Y. Tang, N. Gandotra, G. M. Enns, T. M. Cowan, H. Zhao, and C. Scharfe. 2020. Ethnic variability in newborn metabolic screening markers associated with false-positive outcomes. *Journal of Inherited Metabolic Disease* 43:934-943.

Presidential Commission for the Study of Bioethical Issues. 2013. *Safeguarding children: Pediatric medical countermeasure research.* Washington, DC: Presidential Commission for the study of Bioethical Issues. https://bioethicsarchive.georgetown.edu/pcsbi/node/833.html (accessed January 9, 2025).

President's Council on Bioethics. 2008. *The changing moral focus of newborn screening: An ethical analysis by the President's Council on Bioethics.* Washington, DC: President's Council on Bioethics.

Ram, N. 2022. America's hidden national DNA database. *Texas Law Review* 100(7):1253-1325.

Ram, N. 2024. *Reflections on the mission of NBS programs.* PowerPoint Presentation and discussion, National Academies Committee on Newborn Screening: Current Landscape and Future Directions Meeting 2, Washington, DC, March 26, 2024. https://www.nationalacademies.org/event/42052_03-2024_newborn-screening-current-landscape-and-future-directions-meeting-2 (accessed March 10, 2025).

Rawls, J. 2001. *Justice as fairness: A restatement.* Cambridge, MA: Harvard University Press.

Ross, L. F. 2010. Mandatory versus voluntary consent for newborn screening? *Kennedy Institute of Ethics* 20(4):299-328.

Ross, L. F. 2019. Better than best (interest standard) in pediatric decision making. *Journal of Clinical Ethics* 30(3):183-195.

Ross, L. F., and E. W. Clayton. 2019. Ethical issues in newborn sequencing research: The case study of BabySeq. *Pediatrics* 144(6):e20191031.

Roy, M. C., B. Knoppers, V. Ravitsky, and E. Kleiderman. 2021. A 'serious' threshold for genomic technologies – context counts! *BioNews* 1121. https://www.progress.org.uk/a-serious-threshold-for-genomic-technologies-context-counts/ (accessed September 12, 2024).

RWJF (Robert Wood Johnson Foundation). 2021. *The public's perspective on the United States public health system.* Harvard T.H. Chan School of Public Health. https://www.rwjf.org/en/insights/our-research/2021/05/the-publics-perspective-on-the-united-states-public-health-system.html (accessed January 9, 2025).

Salter, E. K., D. M. Hester, L. Vinarcsik, A. H. M. Antommaria, J. Bester, J. Blustein, E. W. Clayton, D. S. Diekema, A. S. Iltis, L. M. Kopelman, J. R. Malone, M. R. Mercurio, M. C. Navin, E. T. Paquette, T. M. Pope, R. Rhodes, and L. F. Ross. 2023. Pediatric decision making: Consensus recommendations. *Pediatrics* 152(3):e2023061832.

Schieve, L. A., G. M. Simmons, A. B. Payne, K. Abe, L. L. Hsu, M. Hulihan, S. Pope, S. Rhie, B. Dupervil, and W. C. Hooper. 2022. Vital signs: Use of recommended health care measures to prevent selected complications of sickle cell anemia in children and adolescents — selected U.S. States, 2019. *Morbidity and Mortality Weekly Report* 71(39):1241-1246.

Schott, S. L., A. Adams, R. J. Dougherty, T. Montgomery, F. C. Lapite, and F. E. Fletcher. 2023. Renewed calls for abortion-related research in the post-*Roe* era. *Frontiers in Public Health* 11:1322299.

Shi, Z., J. Wei, R. Na, W. K. Resurreccion, S. L. Zheng, P. J. Hulick, B. T. Helfand, M. S. Talamonti, and J. Xu. 2021. Cystic fibrosis F508del carriers and cancer risk: Results from the UK biobank. *International Journal of Cancer* 148(7):1658-1664.

Singh, S. 2022. *Health equity in newborn screening*. Presented at the Advisory Committee on Heritable Disorders in Newborn and Children Meeting, Washington, DC, February 11, 2022. https://www.hrsa.gov/advisory-committees/heritable-disorders/meetings/feb-10-2022 (accessed January 24, 2025).

Sobotka, S., and L. F. Ross. 2023. Newborn screening for neurodevelopmental disorders may exacerbate health disparities. *Pediatrics* 142(4):e2023061727.

Sohn, H., and S. Timmermans. 2019. Inequities in newborn screening: Race and the role of medicaid. *SSM - Population Health* 9:100496.

Solomon S. R. 2013. Protecting and respecting the vulnerable: Existing regulations or further protections? *Theoretical Medicine and Bioethics* 34(1):17-28.

Sterman, J., and D. Molina. 2023. Tasked with critical testing, newborn screening programs feel pinch of funding struggles. *InvestigateTV*. https://www.investigatetv.com/2023/05/22/tasked-with-critical-testing-newborn-screening-programs-feel-pinch-funding-struggles/ (accessed January 9, 2025).

Stoller, J. K. 2018. The challenge of rare diseases. *Chest* 153(6):1309-1314.

Susanna Haas Lyons Engagement Consulting. 2024. *What we heard: Newborn screening in the United States*. Presented to the Committee on Newborn Screening: Current Landscape and Future Directions at the National Academies of Sciences, Engineering, and Medicine. https://www.nationalacademies.org/documents/embed/link/LF2255DA3DD1C41C0A42D3BEF0989ACAECE3053A6A9B/file/D35FB72C883DD3F3496A747004FB20B434E54764D1D0?noSaveAs=1 (accessed December 18, 2024).

Swain, G. R., K. A. Burns, and P. Etkind. 2008. Preparedness: Medical ethics versus public health ethics. *Journal of Public Health Management and Practice* 14(4):354-357.

Tanksley, S. 2024. *Panel reflections and discussion on public trust, May 16, 2024*. Presentation and discussion to the Committee on Newborn Screening: Current Landscape and Future Directions. https://www.nationalacademies.org/event/42550_05-2024_newborn-screening-current-landscape-and-future-directions-meeting-3 (accessed March 4, 2025).

Tarini, B. A. 2007. The current revolution in newborn screening. *Archives of Pediatrics & Adolescent Medicine* 161(8):767-772.

Tarini, B. A., and A. J. Goldenberg. 2012. Ethical issues with newborn screening in the genomics era. *Annual Review of Genomics and Human Genetics* 13(1):381-393.

Tarini, B. A., N. J. Simon, K. Payne, A. Gebremariam, A. Rose, and L. A. Prosser. 2018. An assessment of public preferences for newborn screening using best-worst scaling. *Journal of Pediatrics* 201:62-68.e1.

Taylor, L. A., M. Z. Solomon, and G. E. Kaebnick. 2023. Trust in health care and science: Toward common ground on key concepts. *Hastings Center Report* 53(S2):S2-S8.

Therrell, B. L., Jr., W. H. Hannon, D. B. Bailey, Jr., E. B. Goldman, J. Monaco, B. Norgaard-Pedersen, S. F. Terry, A. Johnson, and R. R. Howell. 2011. Committee report: Considerations and recommendations for national guidance regarding the retention and use of residual dried blood spot specimens after newborn screening. *Genetics in Medicine* 13(7):621-624.

Thomas, J. C., M. Sage, J. Dillenberg, and V. J. Guillory. 2002. A code of ethics for public health. *American Journal of Public Health* 92(7):1057-1059.

Timmins, G. T., J. Wynn, A. M. Saami, A. Espinal, and W. K. Chung. 2022. Diverse parental perspectives of the social and educational needs for expanding newborn screening through genomic sequencing. *Public Health Genomics* 1-8.

Tluczek, A., A. L. Ersig, and S. Lee. 2022. Psychosocial issues related to newborn screening: A systematic review and synthesis. *International Journal of Neonatal Screening* 8(4):53.

Varkey, B. 2021. Principles of clinical ethics and their application to practice. *Medical Principles and Practice* 30(1):17-28.

Von Der Lippe, C., I. Neteland, and K. B. Feragen. 2022. Children with a rare congenital genetic disorder: A systematic review of parent experiences. *Orphanet Journal of Rare Diseases* 17(1):375.

Wallis, H. 2024. *Panel reflections and discussion on public trust, May 16, 2024*. Presentation and discussion to the Committee on Newborn Screening: Current Landscape and Future Directions. https://www.nationalacademies.org/event/42550_05-2024_newborn-screening-current-landscape-and-future-directions-meeting-3 (accessed March 4, 2025).

Warren, R. C., L. Forrow, D. A. Hodge, Sr., and R. D. Truog. 2020. Trustworthiness before trust - Covid-19 vaccine trials and the black community. *New England Journal of Medicine* 383(22):e121.

Watson, M. S., M. A. Lloyd-Puryear, and R. R. Howell. 2022. The progress and future of US newborn screening. *International Journal of Neonatal Screening* 8(3):41.

Wertz, D. C., and B. M. Knoppers. 2002. Serious genetic disorders: Can or should they be defined? *American Journal of Medical Genetics* 108(1):29-35.

Wilson, J. M. G., and G. Jungner. 1968. Principles and practice of screening for disease. *Public Health Papers* 34.

Wong, K. N., M. McIntyre, S. Cook, K. Hart, A. Wilson, S. Moldt, A. Rohrwasser, and R. J. Butterfield. 2024. A five-year review of newborn screening for spinal muscular atrophy in the state of Utah: Lessons learned. *International Journal of Neonatal Screening* 10(3):54.

4

Supporting and Sustaining High-Performing NBS Programs

"We need to figure out ways to maintain the benefits of really one of the most successful public health programs ever while also meeting the challenges of an evolving system. How do we maintain those benefits for families and for future generations?" – Bioethics researcher

Central to public health newborn screening (NBS) are the 56 programs established by states and territories to deliver on the aim of improving health outcomes by screening at birth for certain serious, urgent, and treatable conditions. This chapter focuses on the essential functions these programs fulfill and articulates a vision for supporting and sustaining excellence through performance management systems and shared resources. This chapter ends by discussing considerations for program sustainability including family and provider education, storage and reuse of dried blood spots, long-term follow-up after screening, and workforce development.

NBS PROGRAMS AT THE CORE OF THE PUBLIC HEALTH NBS EFFORT

The mission of public health newborn screening is to reduce morbidity and mortality for affected infants (see Chapter 3), and NBS programs are responsible for detecting and connecting those infants with clinical care. Each of the 56 state and territorial NBS programs operates according to its own processes and requirements for undertaking the routine screening of blood collected from babies shortly after birth, drawing on national guidance while following state-level policies, mandates, and choices around specific conditions screened, technologies used, and the design and implementation of program elements.[1] See Chapters 1 and 2 for a fuller description of public health newborn screening in the United States and how it operates.

While respecting the needs and opportunities for each state and territory to implement its NBS program to meet the needs of its population and align with its circumstances and priorities, all 56 programs need to perform certain essential functions. These include ensuring that all babies born in the state have the opportunity to receive accurate and timely screening; that screening results are communicated to enable babies at risk for identified conditions to receive suitable confirmatory testing, care, and other services; that parents and providers in the state receive accurate information and education about newborn screening; and that the program operates with appropriate quality assurance and performance management.

As NBS programs work to achieve these essential functions, they intersect with and depend on many other partners in the NBS system to achieve the mission of reducing morbidity and mortality for affected infants. For example, ensuring that blood spots are collected in a manner meeting quality and timeliness goals depends on all birth providers and facilities to collect samples, complete paper and/or electronic sample documentation, and return blood spots to the state-designated laboratory. Ensuring that parents understand public health newborn screening and their options regarding participation relies on having effective educational materials for all of a state or territory's communities as well as needing care providers, counselors, and families to engage in these conversations. Although NBS programs do not have direct authority over every one of their critical NBS partners, the programs need to understand whether essential functions are being met, recognize challenges or issues that arise, and work with public and private partners, policy makers, and others to develop solutions.

SCREENING AND CASE MANAGEMENT

Screening babies born in their respective jurisdictions in a timely manner and connecting at-risk infants with clinical care are essential priorities for NBS programs. This entails collecting newborn dried blood

---

[1] Shortly after birth, babies generally receive several forms of screening, including blood spot collection as well as hearing and pulse oximetry testing. This report focuses only on blood spot screening.

spots, accurately testing these samples, and following up on the results. As Chapter 2 described, NBS programs differ in screening assays and methodology used for a given screened disease. Programs also vary in operational details, including their associated fees and fee structures, hours of operation, and laboratory systems. Some NBS programs test their jurisdiction's newborn blood spot samples in state-run public health laboratories, some rely on laboratories housed within universities, some contract with private-sector testing laboratories, and some establish partnerships with other state NBS programs to undertake some or all of their blood spot testing. Programs also vary in terms of how they receive guidance, with many states and territories instituting advisory committees; committees may be voluntary or mandated in statute and contain different balances of expertise.[2]

This federated approach to newborn screening in the United States has both strengths and limitations. NBS programs can implement innovative practices from which peer programs may draw lessons. For example, Iowa's NBS program served as an early example of meeting timeliness goals through innovative practices such as tracking individual hospital performance, implementing a courier service, and keeping the laboratory open every day of the year (Gabler et al., 2013). When the potential application of tandem mass spectrometry first challenged programs to consider expansion, the Massachusetts Department of Public Health (DPH) developed an optional pilot program of 20 disorders to address this challenge (Atkinson et al., 2001); Massachusetts DPH still employs this model to pilot test conditions considered for inclusion on its state panel.[3] Community involvement is foundational to guiding the activities of Hawaii's NBS program. As such, their NBS advisory committee conducts surveys, focus groups, and interviews to ensure that decisions about newborn screening are community driven and serve as a model for how to incorporate community engagement into decision making (Mann, 2015).

Different NBS programs can also demonstrate areas of excellence that may serve as resources to other programs. Wisconsin's NBS laboratory has implemented DNA sequencing as a second-tier screening tool for conditions such as cystic fibrosis (Rock et al., 2023). Rather than independently perform this screening, some programs (e.g., North Carolina) choose to partner with Wisconsin, enabling them to send their samples for specialized second-tier testing as appropriate (Zimmerman, 2016). Tennessee's

---

[2] See https://www.newsteps.org/resources/data-visualizations/newborn-screening-advisory-committees (accessed September 26, 2024) for up-to-date information on whether programs currently have an advisory committee, if the advisory committee is mandatory or voluntary, meeting frequency, and other details.

[3] See https://nensp.umassmed.edu/sites/nensp.umassmed.edu/files/English.pdf (accessed December 19, 2024).

NBS program serves babies from bordering states by managing follow-up for those screened in Tennessee, sharing results with home state programs, and closing cases if care transfers back to the home state. If the child continues care in Tennessee or their care is transferred to Tennessee, the NBS program ensures follow-up until diagnosis or treatment and maintains communication with other state programs through email, phone, and shared portals.[4] State and territorial NBS programs also establish regional partnerships to ensure continued, timely screening for all babies, should operational disruptions occur (e.g., among the NBS programs in Florida, South Carolina, and Tennessee) (Dorley et al., 2024). Other examples of strengths and partnerships abound.

On the other hand, NBS program variability can lead to differences in burdens placed on birth providers or families, including disparities in the effectiveness of screening for a given condition among the full range of a state or territory's population. Box 4-1 describes an example of the implications of this variability in the context of cystic fibrosis newborn screening.

The case management necessary to track and analyze blood spot samples and accurately follow up from screening to communication of results and/or confirmatory testing (referred to as short-term follow-up) is a core responsibility of NBS programs. This process entails a handoff of a baby's screening information from the public health system to the clinical care system. NBS programs vary in length of follow-up time and involvement past confirmatory testing. An essential aim of NBS programs, given the urgent and serious nature of the conditions for which these programs screen, is avoiding the loss or delay of samples, avoiding gaps in communication about results, and avoiding the loss of at-risk babies and families to confirmatory testing and care.

To help safeguard the health of infants, national timeliness goals call for communication of at-risk screening results for time-critical conditions within 5 days of birth, and for all NBS tests to be completed within 7 days (HRSA, 2017). State programs have taken a variety of steps to support timeliness, such as extending NBS laboratory operating hours and giving birth providers free return shipping labels for blood spot samples (Sontag et al., 2020), but ongoing needs and challenges in meeting screening time benchmarks represent another illustration of the implications of program-to-program operational variability (see Box 4-2).

Opportunities to support and enhance program excellence include additional guidance, support, and partnerships aimed at fostering more standardized follow-up processes for screening results that are out of

---

[4] Personal communication from Amanda Ingram, Tennessee Department of Health, December 19, 2024.

BOX 4-1
State and Territorial-Level Differences in Screening for Cystic Fibrosis Variants and Their Effects on Perpetuating Health Disparities

Understanding how screening tests perform for all babies and identifying solutions to mitigate differences in screening effectiveness are important to achieve the mission of public health newborn screening. Differences in screening practices for cystic fibrosis (CF) across newborn screening (NBS) programs provide an illustrative example of how screening performance differences can translate to disparities in health outcomes for certain populations.

CF is an inherited genetic disorder of the cystic fibrosis transmembrane conductance regulator (CFTR) protein that causes mucous in the body to become thick and viscous, resulting in severe damage to the lungs and digestive system. It is a pervasive misconception that CF only affects individuals who are Caucasian; individuals of any racial or ethnic background can be diagnosed with CF (Rubin, 2021). Though there is no cure, early detection and intervention is essential for treating CF, and all 50 states, Puerto Rico, Guam, and the District of Columbia perform screening for CF as a part of their NBS program (NewSTEPs, n.d.). During first-tier biochemical screening, dried blood spots are tested for levels of immunoreactive trypsinogen (IRT), a protein made by the pancreas that is elevated in those with CF (North Carolina Department of Health and Human Services, n.d.). If elevated IRT levels are detected, second-tier molecular screening is performed to detect variants in the *CFTR* gene that cause CF; if a CF variant is detected, a sweat chloride test is performed to formally diagnose CF (Mt. Sinai, n.d.; Nemours Children's Health, 2015).

There are many different genetic variants of the *CFTR* gene that cause CF, some more common than others. State and territorial NBS programs vary widely in how many of these genetic variants are tested. Some programs test for only one variant whereas others test for hundreds (Rehani et al., 2023). States that only test for one or a few variants tend to test for the most common ones, which are most prevalent among people with northern European ancestry. Testing for fewer variants runs the risk of missing less-common variants, resulting in false negatives and delayed treatment for CF. Rarer mutations are more likely to be present in babies of non-European ancestry. Thus, in testing for fewer variants, populations from other ancestral backgrounds are at a higher risk of receiving false-negative results for CF and delays in essential intervention (McGarry et al., 2023).

The variability in testing for *CFTR* gene variants across states has a negative effect on CF patient outcomes. States with greater racial and ethnic diversity have lower overall detection rates for CF (McGarry et al., 2023). Overall, approximately 11 percent of people with CF have a delayed diagnosis, with Black, Hispanic, and mixed-race people being overrepresented (McGarry et al., 2023). These delayed diagnoses result in delayed crucial early intervention for CF among minoritized groups and perpetuate already existing health disparities.[a]

Strategies to document and analyze screening performance and national or regional approaches to share resources and expertise can support the ability of state and territorial NBS programs to provide a high-quality service for all members of their population.

---

[a] Race and ethnicity can be conflated with ancestry. Guidance indicates that racial and/or ethnic descriptors can be misleading and harmful when used to describe population genetic differences (NASEM, 2023). However, it is unlikely that the authors would have had access to ancestral descriptors for this study.

> **BOX 4-2**
> **Timeliness in Public Health Newborn**
> **Screening of Dried Blood Spots**
>
> Effective collection and analysis of data can inform NBS programs and other partners to proactively address emerging challenges in the NBS system. Ongoing challenges with timeliness related to public health newborn screening provide an illustrative example.
>
> In late 2013, the *Milwaukee Journal Sentinel* conducted an investigation that uncovered problems with the timeliness of public health newborn screening across the country. The investigative reporting identified hospital procedures, transportation issues, and laboratory processing times as factors that contributed to this problem, emphasizing that delays could contribute to the risk of death or lifelong health problems for a child (Fauber, 2013; Gabler et al., 2013; Johnson, 2013). This reporting contributed to national attention that ultimately prompted the Newborn Screening Saves Lives Reauthorization Act of 2014 (P.L. 113-240) to specify improved timeliness as an explicit goal; empowered the federal Advisory Committee on Heritable Disorders in Newborns and Children (ACHDNC) to create timeliness goals; and included a provision for the Government Accountability Office (GAO) to audit the timeliness of state-run programs.[a]
>
> Long before timeliness received national media attention, partners within the NBS system were aware and concerned. The American College of Medical Genetics and Genomics (ACMG) report on newborn screening that informed the creation of the Recommended Uniform Screening Panel identified variation of timeliness across states as an issue and made recommendations for the return of results for time-critical conditions and improvements for executing those goals, including overnight courier services. Issues around "unacceptable delay[s]" caused by weekend closures, courier issues, and hospitals batching their samples were also mentioned at ACHDNC meetings as early as 2008 (ACHDNC, 2008; ACMG Newborn Screening Expert Group, 2006).
>
> In response to the concerns and resulting language in the 2014 Act, ACHDNC developed timeliness goals for communicating NBS results, collecting specimens, and transporting those specimens to the laboratory, established in 2015 (HRSA, 2017). A 2016 GAO report, using data collected from 38 states, found that nearly all participating programs failed to meet the recommended timeliness goals (GAO, 2016). More recent data collected from 25 state-run programs indicate improvement in timeliness metrics, especially for programs open 7 days per week; however, timeliness goals are not being universally met (Sontag et al., 2020). The reasons for ongoing program challenges in meeting timeliness goals are likely complex.
>
> ---
>
> [a] At the September 2013 ACHDNC meeting, just before the *Milwaukee Journal Sentinel*'s articles were published, a parent shared the story of her son, Noah, who died of undiagnosed medium-chain acyl-CoA dehydrogenase deficiency (MCADD). Noah's newborn screening results were communicated the day after his death. Following this public comment, the ACHDNC discussed whether timeliness was in its purview, and ultimately decided to ask its Laboratory Subcommittee to investigate this issue (ACHDNC, 2013). Whether more action would have been taken without the *Sentinel*'s reporting and subsequent Congressional request cannot be said.

range and need confirmation and diagnosis, thus building on best practices among high-performing state programs and encouraging adoption across NBS programs to minimize babies and families lost to follow-up.

NBS PROGRAM DATA COLLECTION AND PERFORMANCE MANAGEMENT

"We currently cannot assess whether [the proposed benefits of screening] were realized or not because we do not have the structures and processes to assess performance" – NBS public health professional

Achieving and maintaining excellence in core performance requires each NBS program to implement performance management systems. Collecting and analyzing performance data is essential to drive meaningful improvements in the provision of newborn screening as a public health service. Frameworks supporting quality improvement, such as the one proposed by Donabedian (1966), may help inform this process through their emphasis on incorporating measures for structure, process, and outcomes around the laboratory, technological, follow-up, and other capabilities needed by NBS programs, as well as measuring what successful high performance entails (Donabedian, 1966). The value of establishing a system that can learn has been articulated by the National Academy of Medicine and others; a key attribute of such systems is their ability to integrate information from multiple sources to support continuous improvement to practice.[5]

NBS data collection and analysis fulfills several purposes. It allows state and territorial programs to monitor local operations and performance and identify emerging issues and areas for improvement. Programs establish quality control and quality assurance efforts to monitor adherence to defined criteria across their core processes, such as around sample screening times, assay performance measures, and follow-up.

State and national data can be used in multiple ways, including improving existing testing performance (e.g., refining assay cutoff values and false-positive and false-negative targets based on their relationship to outcomes data), identifying disease outcomes or efficacy of treatments, and assessing outcomes and potential disparities across populations. Through comparison with peer NBS programs, data collection, benchmarking, and performance management can also encourage excellence and provide an opportunity for collaborative learning. Because conditions screened by NBS programs are individually rare with each affecting only

---

[5] See, for example, National Academy of Medicine learning health series and core principles at https://nam.edu/programs/value-science-driven-health-care/lhs-core-principles/ (accessed December 30, 2024).

a small number of babies and families in a state or territory, combining data across jurisdictional boundaries on shorter- and longer-term health outcomes is important for understanding the effectiveness of screening and interventions (Minear et al., 2022; Pizzamiglio et al., 2022). The needs and challenges associated with rare disease were also motivating factors in the Food and Drug Administration's (FDA's) recent establishment of the Rare Disease Innovation Hub to enhance collaboration and regulatory science to facilitate the development of disease therapies (FDA, 2024). Further discussion of long-term follow-up is found below and in Chapter 6, which describes longitudinal research.

NBS programs design and operate their own performance management systems and may implement their own data-sharing arrangements with in-state and/or out-of-state partners. The Newborn Screening Technical assistance and Evaluation Program (NewSTEPs), a program through the Association of Public Health Laboratories (APHL) developed with a grant from the Health Resources and Services Administration (HRSA), represents the current primary mechanism for collecting and sharing data across NBS programs.[6] Participating in the NewSTEPs data repository is voluntary and not incentivized. Programs submitting data can access their own information and receive aggregated data from other participating programs. For many metrics, only 19 programs submitted data in 2022, and as few as 8 programs submitted data on certain quality indicators (NewSTEPs, 2023).

Implementing more strategic and systematic data collection among NBS programs can serve as a valuable opportunity to enhance decision making but would require collection efforts to be structured. Programs would need to commit to collecting a subset of common data elements and establishing certain common processes, while preserving necessary state and territorial authorities, variation, and flexibility. The level and depth of data sharing would likely vary across NBS programs, but some level of minimum data-sharing requirements must be met.

One possible starting point is a subset of measures tied directly to performance excellence in the essential NBS program functions described above. The following three questions are potential areas for more systematic NBS program and cross-program data analysis efforts:

1. *Which infants are missed by public health newborn screening?* Births can occur in a variety of settings through hospitals, community birth centers, and at home, and not all states and territories are currently able to connect NBS records to vital records that record births.[7] Connecting NBS records to vital records would enable

---

[6] See https://www.newsteps.org/ (accessed December 30, 2024).
[7] See https://mchb.tvisdata.hrsa.gov/DataAccessLinkage/ByDataSource (accessed December 18, 2024).

NBS program directors or other public health decision makers to cross-check whether every recorded birth has a matching NBS screening record, identify missed babies, support further analysis to understand reasons behind missed screening, and provide a basis for developing targeted educational, financial, or policy options to address underlying causes.

2. *Do screening assays perform differently among infants from different ancestral backgrounds?* As illustrated in Box 4-1, the ability of screening assays to identify a condition can differ for babies having different ancestral backgrounds. Understanding performance differences and identifying solutions to mitigate these issues is important for sustaining NBS programs that are high quality across all populations and for achieving the central aim of public health newborn screening to reduce babies' morbidity and mortality.

3. *Which infants identified through public health newborn screening as being at risk are not connected with clinical care?* Infants, especially those from underserved backgrounds, can experience delays in confirmatory testing and be lost to follow-up care (Kemper et al., 2010; McColley et al., 2023; Schieve et al., 2022). Understanding whether there was a handoff between public health and clinical care ensures that programs deliver on their promise of connecting infants with early treatment and intervention and provides opportunities for programs to learn where there are gaps in the achievement of this mission. Not all state and territorial NBS programs are currently able to transmit or receive electronic messages.[8] Updating information management systems and implementing electronic messaging would enable more rapid and effective communication and can permit more timely connection to clinical care (Abhyankar et al., 2016; GAO, 2016).

Selected examples of data that could be collected by NBS programs are shown in Table 4-1. Accountability for achieving performance goals and metrics falls to both NBS programs and to other actors in the NBS landscape; for each illustrative goal, the table identifies examples of data sources and responsible parties. Given differing state and territorial NBS policies and requirements, the director of each NBS program may need to work with other public health and clinical leaders and policy makers to implement needed authorities and processes in each state or territorial context.

---

[8] See https://www.newsteps.org/resources/data-visualizations/newborn-screening-electronic-messaging (accessed January 30, 2025) for up-to-date information on electronic messaging for each state or territory's NBS program.

TABLE 4-1 Examples of Data NBS Programs Could Commit to Collect to Understand Performance Around Selected Performance Goals

Goal	Performance Metrics	Data Sources	Accountable Parties
All infants should receive newborn screening. Information should identify any babies missed.	Infants born and infants screened; demographic details on any who are not screened and documentation on why they were not screened	Vital records, state and territorial NBS program records (may require manual data entry from handwritten blood spot cards), hospital or birth center records	State and territorial NBS programs and public health departments (connect and analyze birth and NBS screening records); hospitals/birth centers (data collection/provision)
All screening results should be communicated to the infant's clinical provider, and ultimately to their family/caregiver.	Evidence of NBS outreach provided to families and to providers; documentation that screening results were received	State and territorial NBS program records documenting communication of results; clinical EHR records	State and territorial NBS programs
All infants identified through screening should receive confirmatory testing and connection to care.	Documentation of confirmatory testing; documentation of visits with primary, specialty, and/or genetic counseling care	State and territorial NBS program records; clinical EHR records	State and territorial NBS programs to establish an appropriate connection; clinical care system (hospital or other provider) to establish clear handoff

NOTE: EHR = electronic health record; NBS = newborn screening.

ENSURING NBS PROGRAM EXCELLENCE IN A PERFORMANCE FRAMEWORK

High-performing state and territorial NBS programs advance the public health goals of newborn screening, foster effective identification and diagnosis of screened conditions across all populations, and sustain trust in the program's mission and operations. However, newborn screening and public health professionals also report concerns that they will fall short of achieving their goals. During the committee's information-gathering efforts, NBS laboratory and follow-up professionals reflected on the substantial resources, expertise, and time required to establish laboratory operations, informatics, clinical care relationships, and project management to add each new condition to a state's program, all in resource-constrained environments (Comeau, 2024; Mann, 2024;

Simonetti, 2024; Susanna Haas Lyons Engagement Consulting, 2024). NBS programs rely on a variety of financial and nonfinancial support to achieve and maintain excellence in their daily operations for current conditions, to address new conditions, and to enhance needed efforts and partnerships around longer-term follow-up.

Multiple mechanisms support state and territorial NBS programs in meeting performance goals; however, resources are unevenly allocated, with more support for laboratory functions and fewer mechanisms providing guidance and assistance with short- or longer-term follow-up after screening. Available federal resources are often ad hoc or grant based, requiring NBS program staff to identify challenges, locate prospective resources, draw on personal networks and contacts, and prepare competitive grant applications. Grant-based funding can end as budgets and priorities shift at the federal level. This approach places a burden on resource-constrained NBS programs and can perpetuate and exacerbate existing disparities across programs.

Table 4-2 conveys the general nature and scale of federal agency support to assist state-level NBS programs with their major functions. Additional funding toward research, education, disease treatment, and other dimensions that intersect with newborn screening is also provided by agencies such as the National Institutes of Health, disease support and advocacy organizations, philanthropic funders, and industry and are not included here. See Chapter 6 for additional discussion of support for NBS and rare disease research.

These HRSA and Centers for Disease Control and Prevention (CDC) investments address important dimensions and represent roughly $30–$40 million per year to support newborn screening. A relatively larger number of programs and supports are associated with the laboratory screening functions of state-level NBS programs, including trainings through APHL,[9] quality assurance through CDC,[10] and nonregulatory site visits through CDC and APHL,[11] whereas less federal support is directed toward short-term and longer-term NBS follow-up. Support from HRSA Propel and Co-Propel grants assist some NBS programs to engage in or enhance longer-term follow-up, and others in the NBS system have also made initial investments in this space (HRSA, 2024b,c; Kellar-Guenther et al., 2024). Current support mechanisms are less likely to provide direct technical assistance and practical guidance for states and territories in

---

[9] See https://www.aphl.org/programs/newborn_screening/training/Pages/default.aspx (accessed December 30, 2024).

[10] See https://www.cdc.gov/laboratory-quality-assurance/php/newborn-screening/index.html (accessed December 30, 2024).

[11] See https://www.aphl.org/programs/newborn_screening/pages/molecularassessment-program.aspx (accessed December 30, 2024).

TABLE 4-2 Support from HRSA and CDC for State and Territorial Public Health NBS Programs

Program/Initiative	FY 2021	FY 2022	FY 2023	FY 2024
HRSA				
National Center for Newborn Screening System Excellence (NBS Excel)	$1,500,000	$1,500,000	$2,650,000	$2,300,000
Regional Genetic Networks Program	$4,261,786	$4,285,116		
Long-Term Follow-Up for Severe Combined Immunodeficiency and Other NBS Conditions Program	$2,773,019	$3,619,319		
Quality Improvement in NBS Program	$3,835,000	$3,300,000		
NBS Family Education Program	$400,000	$400,000		
Innovations in NBS Interoperability	$1,271,627	$1,258,809		
Clearinghouse of NBS Information	$421,854	$420,830	$498,117	$497,266
State NBS System Priorities Program (NBS Propel)			$9,476,531	$9,956,080
Cooperative NBS System Priorities Program (NBS Co-Propel)				$3,529,813
Total HRSA Funding	$14,463,286	$14,784,074	$12,624,648	$16,283,159
CDC				
Laboratory Quality and Surveillance	$18,000,000	$19,000,000	Not available	Not available
National Contingency Plan for Newborn Screening		$30,000	Not available	Not available
Total CDC Funding	$18,000,000	$19,030,000	Not available	Not available

NOTES: This list may not be comprehensive. Grey squares indicate the program no longer exists (e.g., Regional Genetics Networks program) or had not yet started yet (e.g., NBS Propel). "Not available" indicates the data were not publicly available as of December 2024. NBS Excel was previously known as the Newborn Screening Data Repository and Technical Assistance Program and funds the Newborn Screening Technical assistance and Evaluation Program (NewSTEPs). CDC = Centers for Disease Control and Prevention; HRSA = Health Resources and Services Administration; NBS = newborn screening.
SOURCES: HRSA 2024a; Email transmitted by Alisha Keehn, HRSA, December 11, 2024, providing FY 2023 and FY 2024 grant funding amounts.

operating and strengthening their follow-up programs. Funding opportunities evolve with agency budgets and priorities; for example, the period of performance for the NBS Propel/Co-Propel awards will end in 2028.

Current support mechanisms rely heavily on grants provided to individual states (i.e., NBS Propel and Co-Propel), as well as information clearinghouses and community listservs (e.g., NewSTEPs Community Discussion) aimed at fostering greater coordination, but often without incentives or requirements for programs to participate. NBS programs may need not only coordinators, but also "do-ers" to directly assist programs with solving their challenges. With an onus largely on state and territorial NBS programs to see where they are struggling and reach out, program staff also rely on their informal networks of colleagues and contacts when they have questions or need assistance. A divergence in capacities and performance between different state programs persists and appears to be widening.

Supporting High Performance of All NBS Programs: What Is Needed

Ensuring that all 56 state- and territorial-run NBS programs achieve and sustain excellence is important to the value proposition of newborn screening. Those involved throughout the landscape of newborn screening are approaching this challenge with good intentions and are striving to deliver a public health service to all babies. In the face of program-to-program variability and geographic disparities, however, strengthening the network of programs so all 56 have what they need to achieve excellence in their essential functions will require aligning both financial and nonfinancial supports and incentives in a more strategic way. This approach will likely require a mix of federal, state, and nonprofit or private support, with buy-in from multiple stakeholders and decision makers.

A more holistic approach to investing in the excellence of NBS programs would include

- a level of core support in nationally identified priority areas to enable all state and territorial programs to achieve a foundational, baseline level of excellence;
- incentives for NBS programs to participate in performance measurement, analysis, and improvement activities;
- a continued role for competitive grant opportunities that enable different NBS programs to address their unique needs and gaps and to capitalize on their specific strengths and opportunities;
- a coherent way for NBS programs to work together on common goals and priorities (participating in a networked approach would

also enable NBS programs to share and implement learning and best practices); and
- a mechanism for greater shared, strategic data and trends analysis, going beyond current data repositories.

Mechanisms for enhancing data collection, analysis, and learning, as well as for providing targeted technical assistance and core financial support, could adapt or draw on existing models. One option to implement this system could be to augment NewSTEPs, operated under APHL, by incentivizing NBS program participation, identifying and collecting agreed metrics across all NBS programs, and ensuring the data are used to provide responsive funding and technical assistance. NewSTEPs has operated a quality improvement program, supported through an award from HRSA, in which state public health programs apply for support for quality improvement efforts they have identified. A total of 14 proposals received support in 2019 and 7 proposals in 2020.[12] It appears these efforts are no longer funded (see Quality Improvement in NBS Program in Table 4-2). The NewSTEPs information repository includes technical assistance resources, and it may provide consultative services at the request of state NBS programs.

CDC's Newborn Screening and Molecular Biology Branch has also been developing and pilot testing the Enhancing Data-driven Disease Detection in Newborns (ED3N) program as a data collection and analysis platform.[13] ED3N is currently focused on the development of modules for biochemical and molecular screening data from state and territorial NBS programs, including analysis tools to help improve screening assay detection algorithms and the interpretation of disease variants. The usefulness and feasibility of developing modules that would share and analyze clinical data from diagnosis and longer-term follow-up care is also being considered, although these are not yet deployed (Cuthbert and Gaviglio, 2023). ED3N is anticipated to be up and running in 2028 (Cuthbert and Gaviglio, 2023).

These existing foundations could be built on and expanded to ensure a performance excellence approach and infrastructure that encompasses all programs in a structured and strategic way. Two other potential examples of models for enhancing systematic data collection and performance excellence—an example of an expanded federal cooperative assistance program and a public–private network—are provided in Box 4-3; other

---

[12] See https://www.aphlblog.org/aphl-newborn-screening-systems-quality-improvement-projects-award-recipients-announced/ for 2019 awardees and https://www.globenewswire.com/news-release/2020/02/25/1990269/0/en/APHL-Announces-Newborn-Screening-Systems-Quality-Improvement-Projects-Second-Cohort-Award-Recipients.html for 2020 awardees (both accessed December 30, 2024).

[13] See https://www.cdc.gov/newborn-screening/php/about/ed3n-project.html (accessed January 16, 2025).

> **BOX 4-3**
> **Two Examples of Models to Support Excellence in Public Health Newborn Screening**
>
> Robust approaches to data collection, analysis, and learning, as well as technical and financial assistance, can support excellence across state and territorial NBS programs. Two examples of potential models or approaches that could be drawn on or adapted to fulfill these aims include (1) a federal cooperative grant program supporting activities helping to sustain and build all states' capacity to address infectious diseases (such the Centers for Disease Control and Prevention [CDC] Epidemiology and Lab Capacity program); and (2) an arrangement in which a private or nonprofit organization supports and coordinates quality improvement efforts (such as the California Perinatal and Maternal Quality Care Collaborative).
>
> **CDC Epidemiology and Lab Capacity (ELC) Program**
>
> Established in 1995, CDC's ELC program has provided funding to health departments across the United States to detect, prevent, and respond to infectious disease outbreaks. The program funds an ELC cooperative agreement, which awards funding to 65 U.S. state, local, territory, and affiliate health departments.
>
> Flexible funding allows recipients to meet their unique needs instead of relying on a one-size-fits-all approach. Projects targeting specific diseases, such as rabies surveillance or vaccine-preventable diseases, allow different areas or populations to focus on their priority health topics. The ELC program also distributes supplemental funding on behalf of CDC for emergency response efforts, such as those for H1N1, Zika, Ebola, and COVID-19.
>
> SOURCES: https://www.cdc.gov/epidemiology-laboratory-capacity/media/pdfs/2023-2024-ELC-Fact-Sheet.pdf;
> https://www.cdc.gov/epidemiology-laboratory-capacity/php/our-work/index.html (both accessed January 16, 2025).
>
> **California Perinatal and Maternal Quality Care Collaborative**
>
> The California Perinatal and Maternal Quality Care Collaborative (CPQCC/CMQCC), housed at Stanford Medicine, unites nearly all of California's birth hospitals and neonatal intensive care units in a multistakeholder, public–private network focused on enhancing health care quality and equity. It achieves its goals through key activities that include the following:
>
> - Collection and reporting of standardized, real-time data, generating clinical reports and dashboards that allow hospitals to track performance over time and benchmark against peers;
> - Collaborative quality improvement initiatives driven by member feedback to align with clinical or health policy priorities;
> - Provision of in-person and online educational resources to promote potentially better practices and professional development, giving practitioners access to tools that enable them to deliver high-quality care, support optimal patient outcomes, and help combat burnout;

> **BOX 4-3 Continued**
>
> - Contributions to research advancing knowledge in perinatal and maternal health care;
> - Partnerships between CPQCC/CMQCC and state agencies, families, community organizations, and professional associations to increase effectiveness; and
> - Member-driven, bottom-up philosophy harnessing professionalism coupled with incentives to encourage participation.
>
> SOURCES: www.cpqcc.org; www.cmqcc.org (both accessed January 16, 2025).

approaches could also be taken. Under whichever implementation mechanism is selected, creating a universal system with the active engagement of all state and territorial NBS programs is likely to require some level of incentives to NBS programs, beyond current ad hoc grants.

State and territorial NBS programs may be able to share scarce or specialized resources in a more comprehensive and systematic way to support their collective high performance. Each of the 56 individual NBS programs does not need to duplicate all capacities and types of expertise, but all programs need a way to access these resources when needed. Two examples follow

- *Certain technical capacities*: Each NBS program does not necessarily need to develop and house the full suite of instrumentation and expertise required to undertake DNA sequencing and analysis, which is currently used for certain second- and third-tier testing when initial screening results warrant. Similarly, each program does not need to duplicate the specialized technical expertise involved in developing and improving laboratory assays for screened conditions, as long as all programs have a way to make use of such expertise when they need to implement new screening or access technical assistance when performance issues arise.
- *Certain specialized expertise areas:* Genetic counselors work with families and care providers to help them understand NBS results. Genetic counselors are specially trained to deliver complex health information to families, but there is a shortage of counselors to provide this service after newborn screening. Available providers are concentrated in metropolitan areas and some states and territories have few to no practitioners (Jenkins et al., 2021; NSGC, 2020; Vockley, 2021). Genetic counselors may be able to practice across state lines, but geography is not the only impediment to access as availability of state-recognized licensure and billing practices also pose challenges (Boothe et al., 2020;

Roberts et al., 2017; Tschirgi et al., 2021). Telehealth, distributed systems of clinical expertise, or other mechanisms may be necessary to engage families and connect them to evidence-based care.

Supporting all 56 NBS programs to achieve high performance in their essential functions will require flexibility. Each program needs different things and will have different expertise to contribute to its peers. A useful first step would be identifying the resources and knowledge available among the network of NBS programs, including which state programs have advanced capabilities in which areas. This effort would assist peer programs in knowing where to look or who to ask for help in particular areas when they have gaps and needs and would help maximize the value of expertise that is unevenly distributed across the United States.

Another option to address variability in state capacities for scarce or advanced resources and expertise could be to develop centers for expertise that provide a layer of support to state-run programs within their network. Such centers could expand on the existing CDC-funded Center of Excellence to Enhance Disease Detection in Newborns (award period 2024–2028),[14] which is focused on positioning NBS programs to adapt to advanced technologies and meet increasing demands. Centers for expertise could provide mentorship or direct services to enable state programs to perform existing screening at the highest quality and more quickly add new conditions. Such centers could also house or facilitate connections with genetic counseling services (with the appropriate licensing to work across state lines) to assist states with results interpretation and family communication. Although establishing or designating centers for specialized expertise could help foster greater harmonization of capacities across states and territories, there is a risk that they could deepen geographic disparities by directing resources toward strong programs.

PROGRAM SUSTAINABILITY

"The biggest issue facing newborn screening programs is sustainability."
– NBS public health professional

Supporting and sustaining NBS program excellence relies not only on program resources and performance management, but also on the state, community, and legal contexts in which these programs operate. Maintaining relationships with perinatal care providers, ensuring that these professionals have accurate resources and information about public health

---

[14] See https://www.cdc.gov/newborn-screening/php/about/state-newborn-screening-laboratories.html (accessed December 30, 2024).

newborn screening, and addressing current workforce challenges and future needs are all required for effective program implementation. Similarly, the continued existence of NBS programs to provide a public health service for all babies and families relies on public agreement and trust in their mission. Family education and engagement are important elements in sustaining NBS programs, as are state and territorial program awareness of and attention to the many views and evolving legal landscape around storage and use of NBS dried blood spot samples after screening. Further, the collection and analysis of long-term follow-up data are necessary to achieve NBS programs' aim of improving affected babies' health, and this is an area that bridges public health, clinical care, and research. These key areas for program success are briefly explored in the sections below.

The national context in which NBS programs operate also contributes to their operations and sustainability. Federal support to programs is discussed above. Important federal guidance is also provided to NBS programs through the Recommended Uniform Screening Panel (RUSP) and activities of the Advisory Committee on Heritable Disorders in Newborns and Children (ACHDNC); see Chapter 7 for a discussion of needs and opportunities for federal coordination, input, and priority-setting and to optimize RUSP decision making.

Professional Information and Training

NBS programs must provide clear and accurate information to the many providers and health facilities that speak with prospective parents about screening, collect and return samples, and receive and communicate results. This includes ensuring provider awareness of their state's requirements and obligations and ensuring providers have the necessary materials and information to complete the required sample documentation. This responsibility can also entail outreach more generally to ensure that providers and facilities are prepared to share accurate information with families about what will happen during newborn screening and why, and to communicate with families when screening results are returned. The need for NBS programs to educate perinatal health care providers about newborn screening was recognized and called for by ACHDNC over a decade ago (Therrell et al., 2011). Voluntary guidance from the Clinical and Laboratory Standards Institute (CLSI) also discusses the need for and scope of communication and education around newborn screening (CLSI, 2023).

Professional education and training are important to the success of newborn screening, and providers do not always feel sufficiently informed about the rare diseases covered by newborn screening nor do they feel equipped to interpret and communicate results effectively (Evans et al.,

2019; Kemper et al., 2006; Raia et al., 2024). Providers may also use outdated terminology, such as referring to public health newborn screening as a "PKU test," which can confuse families.[15] Comments shared during information-gathering and listening sessions reinforced and echoed persistent calls for the need for additional NBS education; for practical tools to support providers across the prenatal, perinatal, and postnatal periods; and for greater consistency in this area (Clayton, 2024; Hassan, 2024; Susanna Haas Lyons Engagement Consulting, 2024; Tanksley, 2024; Wallis, 2024). Public health programs, in partnerships with professional associations and programs that train care providers, can assume responsibilities, provide guidance, and facilitate professional awareness and preparation by disseminating effective materials and resources.

Engaging with Families About Newborn Screening

"Clear communication, openness, and transparency would help build trust."
– Parent

More proactive, multifaceted, and robust engagement with families around newborn screening is needed and was raised as a central theme during the committee's information-gathering efforts. Public health NBS programs assume various roles in collaboration and partnership with others. Information about newborn screening is needed not only during blood spot collection at birth but also during pregnancy, and earlier receipt of this information from a heath care provider has been associated with greater parent satisfaction (Araia et al., 2012; Raia et al., 2024).

Current strategies for family awareness and engagement about newborn screening have both strengths and shortcomings. Best practices for engaging families have been elucidated and vetted, multiple research-based educational materials are already available, and refusal rates for newborn screening are generally very low (Evans et al., 2019; Raia et al., 2024).[16] However, the current NBS system is not effectively engaging all families. Many parents report being unaware of newborn screening until a nurse comes to take a blood sample, whereas others do not recall that their infant ever received newborn screening (Bellamy, 2024; Campbell and Ross, 2004; Clayton, 2024; Hassan, 2024; Hoffman, 2024; Kusyk et al., 2013; Rink, 2024; Susanna Haas Lyons Engagement Consulting, 2024; Tanksley, 2024; Wallis, 2024; Williams, 2024).

---

[15] See https://www.newsteps.org/about/screening-successes/north-dakota-newborn-screening-more-pku (accessed March 3, 2025).
[16] A number of resources are also available through the Baby's First Test website; see https://www.babysfirsttest.org/ (accessed November 27, 2024).

When families are unaware of screening until late in the process, they may lack an adequate understanding of what screening means, what is being screened for, or the benefits of screening. Feeling blindsided by this process can undermine trust, lead to confusion or fear, and potentially impede transition to follow-up testing and care for infants identified as at risk through screening. On the other hand, prenatal awareness and engagement has been linked to increased support for the program (Botkin et al., 2016).

Viewing Families as Partners in the Dynamic NBS Landscape

Engaging with families is most effective when done via multiple channels and at multiple time points; this helps to increase retention and understanding and ensure all families encounter information at some point even if there are gaps in their access to care (Tluczek et al., 2009, 2022; WHO, 2017). Multiple actors can and should play roles in this effort. Obstetricians, midwives, maternal care nurses, and family practitioners have a critical opportunity to share information about newborn screening during the prenatal period, a time when pregnant people are already participating in many health screens and are focused on planning for their baby's birth. While engagement about newborn screening can happen during the course of prenatal care, it may be most effective if it is delivered more than once and if there are systems in place to ensure it is consistently delivered. In particular, parents and providers have identified the third trimester as one important window for such information (ACOG Committee on Genetics, 2019; Davis et al., 2006).

The time around birth is another critical period when clinicians can reinforce awareness and understanding of newborn screening by clearly communicating what is happening when a sample is taken and reminding families about the next steps in the process when the family is discharged home. During this period, it is especially helpful to provide simple, action-oriented information (Davis et al., 2006; Tluczek et al., 2022). After birth, pediatricians, pediatric nurses, family physicians, and advance practice nurses also have key roles. Their primary responsibility is to close the loop on reporting results to families, even when the screening results are in range. Pregnant people and their families support awareness and engagement as well, by actively seeking out information about newborn screening, asking questions, engaging in conversations with care providers, and sharing information within their own networks.

Engagement needs to be a two-way street, working with families as partners within the NBS landscape. Family awareness and engagement around newborn screening ties into interrelated ethical issues and can help support the overall success of NBS programs. In keeping with public health ethical principles, newborns and their families should be treated as partners—not passive recipients—in newborn screening (see Chapter 3).

To build and maintain trust, the NBS system must demonstrate that it is trustworthy, and engagement contributes to this aim.

Public trust in NBS programs cannot be taken for granted, particularly as conversations continue around complex issues such as the use of genome sequencing and blood spot storage and use. A lack of transparency around the NBS process or a lack of awareness of its benefits and parental options can lead to backlash. Several lawsuits have already been filed by parents in multiple jurisdictions over policies concerning residual dried blood spots (Hughes et al., 2022). Finally, family engagement can help the NBS system work better. By knowing how the process should work and when they should expect to receive results, families become another check in the process to ensure results are reported and follow-up occurs.

Goals and Resources

Achievable goals can help guide communication with parents about newborn screening. First, it is important for families to be aware that newborn screening happens. This ideally includes awareness that newborn screening will happen (before birth), that it is happening (heel stick to collect newborn blood spot), and that it has happened (results are reported back to the family). Second, families need to have a basic understanding of what newborn screening entails and their options, including both the initial screening and any subsequent storage and use of the blood spot. They should have opportunities to ask questions and get additional information if they want to learn more. Third, families need to have a basic understanding of why newborn screening is done. This includes awareness of the benefits of detecting urgent and serious health conditions before symptoms develop at a stage when interventions can substantially improve a baby's lifelong health. This awareness can reinforce the importance of engaging with providers to facilitate follow-up testing and treatment as appropriate.

Education and engagement around newborn screening can take varied forms, and many NBS educational resources exist, developed by family support and advocacy organizations, professional associations, government agencies, and others.[17] Pamphlets, posters, and other printed materials can be especially useful for conveying information without adding burdens to a provider's time with patients because they can be displayed or distributed

---

[17] Links to multiple resources and materials on newborn screening are available through the HRSA's Newborn Screening Resources page (https://newbornscreening.hrsa.gov/about-newborn-screening/newborn-screening-resources; accessed November 27, 2024), through Baby's First Test (https://www.babysfirsttest.org/newborn-screening/resources; accessed November 27, 2024), through Expecting Health (https://expectinghealth.org/programs/newborn-screening-family-education-program; accessed February 4, 2025), and through multiple other sources.

in the waiting room before a prenatal visit or given as a resource for families to review at home. Electronic resources such as videos, images, and websites can be helpful within and outside of health care contexts. They can be well suited for reaching people in the online spaces where they already spend time, such as through social media campaigns or prenatal education classes held online. Finally, conversations with care providers and educators can help to deliver information while giving families a chance to express concerns or ask questions (Bellamy, 2024; Raia et al., 2024).

The existence of best practices and educational resources has not consistently translated into effective family engagement and awareness around newborn screening, however. One important barrier is that responsibilities for communicating with parents and families are diffuse and there is a general lack of clarity about whose responsibility it is to deliver this information to parents, how available materials can be obtained, and when and how they should be communicated (Davis et al., 2006; Evans et al., 2019; Faulkner et al., 2006; Raia et al., 2024). A "no wrong door" approach may be an effective strategy for empowering providers to educate parents about newborn screening. Multiple providers may be involved in perinatal care, and the role of these practitioners may differ across communities. For example, community pharmacists are often the most accessible providers in rural or frontier communities (Berenbrok et al., 2020, 2022; San-Juan-Rodriguez et al., 2018). All providers interfacing with families during the perinatal period can play a key role in educating parents or directing parents to trusted resources about newborn screening.

Language and health literacy can also pose barriers if materials are not well matched with the intended populations. Whatever form engagement takes, information must be delivered in ways that are accessible, digestible, and linguistically and culturally appropriate. Additional investment may be needed to tailor existing materials or develop further materials for communicating effectively with all members of a state or territory's population, including those from medically underserved communities (Davis et al., 2006; Evans et al., 2019, 2020; Tluczek et al., 2022). Translating into practice these calls for more systematic and effective engagement with parents and families about newborn screening may require efforts among relevant provider communities to issue or update practice guidance. In addition, provision and reimbursement of health-related services is affected by the existence and use of codes through the Healthcare Common Procedure Coding System (HCPCS).[18] Such codes include Current Procedural Terminology codes overseen by the American Medical Association and additional HCPCS codes established by the Centers for

---

[18] See https://www.cms.gov/medicare/coding-billing/healthcare-common-procedure-system (accessed January 2, 2025).

Medicare & Medicaid Services. Further discussions among care providers and public and private health payors may be needed regarding the applicability and reimbursement of NBS education under current coding.

Storage and Reuse of Residual Dried Blood Spots

> *Understand that the majority of end-users of the newborn screening system are not rare disease patients, but instead patients with negative test results. Given that their children did not have a disease identified, their main concerns and considerations may not be related to diagnosis and care, but instead privacy, consent for the use of samples, and why their child may need to be screened in the first place. – NBS public health professional*

Extra or "residual" dried blood spots exist after public health NBS tests are completed (Ram, 2022). What happens to infants' collected blood spots after screening is another issue important to the sustainability and future effectiveness of NBS programs. All states need to maintain screened dried blood spots for some period of time during which these samples are available for additional testing if initial screening results are out of range, and to enable NBS programs to use deidentified dried blood spots in quality control and assurance efforts. These types of uses are fundamental—generally not controversial—and essential parts of operating a functioning NBS program (Botkin et al., 2013). It is critical to distinguish these core program uses from other types of potential uses such as research or forensics.

Using dried blood spots for health research can offer benefits for future infants, pregnant people, and the public health (Botkin et al., 2013), leading the American College of Medical Genetics and Genomics (ACMG) to describe dried blood spots as a "valuable national resource" (ACMG, 2009, p. 2). This kind of research can include "toxicology, environmental exposure, or vaccine studies" (Preslan and Mathews, 2013, p. 27) or "state-level concerns over infectious agents, environmental exposures, and population genetics" (Botkin et al., 2013, p. 122). In 2013, a study found that 26 states allowed research use of dried blood spots, while 12 prohibited it. Only a few states have specifically prohibited types of research including research related to the military and "cosmetics, abortion, or nonhealth topics" (Preslan and Mathews, 2013, p. 27). In addition, the Texas legislature amended the statutory framework governing newborn screening to prohibit use of dried blood spots for "forensic science"[19] following *Beleno v. Lakey*, described below (Ram, 2022).

Forensic or police use of dried blood spots might include identifying a child postmortem (Botkin et al., 2013), or even for criminal prosecution.

---

[19] Tex. Health & Safety Code Ann. § 33.018(f)(2).

These broad and important uses led Jeffrey Botkin and colleagues to "encourage states to consider the retention of residual NBS specimens and to make retained specimens available to qualified investigators. . ." within parameters (Botkin et al., 2013, p. 122). This section describes the current landscape of policies concerning dried blood spots, court cases, and areas of specific consideration moving forward.

Policies for Use

Despite these broad and important potential uses of dried blood spots, there are few consistent policies at the federal, state, or laboratory level setting rules or expectations (Lewis et al., 2011). In 2008 Congress passed the Newborn Screening Saves Lives Act (P.L. 110-204) to "promote and improve newborn screening for heritable disorders, develop population research surveillance and epidemiology, and expand research partnerships within the government as well as academic and private institutions" (Drabiak-Syed, 2011, p. 9). Section 1116 of the Act (Hunter Kelly Research Program) states that the "Secretary, in conjunction with the Director of the National Institutes of Health and taking into consideration the recommendations of the Advisory Committee, may continue carrying out, coordinating, and expanding research," including "for additional newborn conditions, and other genetic, metabolic, hormonal, and or functional conditions that can be detected through newborn screening" (P.L. 110-204, Sec. 1116).

In 2009 the U.S. Secretary of Health and Human Services ACHDNC made recommendations regarding dried blood spot retention and use, including that all states should have a related policy. ACHDNC recommended that such policies should ensure respect for the privacy and confidentiality of families, promote public trust, and emphasize transparency. Such policies should also help support informed public participation (ACHDNC, 2010). The following year ACHDNC also added that the retention and use of dried blood spots for "nonstandard uses such as research may not be adequately addressed in current state laws or policies" (Therell et al., 2011, p. 624). The same year, a workshop convened by the Institute of Medicine (IOM) explored calls for more transparency and accountability in this space (IOM, 2010).

In 2014, amendments to the Public Health Service Act (Newborn Screening Saves Lives Reauthorization Act, P.L. 113-240) required two new elements regarding research use of dried blood spots acquired during public health newborn screening. First, the amendments required that research with dried blood spots be understood to meet the definition of human subjects research, even if the spots were deidentified. Typically, the definition of "human subject" in the Common Rule (45 CFR 46) is limited to interventional research or research with *identified* data or specimens. Second, the amendments prohibited an institutional review board (IRB) waiver of informed consent for research with dried blood spots. Typically, an IRB could offer a waiver for research that was low risk where consent was impracticable to obtain (as well as several other metrics) (Rothwell et al., 2019). This Act lapsed in 2019 with the revisions to the Common Rule, and current research with dried blood spots is now governed by the standard metrics (Ram, 2022).

Parental Education and Consent for the Retention and Use of Dried Blood Spots

Disclosure of retention and future research use of dried blood spots is not mandated in most states. Policies vary widely regarding disclosure, types of research use, destruction of retained dried blood spots, or potential return of clinical results (Lewis et al., 2011). That said, a 2019 study of research publications using dried blood spots found that the majority of papers obtained informed consent and/or used deidentified or anonymous samples (Rothwell et al., 2019). However, many parents report a preference for being given a choice whether their child's dried blood spots be used for things other than the clinical testing, quality assurance, and quality improvement. Thus, while the public health component of NBS is often justified by the state's interest in protecting the health of newborns, assuming that state interest can be extended to also doing research with the dried blood spots is controversial (Suter, 2022). Nevertheless, when given a choice, 76 percent of parents in a survey reported being very or somewhat willing to consent to research (Tarini et al., 2010). Whether this percentage would differ today as trust in research and public health has evolved is unknown.

Two general approaches to informed consent particularly relevant to the newborn screening context have been described in the literature. In an opt-in approach, parents affirmatively sign a consent form to allow dried blood spots to be used for research. As Botkin et al. have argued, "The major advantage of the opt-in approach is that it requires an interaction with parents to obtain a signature and therefore enhances the possibility that parents would make an informed choice" (Botkin et al., 2013). Parental preferences are also consistent with this approach (Botkin et al., 2012). Opt-in, however, has been criticized as potentially being too burdensome for hospitals to implement given the number of clinical needs in the peripartum time period. The concern is that hospitals would not bother to ask for consent, severely limiting the supply of dried blood spots for research—even from parents that would have otherwise consented (Drabiak-Syed, 2011; SACHRP, 2015).

On the other hand, in an opt-*out* approach, parents would be informed about the future potential retention and use of their children's dried blood spots and their right to not consent to that use. But, unless the parent affirmatively signs an opt-out form, the default will be that the dried blood spot *can* be used for research. This switch in administrative burden has, in other contexts, demonstrated increased participation rates (Davidai et al., 2012). Botkin et al. therefore argued that opt-out was the better policy choice, assuming:

> (1) parents are informed about the retention and use of residual samples in a meaningful way that permits an informed decision, (2) parents understand that they have the option to refuse, and (3) the ability to opt-out entails a process that is not unduly burdensome (Botkin et al., 2013, p. 124).

In 2009, Michigan was the first state to develop a comprehensive opt-in approach for research use of dried blood spots along with providing educational materials and trainings through the Michigan BioTrust for Health (Michigan BioTrust). The majority of adults in Michigan were found to be supportive of research with dried blood spots. In early implementation, hospitals reported that in the vast majority of cases, the consent process required less than 5 minutes (Duquette et al., 2011, 2012). In 2010–2012, almost 60 percent of parents affirmatively opted in to such research (only 16 percent actually declined; the rest were returned blank or not at all). This was a significant reduction in dried blood spots being available for research; however, the Michigan BioTrust saw the program design as a reasonable public health trade-off. Overall, the Michigan BioTrust did not observe a substantial increase in parent refusal for public health newborn screening itself (Langbo et al., 2013). That said, the Michigan BioTrust is involved in an ongoing court case regarding the legality of their approach (see below).

Selected Court Cases Challenging Newborn Screening and Their Implications

There have been several past and ongoing court cases regarding the storage and use of dried blood spots collected through public health newborn screening. Brief summaries of four court cases are provided to give context for considerations on standards for storage, retention, and reuse policies.

Beleno v. Lakey *(Texas, 2009)*

In *Beleno*, several parents sued the Texas Department of State Health Services for storing their children's dried blood spots indefinitely for research purposes without explicit parental consent. Parents argued that this was *federally* unconstitutional under the Fourth Amendment (prohibiting unreasonable searches and seizures) and the Fourteenth Amendment (prohibiting the deprivation of liberty without due process).[20] Texas requested that the case be dismissed, but the court declined to do so for the majority of claims.[21] As the parties were amending their complaints, it was revealed that the Texas Department of State Health Services had also shared approximately 800 dried blood spots to the U.S. Armed Forces Pathology Laboratory for forensic use. The plaintiffs filed an additional lawsuit (Ramshaw, 2010). Texas decided to settle the case and agreed to destroy five million dried blood spots. A more protective state law also took effect around the same time (Lewis et al., 2011).

Bearder v. State *(Minnesota, 2011)*

In *Bearder*, several parents sued the state of Minnesota for retaining their children's dried blood spots indefinitely for research without parental consent. The parents argued that, unlike in *Beleno*, this was a violation of Minnesota law—a section of the Minnesota Government Data Practices Act that required written informed consent for genetic testing.[22] While a lower court held that the Minnesota Genetic Privacy Act did not apply to the case because testing of biological specimens was not genetic information and that the state health commissioner had express authority to conduct health studies with the specimens,[23] the Minnesota Supreme Court concluded otherwise. The court held that "biological information includes blood samples"[24] and that, while the collection and use of dried blood spots for public health newborn screening was expressly allowed by law, use for *research* required consent.[25] The state was ordered to destroy one million samples (Wadman, 2012).

Kanuszewski v. Michigan *(Michigan, 2023)*

In *Kanuszewski*, several parents sued the Michigan Department of Health and Human Services and Neonatal Biorepository for retention of their children's dried blood spots without informed consent. Like in *Beleno*, parents argued that this was federally unconstitutional under the Fourth and Fourteenth Amendments.[26] The Sixth Circuit Court noted that, while the U.S. Supreme Court had not weighed in on whether parents have

---

[20] *Beleno v. Lakey.* 306 F. Supp. 3d 930 (W.D. Tex. 2009).
[21] *Beleno v. Lakey.* 306 F. Supp. 3d 930 (W.D. Tex. 2009).
[22] Minn. Stat. §13.386 (2010) on the treatment of genetic information, which has been referred to as the Genetic Privacy Act.
[23] *Bearder v. State*, 788 N.W.2d 144, 149 (2010).
[24] *Bearder v. State*, 806 N.W.2d 766, 773 (2011).
[25] *Bearder v. State*, 806 N.W.2d 766 (2011).
[26] *Kanuszewski v. Mich. HHS*, 927 F. 3d 396 (2019).

a "fundamental right" to direct their child's medical care, the Supreme Court had found that parents have the right to direct their education and religious upbringing. Therefore, the Sixth Circuit reasoned, the direction of medical care must also be a fundamental right.[27] Any limitation on a fundamental right warrants "strict scrutiny," meaning the government has to demonstrate that the limitation is "narrowly tailored" in response to a "compelling government interest."[28] While acknowledging that public health dried blood spots might meet a strict scrutiny standard because of the state's *parens patriae* interest in keeping children alive,[29] the court was skeptical about the state's extension of it to the retention of specimens "after [the state] has finished screening the samples for diseases."[30]

On remand from the Sixth Circuit, the lower court held that the state was liable for Fourth Amendment violations as the "seizure" of the blood spots was unreasonable. While the seizure of dried blood spots for public health purposes related to newborn screening might be a compelling interest, it held that indefinite retention of dried blood spots was *not* narrowly tailored to achieve it.[31] The district court also concluded that law enforcement use of dried blood spots would violate the Fourth Amendment.[32] The court directed the state to either gather informed consent for each retained blood spot or destroy them within 1 year; Michigan destroyed over three million dried blood spots (White, 2022).[33] It has been appealed again to the Sixth Circuit and oral arguments are scheduled for March 2025.

Lovaglio v. Baston *(New Jersey, 2023)*

In *Lovaglio,* parents sued the New Jersey Department of Health under federal constitutional arguments,[34] like in *Beleno* and *Kanuszewski.* New Jersey has a known record of law enforcement using dried blood spots in at least several cases. In 2024, the state of New Jersey released a new directive requiring "genuinely exceptional circumstances" for approval of law enforcement use.[35] Whether this new directive is constitutionally satisfactory remains pending before the New Jersey Court (Difilippo, 2023).

---

[27] *Kanuszewski v. Mich. HHS*, 927 F. 3d 396, 411 (2019).
[28] *Kanuszewski v. Mich. HHS*, 927 F. 3d 396, 419 (2019).
[29] *Kanuszewski v. Mich. HHS*, 927 F. 3d 396, 420 (2019).
[30] *Kanuszewski v. Mich. HHS*, 927 F. 3d 396.
[31] *Kanuszewski v. Mich. HHS*, 684 F. Supp. 3d 637, 652 (2023).
[32] *Kanuszewski v. Mich. HHS*, 684 F. Supp. 3d 637, 652–53 (2023).
[33] *Kanuszewski v. Mich. HHS*, 684 F. Supp. 3d 637, 660 (2023).
[34] *Lovaglio v. Baston*, No. 3:23-cv-21803-GC_RLS.
[35] State of New Jersey Office of the Attorney General, *Investigatory Use of Documentary Records and Physical Blood Samples Maintained by the Newborn Screening Program*, Attorney General Law Enforcement Directive No. 2024-03 (Trenton, NJ: OAG, 2024), https://www.nj.gov/oag/dcj/agguide/directives/ag-Directive-2024-03_Physical-Blood-Samples.pdf (accessed March 18, 2025).

Policy Areas to Consider for Storage and Reuse of Dried Blood Spots

Many professional organizations and experts have recommended that states should establish consistent policies regarding secondary dried blood spot (DBS) use (Botkin et al., 2012, 2013). Building and maintaining trust is critical to any public health program because so many public health programs rely on the community to voluntarily engage (Ram, 2022). Whereas a lack of explicit consent or more education has sometimes been justified by the importance of the NBS program, as the cases above demonstrate, overstepping the legal bounds of that program not only can undermine trust but can also lead to the destruction of entire research biobanks (including samples for which parents might have consented in the first place) (Lewis et al., 2011). A recent white paper from the National Organization for Rare Disorders (NORD) describes public, policy-maker, and legal attention to this question, and highlights the importance of maintaining trust and transparency while preserving the ability of programs to carry out their essential functions (NORD, 2025). There are several specific areas for consideration in the development of such policies.

Duration of Retention

As discussed in several of the dried blood spot court cases, duration of retention of dried blood spots is a critical component of assessing whether government collection of dried blood spots is appropriate to achieve the public health goals of newborn screening. A 2019 study found that whereas some states only retain dried blood spots for 3–6 months to complete public health screening, three states store them for 10–20 years, eight store them for 21–30 years, and six store them indefinitely (Rothwell et al., 2019). Therefore, while dried blood spots might be valuable to research for decades (Botkin et al., 2013), there is no state-level consensus on how long to retain specimens either for public health or research purposes (Botkin et al., 2012). In 2013, Botkin et al. recommended that states retain dried blood spots for at least 3 months for public health screening purposes and true positive specimens as long as target analytes are stable. They also recommended that dried blood spots should be retained until the legal age of adulthood for the child, but that parents should have the right to have them destroyed prior to that as well (Botkin et al., 2013).

Use of Genomic Sequencing

Retention and use of dried blood spots might also be affected by evolving technologies and the use of genomic sequencing in particular. While the Michigan BioTrust in the *Kanuszewski* case argued that the retention of blood spots was unlikely to carry a high risk of reidentification, the court dismissed this claim because, it noted, that an argument that something does not currently happen does not mean it cannot happen in the future. In fact, the National Human Genome Research Institute has concluded publicly that "genome sequencing [in newborn screening] will eventually happen" (Ram, 2022, p. 1266). As Natalie Ram has argued, "The push toward generating broader swaths of genetic sequence data as part of newborn screening may make those subsequent uses much broader—and perhaps more controversial, too" (Ram, 2022, p. 1268).

Access to Dried Blood Spots by the Criminal Justice System

A third important consideration is access and use of dried blood spots by the criminal justice system. Dried blood spots have been used for criminal investigation, including in California and New Jersey, which made arrests on the basis of dried blood spots (Biryukov, 2022; Ram, 2022). Some states, like Iowa,[36] have clear protections against law enforcement use of residual dried blood spots,[37] but most states do not. Experts including Botkin et al. and Ram have argued strongly against this use of dried blood spots, and courts, such as the one in Michigan, have used law enforcement's use of dried blood spots as an example of why retention programs can violate the Fourth Amendment (Botkin et al., 2013; Ram, 2022).[38] As Ram has argued, "... it is nonsensical to imagine that the state can, in the exercise of its *parens patriae* power, consent to law enforcement searches for ordinary crime-detection purposes (Ram, 2022, p. 1311)." As Sonia Suter has added:

> If the state usurps control over intimate personal biological samples and associated medical information by stepping in as "parents of the country" and then uses those involuntarily collected samples for its own surveillance, that is worse than "overweening government power." It is akin to abuse of power. (Suter, 2022, p. 15)

Connecting Newborn Screening to Health Outcomes: An Ongoing Challenge

"While infants are generally screened universally, the system for follow-up and treatment for screen positive infants mirrors our healthcare system. [Some] infants are lost to follow-up or don't receive treatment in a timely manner."
– Health care provider

---

[36] Iowa Admin. Code r. 641-4.3(8)(e)(2022).
[37] Although Iowa's regulatory framework clearly bars law enforcement use of NBS dried blood spots, law enforcement use of data derived from newborn screening may be permitted (Ram, 2022). See Iowa Admin. Code r. 641-4.3(7)(b)(3) (2021).
[38] *Kanuszewski v. Mich. HHS*, 684 F. Supp. 3d 637, 660 (2023).

A key motivation for undertaking at-birth, population-level newborn screening is to support improved health outcomes for babies through early detection and intervention. Longer-term follow-up in the context of newborn screening generally refers to activities after confirmatory testing is completed (Hinton et al., 2014; Kemper et al., 2008). After state NBS programs document the transition of an identified baby and their family to the clinical care system for follow-up and ongoing care, the baby's subsequent record largely falls outside the capacity of most NBS programs to monitor.

Information on long-term care, services, and health outcomes for the individuals and families diagnosed with a screened condition thus involves medical records located in hospital or clinician electronic health records, public or private health insurance records—whether through private insurance plans or public plans such as Medicaid, and a range of potential disease-specific registries, some operated by agencies such as CDC[39] or by disease advocacy organizations and industry, such as the Cystic Fibrosis Foundation Patient Registry,[40] or the National PKU Alliance Patient Registry.[41] As such, long-term health outcomes data involve multiple personal, state, and federal sources outside the control of state NBS programs. Persistent socioeconomic, geographic, racial, and other disparities associated with the U.S. health care system complicate the ability of all babies identified with a serious condition to receive the care they need, and some babies fall out of the health care system after screening.

Documenting the longer-term effects of newborn screening is important for

- understanding the effectiveness of available treatments on babies' improved health outcomes,
- developing new or improved interventions to fill gaps,
- maintaining public and decision-maker support for newborn screening,
- analyzing health and economic benefits from investing in at-birth screening, and
- learning and improving the overall NBS system.

Effective long-term data collection and outcomes analysis after newborn screening remains challenging and does not have simple or

---

[39] For example, the CDC Sickle Cell Data Collection (SCDC) program, which currently includes 16 states (https://www.cdc.gov/sickle-cell/scdc/index.html; accessed December 30, 2024).

[40] See https://www.cff.org/medical-professionals/patient-registry (accessed December 30, 2024).

[41] See https://www.npkua.org/registry/ (accessed December 30, 2024).

immediate solutions. NBS programs need to be involved in longer-term follow-up efforts after screening, as essential partners with clinical health, information systems, and other collaborators, but such follow-up extends beyond core program functions and is outside the current scope and ability of most state and territorial NBS programs. (See also Chapter 6 for discussion of longitudinal follow-up research).

Workforce Development

"Most lab facilities are underfunded, understaffed, and under-supported."
– NBS public health professional

Sustainability of NBS programs relies on a robust public health workforce. However, public health programs face ongoing workforce challenges related to recruitment and retention. The public health workforce has declined substantially since the 1970s, and between the 2009 Great Recession and the COVID-19 pandemic more than 40,000 state and local public health positions were lost (Leider et al., 2023). Rising workload coupled with insufficient support have resulted in staff burnout, decreased morale, and high turnover across public health and for NBS programs, specifically (Leider et al., 2023; Olney et al. 2023; Susanna Haas Lyons Engagement Consulting, 2024). Labor market competition from the private sector and limited career growth opportunities add to the difficulty of attracting and retaining experienced staff (APHL, 2024; Leider et al., 2023; Susanna Haas Lyons Engagement Consulting, 2024).

There are several possible strategies to sustain and rebuild the NBS public health workforce. Workforce development initiatives, including new approaches to training and education, staff engagement activities, and alternate work schedules have been successful in alleviating some of these challenges (Olney et al., 2023). Loan repayment programs for governmental public health staff, improvements to governmental hiring processes, and expanded internship and mentorship programs are also possible opportunities (Leider et al., 2023; NASEM, 2022). Further discussions on public health workforce development, recruitment, and retention are needed.

CONCLUSIONS

Conclusion 4-1: While respecting the autonomy of each state and territorial public health NBS program to meet the needs of its population, all programs need to be accountable for achieving certain essential functions:

- *Provide every infant born in the state or territory with the opportunity to receive screening for a set of serious, urgent, and treatable conditions.*

- *Provide NBS educational materials to all state/territorial prenatal and birth providers.*
- *Strive for high-quality, timely screening designed to perform accurately for all members of the population.*
- *Ensure high quality and timely case management for every infant screened. This includes directly communicating out-of-range results for infants to their providers, and ultimately to the family/caregiver, as well as confirming those infants are connected to further evaluation or care by documenting diagnoses. This also includes reporting in-range results such that every infant's results are communicated to their provider, and ultimately to the family/caregiver.*
- *Establish and maintain systems for quality assurance, program excellence, and performance improvement.*

Conclusion 4-2: *The ability to document, measure, and evaluate core program functions would enable NBS programs to improve on their performance. Many NBS programs track a variety of metrics, but not all programs collect or report the same metrics and metrics are not always connected with achieving core goals. Establishing a performance-based, learning approach at both state and national levels would support the excellence of this important public health program.*

Conclusion 4-3: *Education about public health newborn screening is haphazard and often nonexistent, leaving many parents unaware that newborn screening has taken place. There are significant gaps in families' interactions with the NBS system, particularly around knowledge that screening occurs and the benefits of screening, as well as the practices around the storage and reuse of dried blood spots. Risks of inadequate education include parents opting their child out of screening, being blindsided by screening results, or having a child fall through the cracks. Engaging with families about newborn screening is essential for an effective and trustworthy system.*

Conclusion 4-4: *Providers can feel ill equipped or unable to engage with families about newborn screening due in part to insufficient knowledge. Education on the mission and practices of newborn screening, how to routinely integrate and disseminate resources on newborn screening into care, and the fundamentals of genetics would prepare providers to responsibly communicate with their patients about newborn screening throughout the prenatal to postanal period.*

Conclusion 4-5: *NBS programs need the authority to retain dried blood spots for at least a limited time for quality assurance and quality improvement activities. These are essential for operating a functional NBS program and maintaining a high-quality public health service.*

Conclusion 4-6: *Long-term follow-up is important to understand the public health impacts of newborn screening and make improvements across the NBS system but requires clinical health and public health partnerships, health information technology infrastructures, and other capacities that are outside the scope and ability of most state and territorial NBS programs.*

Conclusion 4-7: Multiple mechanisms support NBS programs in meeting their goals; however, resources are unevenly allocated and federal programs are often based on competitive grant applications that can burden resource-constrained programs and can perpetuate and exacerbate existing disparities among programs. NBS programs would need responsive financial and nonfinancial supports and incentives to achieve and maintain systemwide excellence and capacity while respecting each program's autonomy, unique challenges, and broader context.

REFERENCES

Abhyankar, S., R. M. Goodwin, M. Sontag, C. Yusuf, J. Ojodu, and C. J. McDonald. 2016. An update on the use of health information technology in newborn screening. *Seminar in Perinatology* 39(3):188-193.

ACHDNC (Advisory Committee on Heritable Disorders in Newborns and Children). 2008. *Transcript, Monday, January 14*. Department of Health and Human Services. https://public3.pagefreezer.com/content/health-resources-and-services-administration/22-08-2022T12:52/https:/www.hrsa.gov/sites/default/files/hrsa/advisory-committees/heritable-disorders/meetings/Heritable%20Disorders%202004-2015/2008/Jan%2014,%202008/transcript.pdf (accessed January 15, 2025).

ACHDNC. 2010. *Letter from R. R. Howell to K. Sebelius, October 13, 2010*. https://www.hrsa.gov/sites/default/files/hrsa/advisory-committees/heritable-disorders/reports-recommendations/letter-sec-dried-blood.pdf (accessed January 15, 2025).

ACHDNC. 2013. *Transcript, Friday, September 20*. Department of Health and Human Services. https://us.pagefreezer.com/en-US/wa/browse/d6b93713-1f22-47f2-a0e2-ce7a6df7744a?find-by-timestamp=2022-08-22T12:52:59Z&url=https:%2Fwww.hrsa.gov%2Fsites%2Fdefault%2Ffiles%2Fhrsa%2Fadvisory-committees%2Fheritable-disorders%2Fmeetings%2FHeritable%20Disorders%202004-2015%2F2013%2FSeptember%2011-12,%202013%2Fdaytwotranscript.pdf&timestamp=2022-08-22T11:59:24Z (accessed January 15, 2025).

ACMG (American College of Medical Genetics) Newborn Screening Expert Group. 2006. Newborn screening: Toward a uniform screening panel and system. *Genetics in Medicine* (Suppl 1):1S-252S.

ACMG. 2009. *Position statement on importance of residual newborn screening dried blood spots*. https://www.acmg.net/PDFLibrary/NBS-Blood-Spot-Retention.pdf (accessed January 15, 2025).

ACOG (American College of Obstetricians and Gynecologists) Committee on Genetics. 2019. Newborn screening and the role of the obstetrician-gynecologist. ACOG Committee Opinion Number 778. *Obstetrics and Gynecology* 133(5):e357-e361.

APHL (Association of Public Health Laboratories). 2024. *2024 laboratory workforce profile: Survey summary report*. https://www.aphl.org/aboutAPHL/publications/Documents/QSA-Workforce-Profile-2024-Survey-Summary.pdf (accessed February 14, 2025).

Araia, M. H., B. J. Wilson, P. Chakraborty, K. Gall, C. Honeywell, J. Milburn, T. Ramsay, and B. K. Potter. 2012. Factors associated with knowledge of and satisfaction with newborn screening education: A survey of mothers. *Genetics in Medicine* 14(12):963-970.

Atkinson, K., B. Zuckerman, J. M. Sharfstein, D. Levin, R. J. R. Blatt, and H. K. Koh. 2001. A public health response to emerging technology: Expansion of the Massachusetts newborn screening program. *Public Health Reports* 116(2)122-131.

Bellamy, C. 2024. *Webinar on family education for newborn screening, October 7, 2024*. Presentation and discussion to the Committee on Newborn Screening: Current Landscape and Future Directions. https://www.nationalacademies.org/event/43820_10-2024_newborn-screening-current-landscape-and-future-directions-webinar-on-family-education-for-newborn-screening (accessed: February 13, 2025).

Berenbrok, L. A., N. Gabriel, and K. C. Coley. 2020. Evaluation of frequency of encounters with primary care physicians vs visits to community pharmacies among Medicare beneficiaries. *Journal of the American Medical Association Network Open* 3(7):e209132.

Berenbrok, L. A., S. Tang, N. Gabriel, J. Guo, N. Sharareh, N. Patel, S. Dickson, and I. Hernandez. 2022. Access to community pharmacies: A nationwide geographic information systems cross-sectional analysis. *Journal of the American Pharmacists Association* 62(6):1816-1822.

Biryukov, N. 2022. Newborn screening program used to aid criminal investigation, public defender says. *New Jersey Monitor*. https://newjerseymonitor.com/2022/07/13/newborn-screening-program-used-to-aid-criminal-investigation-public-defender-says/ (accessed January 29, 2025).

Boothe, E., S. Greenberg, C. L. Delaney, and S. A. Cohen. 2020. Genetic counseling service delivery models: A study of genetic counselors' interests, needs, and barriers to implementation. *Journal of Genetic Counseling* 30(1):283-292.

Botkin, J. R., E. Rothwell, R. Anderson, L. Stark, A. Goldenberg, M. Lewis, M. Burbank, and B. Wong. 2012. Public attitudes regarding the use of residual newborn screening specimens for research. *Pediatrics* 129(2):231-238.

Botkin, J. R., A. J. Goldenberg, E. Rothwell, R. A. Anderson, and M. H. Lewis. 2013. Retention and research use of residual newborn screening blood spots. *Pediatrics* 131(1):120-127.

Botkin, J. R., E. Rothwell, R. A. Anderson, N. C. Rose, S. M. Dolan, M. Kuppermann, L. A. Stark, A. Goldenberg, and B. Wong. 2016. Prenatal education of parents about newborn screening and residual dried blood spots: A randomized clinical trial. *JAMA Pediatrics* 170(6):543-549.

Campbell, E. D., and L. F. Ross. 2004. Incorporating newborn screening into prenatal care. *American Journal of Obstetrics and Gynecology* 190(4):876-877.

Clayton, E. W. 2024. *Panel reflections and discussion on public trust, May 16, 2024*. Presentation and discussion to the Committee on Newborn Screening: Current Landscape and Future Directions. https://www.nationalacademies.org/event/42550_05-2024_newborn-screening-current-landscape-and-future-directions-meeting-3 (accessed March 4, 2025).

CLSI (Clinical and Laboratory Standards Institute). 2023. *Newborn screening follow-up and education*. CLSI guideline NBS02. Berwyn, PA: Clinical and Laboratory Standards Institute.

Comeau, A. M. 2024. *Panel: State/regional NBS programs–Perspectives on the study task, January 26, 2024*. Presentation and discussion to the Committee on Newborn Screening: Current Landscape and Future Directions. https://www.nationalacademies.org/event/41786_01-2024_newborn-screening-current-landscape-and-future-directions-meeting-1b (accessed March 4, 2025).

Cuthbert, C., and A. Gaviglio. 2023. *ED3N: Enhancing Data-Driven Disease Detection in Newborns*. Presentation to a meeting of the Advisory Committee on Heritable Disorders in Newborns and Children, May 4, 2023. https://www.hrsa.gov/sites/default/files/hrsa/advisory-committees/heritable-disorders/meetings/cdc-enhancing-data-driven-disease-detection.pdf (accessed January 21, 2025).

Davidai, S., T. Gilovich, and L. D. Ross. 2012. The meaning of default options for potential organ donors. *Proceedings of the National Academy of Sciences* 109(38):15201-15205.

Davis, T. C., S. G. Humiston, C. L. Arnold, J. A. Bocchini, Jr., P. F. Bass, 3rd, E. M. Kennen, A. Bocchini, D. Williams, P. Kyler, and M. Lloyd-Puryear. 2006. Recommendations for effective newborn screening communication: Results of focus groups with parents, providers, and experts. *Pediatrics* 117(5 Pt 2):S326-S340.

Difilippo, D. 2023. Civil rights group sues New Jersey to stop secret storage, use of baby blood spots. *New Jersey Monitor*. https://newjerseymonitor.com/2023/11/02/civil-rights-group-sues-new-jersey-to-stop-secret-storage-use-of-baby-blood-spots/ (accessed March 18, 2025).

Donabedian, A. 1966. Evaluating the quality of medical care. *Milbank Quarterly* 44(3):166-206.

Dorley, M. C., E. Bair, P. Ryland, A. D. Ingram, E. Reeves, K. J. Levinson, O. O. Adair, J. F. Meredith, and S. Crowe. 2024. Continuity of operations in newborn screening: Lessons learned from three incidents. *International Journal of Neonatal Screening* 10(3):55.

Drabiak-Syed, K. 2011. Legal regulation of banking newborn blood spots for research: How *Bearder* and *Beleno* resolved the question of consent. *Houston Journal of Health Law and Policy* 11:1-46.

Duquette, D., A. P. Rafferty, C. Fussman, J. Gehring, S. Meyer, and J. Bach. 2011. Public support for the use of newborn screening dried blood spots in health research. *Public Health Genomics* 14(3):143-152.

Duquette, D., C. Langbo, J. Bach, and M. Kleyn. 2012. Michigan BioTrust for Health: Public support for using residual dried blood spot samples for health research. *Public Health Genomics* 15(3-4):146-155.

Evans, A., K. LeBlanc, N. Bonhomme, S. M. Shone, A. Gaviglio, D. Freedenberg, J. Penn, C. Johnson, B. Vogel, S. M. Dolan, and A. J. Goldenberg. 2019. A newborn screening education best practices framework: Development and adoption. *International Journal of Neonatal Screening* 5(2):22.

Evans, A., M. Lynch, M. Johnson, and N. Bonhomme. 2020. Assessing the newborn screening education needs of families living in medically underserved areas. *Journal of Genetic Counseling* 29(4):658-667.

Fauber, J. 2013. More than half of state labs do not process newborn samples on weekends, creating critical delays in the process. *Milwaukee Journal Sentinel*. https://archive.jsonline.com/watchdog/watchdogreports/Deadly-Delays-Watchdog-Report-More-than-half-of-state-labs-do-not-process-newborn-samples-on-weekends-creating-critical-delays-in-the-process-228832381.html (accessed January 21, 2025).

Faulkner, L. A., L. B. Feuchtbaum, S. Graham, J. P. Bolstad, and G. C. Cunningham. 2006. The newborn screening educational gap: What prenatal care providers do compared with what is expected. *American Journal of Obstetrics and Gynecology* 194(1):131-137.

FDA (Food and Drug Administration). 2024. FDA takes exciting steps toward establishing the Rare Disease Innovation Hub. *FDA Voices*, November 1, 2024. https://www.fda.gov/news-events/fda-voices/fda-takes-exciting-steps-toward-establishing-rare-disease-innovation-hub (accessed December 30, 2024).

Gabler E., M. Johnson, and J. Fauber. 2013. Deadly delays. *Milwaukee Journal Sentinel*, November 16.

GAO (Government Accountability Office). 2016. *Newborn screening timeliness: Most states had not met screening goals, but some are developing strategies to address barriers*. GAO-17-196. https://www.gao.gov/assets/gao-17-196.pdf (accessed January 15, 2025).

Hassan, S. 2024. *Panel reflections and discussion on public trust, May 16, 2024*. Presentation and discussion to the Committee on Newborn Screening: Current Landscape and Future Directions. https://www.nationalacademies.org/event/42550_05-2024_newborn-screening-current-landscape-and-future-directions-meeting-3 (accessed March 4, 2025).

Hinton, C. F., C. T. Mai, S. K. Nabukera, L. D. Botto, L. Feuchtbaum, P. A. Romitti, Y. Wang, K. N. Piper, and R. S. Olney. 2014. Developing a public health-tracking system for follow-up of newborn screening metabolic conditions: A four-state pilot project structure and initial findings. *Genetics in Medicine* 16(6):484-490.

Hoffman, B. 2024. *Webinar on family education for newborn screening, October 7, 2024*. Presentation and discussion to the Committee on Newborn Screening: Current Landscape and Future Directions. https://www.nationalacademies.org/event/43820_10-2024_newborn-screening-current-landscape-and-future-directions-webinar-on-family-education-for-newborn-screening (accessed: February 13, 2025).

HRSA (Health Resources and Services Administration). 2017. *Newborn screening timeliness goals*. https://www.hrsa.gov/advisory-committees/heritable-disorders/newborn-screening-timeliness (accessed September 18, 2024).

HRSA. 2024a. *Report to Congress: Newborn screening activities fiscal year 2021 and fiscal year 2022*. https://www.govinfo.gov/content/pkg/CMR-HE20_9000-00186876/pdf/CMR-HE20_9000-00186876.pdf (accessed January 15, 2025).

HRSA. 2024b. *Cooperative newborn screening system priorities (NBS Co-Propel) program.* https://mchb.hrsa.gov/programs/cooperative-newborn-screening-system-priorities (accessed September 26, 2024).

HRSA. 2024c. *State newborn screening system priorities (NBS Propel) program.* https://mchb.hrsa.gov/programs/newborn-screening-propel (accessed March 3, 2024).

Hughes, R., IV, S. Choudhury, and A. Shah. 2022. Newborn screening blood spot retention and reuse: A clash of public health and privacy interests. *Health Affairs Forefront.* https://www.healthaffairs.org/content/forefront/newborn-screening-blood-spot-retention-and-reuse-clash-public-health-and-privacy (accessed January 21, 2025).

IOM (Institute of Medicine). 2010. *Challenges and opportunities in using residual newborn screening samples for translational research: Workshop summary.* Washington, DC: The National Academies Press.

Jenkins, B. D., C. G. Fischer, C. A. Polito, D. R. Maiese, A. S. Keehn, M. Lyon, M. J. Edick, M. R. G. Taylor, H. C. Andersson, J. N. Bodurtha, M. G. Blitzer, M. Muenke, and M. S. Watson. 2021. The 2019 US medical genetics workforce: A focus on clinical genetics. *Genetics in Medicine* 23(8):1458-1464.

Johnson, M. 2013. Testing delay puts newborn's life at risk. *Milwaukee Journal Sentinel.* https://archive.jsonline.com/watchdog/watchdogreports/Deadly-Delays-Watchdog-Report-Newborn-screening-testing-delay-puts-newborns-life-at-risk-228832681.html (accessed January 21, 2025).

Kellar-Guenther, Y., L. Barringer, K. Raboin, G. Nichols, K. Y. F. Chou, K. Nguyen, A. R. Burke, S. Fawbush, J. B. Meyer, M. Dorsey, A. Brower, K. Chan, M. Lietsch, J. Taylor, M. Caggana, and M. K. Sontag. 2024. Defining the minimal long-term follow-up data elements for newborn screening. *International Journal of Neonatal Screening* 10(2):37.

Kemper, A. R., R. L. Uren, K. L. Moseley, and S. J. Clark. 2006. Primary care physicians' attitudes regarding follow-up care for children with positive newborn screening results. *Pediatrics* 118(5):1836-1841.

Kemper, A. R., C. A. Boyle, J. Aceves, D. Dougherty, J. Figge, J. L. Fisch, A. R. Hinman, C. L. Greene, C. A. Kus, J. Miller, D. Robertson, B. Therrell, M. Lloyd-Puryear, P. C. van Dyck, and R. R. Howell. 2008. Long-term follow-up after diagnosis resulting from newborn screening: Statement of the US Secretary of Health and Human Services' Advisory Committee on Heritable Disorders and Genetic Diseases in Newborns and Children. *Genetics in Medicine* 10(4):259-261.

Kemper, A. R., L. Ouyang, and S. D. Grosse. 2010. Discontinuation of thyroid hormone treatment among children in the United States with congenital hypothyroidism: Findings from health insurance claims data. *BMC Pediatrics* 10(1):9.

Kusyk, D., K. Acharya, K. Garvey, and L. F. Ross. 2013. A pilot study to evaluate awareness of and attitudes about prenatal and neonatal genetic testing in postpartum African American women. *Journal of the National Medical Association* 105(1):85-91.

Langbo, C., J. Bach, M. Kleyn, and F. P. Downes. 2013. From newborn screening to population health research: Implementation of the Michigan BioTrust for health. *Public Health Reports* 128(5):377-384.

Leider, J. P., V. A. Yeager, C. Kirkland, H. Krasna, R. Hare Bork, and B. Resnick. 2023. The state of the US public health workforce: Ongoing challenges and future directions. *Annual Review of Public Health* 44:323-341.

Lewis, M. H., A. Goldenberg, R. Anderson, E. Rothwell, and J. Botkin. 2011. State laws regarding the retention and use of residual newborn screening blood samples. *Pediatrics* 127(4):703-712.

Mann, S. 2015. Insights in public health: Newborn screening saves babies using public/private partnerships. *Hawai'i Journal of Medicine and Public Health* 74(12):415-418.

Mann, S. 2024. *Panel: State/regional NBS programs–Perspectives on the study task, January 26, 2024.* Presentation and discussion to the Committee on Newborn Screening:

Current Landscape and Future Directions. https://www.nationalacademies.org/event/41786_01-2024_newborn-screening-current-landscape-and-future-directions-meeting-1b (accessed March 4, 2025).

McColley, S. A., S. L. Martiniano, C. L. Ren, M. K. Sontag, K. Rychlik, L. Balmert, A. Ebert, R. Wu, and P. M. Farrell. 2023. Disparities in first evaluation of infants with cystic fibrosis since implementation of newborn screening. *Journal of Cystic Fibrosis* 22(1):89-97.

McGarry, M. E., C. L. Ren, R. Wu, P. M. Farrell, and S. A. McColley. 2023. Detection of disease-causing CFTR variants in state newborn screening programs. *Pediatric Pulmonology* 58(2):465-474.

Minear, M. A., M. N. Phillips, A. Kau, and M. A. Parisi. 2022. Newborn screening research sponsored by the NIH: From diagnostic paradigms to precision therapeutics. *American Journal of Medical Genetics Part C: Seminars in Medical Genetics* 190(2):138-152.

Mt. Sinai. n.d. *Neonatal cystic fibrosis screening test*. https://www.mountsinai.org/health-library/tests/neonatal-cystic-fibrosis-screening-test (accessed January 15, 2025).

NASEM (National Academies of Sciences, Engineering, and Medicine). 2022. *Improving diversity of the genomics workforce: Proceedings of a workshop—in brief*. Washington, DC: The National Academies Press.

NASEM. 2023. *Using population descriptors in genetics and genomics research: A new framework for an evolving field*. Washington, DC: The National Academies Press.

Nemours Children's Health. 2015. *Cystic fibrosis newborn screening information for pediatricians*. https://www.youtube.com/watch?v=2bQ40fKaGMU (accessed January 15, 2025).

NewSTEPs. n.d. *Screened conditions report*. https://www.newsteps.org/data-center/reports/screened-conditions-report (accessed December 30, 2024).

NewSTEPs. 2023. *NewSTEPs 2022 annual report*. newsteps.org/sites/default/files/resources/download/NewSTEPS-2022-Annual-Report.pdf (accessed December 30, 2024).

NORD (National Organization for Rare Disorders). 2025. *Preserving public trust in the U.S. newborn screening system: Policy principles and recommendations on the retention and secondary use of residual dried blood spots*. https://rarediseases.org/wp-content/uploads/2025/02/NRD-2368-Newborn-Screening-Report_FNL.pdf (accessed March 6, 2025).

North Carolina Department of Health and Human Services. n.d. *North Carolina newborn screening program. Elevated IRT and 2 CFTR variants fact sheet for parents*. https://www.ncdhhs.gov/1elevated-irtand2-cftrvariantsparentspdf/download?attachment?attachment (accessed January 15, 2025).

NSGC (National Society of Genetic Counselors). 2020. *Professional status survey 2020: Executive summary*. https://www.nsgc.org/Portals/0/Docs/Policy/PSS%20Executive%20Summary%202020%20FINAL%2005-03-20.pdf (accessed January 15, 2025).

Olney, R. S., J. R. Bonham, P. Schielen, D. Slavin, and J. Ojodu. 2023. 2023 APHL/ISNS newborn screening symposium. *International Journal of Neonatal Screening* 9(4):54.

Pizzamiglio, C., H. J. Vernon, M. G. Hanna, and P. D. S. Pitceathly. 2022. Designing clinical trials for rare disease: Unique challenges and opportunities. *Nature Reviews Methods Primers* 2(1):s43586-022-00100-2.

Preslan, E. D., and D. J. Mathews. 2013. A comparative analysis of the governance and use of residual dried blood spots from state newborn screening programs and neonatal biobanks. *Journal of Empirical Research on Human Research Ethics* 8(3):22-33.

Raia, M. H., M. M. Lynch, A. C. Ward, J. A. Brown, N. F. Bonhomme, and V. L. Hunting. 2024. One size does not fit all: A multifaceted approach to educate families about newborn screening. *International Journal of Neonatal Screening* 10(3):44.

Ram, N. 2022. America's hidden national DNA database. *Texas Law Review* 100(7):1253-1325.

Ramshaw, E. 2010. DNA deception. *The Texas Tribune*. https://www.texastribune.org/stories/2010/feb/22/dna-deception (accessed March 3, 2025).

Rehani, M. R., M. S. Marcus, A. B. Harris, P. M. Farrell, and C. L. Ren. 2023. Variation in cystic fibrosis newborn screening algorithms in the United States. *Pediatric Pulmonology* 58(3):927-933.

Rink, B. 2024. *Webinar on family education for newborn screening, October 7, 2024.* Presentation and discussion to the Committee on Newborn Screening: Current Landscape and Future Directions. https://www.nationalacademies.org/event/43820_10-2024_newborn-screening-current-landscape-and-future-directions-webinar-on-family-education-for-newborn-screening (accessed February 13, 2025).

Roberts, M. C., E. M. Wood, J. B. Gaieski, and A. R. Bradbury. 2017. Possible barriers for genetic counselors returning actionable genetic research results across state lines. *Genetics in Medicine* 19:1202-1204.

Rock, M. J., M. Baker, N. Antos, and P. M. Farrell. 2023. Refinement of newborn screening for cystic fibrosis with next generation sequencing. *Pediatric Pulmonology* 58(3):778-787.

Rothwell, E., E. Johnson, N. Riches, and J. R. Botkin. 2019. Secondary research uses of residual newborn screening dried blood spots: A scoping review. *Genetics in Medicine* 21(7):1469-1475.

Rubin, R. 2021. Tackling the misconception that cystic fibrosis is a "White people's disease". *JAMA* 325(23):2330-2332.

SACHRP (Secretary's Advisory Committee on Human Research Protections). 2015. *Attachment E: Recommendations regarding research uses of newborn dried bloodspots and the Newborn Screening Saves Lives Reauthorization Act of 2014.* https://www.hhs.gov/ohrp/sachrp-committee/recommendations/2015-april-24-attachment-e/index.html (accessed March 3, 2025).

San-Juan-Rodriguez, A., T. V. Newman, I. Hernandez, E. C. S. Swart, M. Klein-Fedyshin, W. H. Shrank, and N. Parakh. 2018. Impact of community pharmacist-provided preventative services on clinical, utilization, and economic outcomes: An umbrella review. *Preventative Medicine* 115:145-155.

Schieve, L. A., G. M. Simmons, A. B. Payne, K. Abe, L. L. Hsu, M. Hulihan, S. Pope, S. Rhie, B. Dupervil, and W. C. Hooper. 2022. Vital signs: Use of recommended health care measures to prevent selected complications of sickle cell anemia in children and adolescents—selected US states, 2019. *Morbidity and Mortality Weekly Report* 71(39):1241-1246.

Simonetti, J. 2024. *Panel: State/regional NBS programs–Perspectives on the study task, January 26, 2024.* Presentation and discussion to the Committee on Newborn Screening: Current Landscape and Future Directions. https://www.nationalacademies.org/event/41786_01-2024_newborn-screening-current-landscape-and-future-directions-meeting-1b (accessed March 4, 2025).

Sontag, M. K., J. I. Miller, S. McKasson, R. Sheller, S. Edelman, C. Yusuf, S. Singh, D. Sarkar, J. Bocchini, J. Scott, J. Ojodu, and Y. Kellar-Guenther. 2020. Newborn screening timeliness quality improvement initiative: Impact of national recommendations and data repository. *PLoS One* 15(4):e0231050.

Susanna Haas Lyons Engagement Consulting. 2024. *What we heard: Engagement summary for committee on newborn screening: Current landscape and future directions.* Washington, DC: National Academies of Sciences, Engineering, and Medicine.

Suter, S. 2022. Mission creep in newborn screening and DNA forensics. *Texas Law Review* 101:8-20.

Tanksley, S. 2024. *Panel reflections and discussion on public trust, May 16, 2024.* Presentation and discussion to the Committee on Newborn Screening: Current Landscape and Future Directions. https://www.nationalacademies.org/event/42550_05-2024_newborn-screening-current-landscape-and-future-directions-meeting-3 (accessed March 4, 2025).

Tarini, B. A., A. Goldenberg, D. Singer, S. J. Clark, A. Butchart, and M. M. Davis. 2010. Not without my permission: Parents' willingness to permit use of newborn screening samples for research. *Public Health Genomics* 13(3):125-130.

Therrell, B. L., Jr., W. H. Hannon, D. B. Bailey, Jr., E. B. Goldman, J. Monaco, B. Norgaard-Pedersen, S. F. Terry, A. Johnson, and R. R. Howell. 2011. Committee report: Considerations and recommendations for national guidance regarding the retention and use of residual dried blood spot specimens after newborn screening. *Genetics in Medicine* 13(7):621-624.

Tluczek, A., K. M. Orland, S. W. Nick, and R. L. Brown. 2009. Newborn screening: An appeal for improved parent education. *Journal of Perinatal & Neonatal Nursing* 23(4):326-334.

Tluczek A., A. L. Ersig, and S. Lee. 2022. Psychosocial issues related to newborn screening: A systematic review and synthesis. *International Journal of Neonatal Screening* 8(4):53.

Tschirgi, M. L., K. M. Owens, M. S. Mackall, J. Allen, and R. Allen. 2021. Easing the burden of multi-state genetic counseling licensure in the United States: Processes, pitfalls, and possible solutions. *Journal of Genetic Counseling* 31(1):41-48.

Vockley, C. W. 2021. *Genetic counselors and newborn screening: Roles, activities and future challenges*. Presentation to Advisory Committee on Heritable Disorders in Newborns and Children, May 14, 2021. https://www.hrsa.gov/sites/default/files/hrsa/advisory-committees/heritable-disorders/meetings/vockley.pdf (accessed December 30, 2024).

Wadman, M. 2012. Minnesota starts to destroy stored blood spots. *Nature*. https://doi.org/10.1038/nature.2012.9971 (accessed December 30, 2024).

Wallis, H. 2024. *Panel reflections and discussion on public trust, May 16, 2024*. Presentation and discussion to the Committee on Newborn Screening: Current Landscape and Future Directions. https://www.nationalacademies.org/event/42550_05-2024_newborn-screening-current-landscape-and-future-directions-meeting-3 (accessed March 4, 2025).

White, E. 2022. Michigan to destroy some blood spots in fight over consent. *Associated Press*. https://apnews.com/article/technology-science-health-lawsuits-michigan-a68becbf0cb78f8e658cfd39e2420a6c (accessed December 30, 2024).

WHO (World Health Organization). 2017. *WHO strategic communications framework for effective communications*. Geneva: WHO. https://www.who.int/docs/default-source/documents/communicating-for-health/communication-framework.pdf (accessed December 18, 2024).

Williams, T. 2024. *Webinar on family education for newborn screening, October 7, 2024*. Presentation and discussion to the Committee on Newborn Screening: Current Landscape and Future Directions. https://www.nationalacademies.org/event/43820_10-2024_newborn-screening-current-landscape-and-future-directions-webinar-on-family-education-for-newborn-screening (accessed: February 13, 2025).

Zimmerman, S. J. 2016. *Cystic fibrosis DNA testing reinstated. Memo to Birthing Centers and Hospitals, Physician Officers from Scott J. Zimmerman, North Carolina State Laboratory of Public Health*. North Carolina Department of Health and Human Services. https://slph.dph.ncdhhs.gov/doc/Memo-CF-DNA-061016.pdf (accessed December 18, 2024).

5

The Responsible Application of Emerging Technologies in Public Health Newborn Screening

"What do these new technologies and the data they will produce really mean for families and what families need to deal with?" – Representative from an organization serving families

The prior chapter describes the report's vision for supporting and sustaining public health newborn screening as it navigates ongoing and nascent challenges. Among these challenges, technologies loom large as tools with the potential to change the way that decision makers, partners in the NBS ecosystem, and the public consider the role of public health newborn screening. One of the technologies garnering the greatest interest, research attention, and momentum is genomic sequencing. This chapter uses genomic sequencing as an illustrative example for considering the novel application of any technology to public health newborn screening, and also discusses the unique technical, operational, and ethical considerations raised by genomic sequencing specifically.

CURRENT LANDSCAPE OF DNA-BASED TESTS IN THE NBS ECOSYSTEM

DNA-based tests encompass a wide range of methodologies and potential screening readouts from those that are highly targeted to those that are more expansive. Different methods have different capabilities regarding the number of genes or genetic variants that can be assessed simultaneously, ranging from a single variant to complete gene

> **BOX 5-1**
> **Genomic Sequencing Defined**
>
> Whole genome sequencing (WGS) is often used to refer to next-generation sequencing (NGS) across the entire genome (Goodwin et al., 2016). This term can be misinterpreted as it suggests that the genome is fully sequenced, analyzed, and reported in its entirety. WGS may generate data across the genome, but not all the sequencing data are typically analyzed and interpreted into reportable results. Throughout this chapter, the term *genomic sequencing* is used to avoid confusion.

sequencing and deletion/duplication analysis. When necessary, DNA can be amplified by polymerase chain reaction (PCR) followed by targeted gene/genetic variant assessment. Next-generation sequencing (NGS) can be used to generate sequences that range from targeted genetic variants, a limited number of targeted genes, exome sequences of the coding regions of all genes, to a genome sequence that includes coding and noncoding regions of all genes. Critically, all sequencing data produced do not need to be analyzed to become reportable information (see Box 5-1) (Goodwin et al., 2016).

Different sequencing collection and analysis approaches are used in clinical care, including for the diagnosis of symptomatic newborns and children (Kingsmore et al., 2024; Retterer et al., 2016; Willig et al., 2015; Yang et al., 2013). Most of these strategies have not been applied to screening healthy infants at birth outside of research contexts (Figure 5-1) (Furnier et al., 2020; NASEM, 2023). This section describes the current status of molecular analysis using DNA-based tests in public health newborn screening as well as in research initiatives within the United States.

Public Health Newborn Screening

Conditions included in NBS panels are largely genetic disorders. Historically, a reliable biochemical marker for a condition has served as the screening test of choice, but for some disorders, including severe combined immunodeficiency and spinal muscular atrophy, DNA-based testing is the only option (see Box 2-4) (ACHDNC, 2011; Almannai et al., 2016; Kraszewski et al., 2018). Heretofore, sequencing across a single gene has been used in a second-tier or reflex test setting to provide independent molecular genetic analysis after a first-tier biochemical or enzymatic testing result is out of range or as additional information to help clinical decision making and patient communication (e.g., sequencing of *CFTR* to screen for

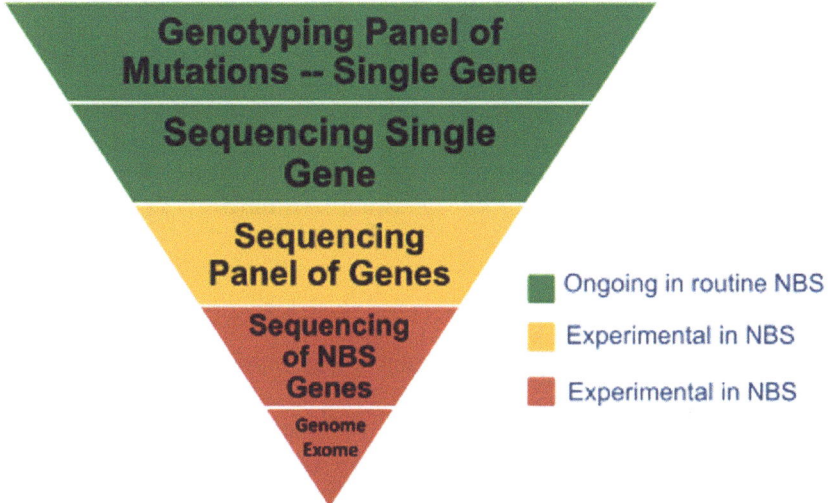

FIGURE 5-1 Staged approach to molecular analysis in public health newborn screening.
NOTE: NBS = newborn screening.
SOURCE: CDC, 2024.

cystic fibrosis) (Furnier et al., 2020). Genomic sequencing that enables more expansive readouts has yet to be applied toward screening for conditions in public health newborn screening (NASEM, 2023).

Research Landscape

Recent advances in sequencing technology, including developments that decrease cost, have attracted large-scale research investment to determine the usefulness and acceptability of genomic sequencing in newborns (Minear et al., 2022). The Newborn Sequencing in Genomic Medicine and Public Health (NSIGHT) program was a research initiative jointly funded by the National Human Genome Research Institute (NHGRI) and the *Eunice Kennedy Shriver* National Institute of Child Health and Human Development (NICHD) from 2013 to 2019, with an initial funding commitment totaling $25 million (NIH, 2022).[1] The consortium was composed of four centers that investigated sequencing in newborns within different contexts, including clinical diagnosis of sick newborns in intensive care

---

[1] https://grants.nih.gov/grants/guide/rfa-files/RFA-HD-13-010.html (accessed March 24, 2025).

unit settings and screening of healthy newborns at birth. Together, the centers aimed to address three research questions:

1. For disorders currently screened in newborns, how can genomic sequencing replicate or augment known NBS results? Can sequencing replace current screening modalities; if so, for which conditions?
2. What knowledge could genomic sequencing provide about conditions not currently screened in newborns?
3. What additional clinical information could be learned from genomic sequencing relevant to the clinical care of newborns (Berg et al., 2017)?

Each center used different approaches with minimal coordination and had a sequencing project, a clinical project, and an ethics project.

The investment in NSIGHT led to several major findings relevant to considering sequencing as a screening tool for healthy newborns. At the time of study publication in 2020, sequencing alone was insufficiently sensitive or specific to replace traditional screening methods (Adhikari et al., 2020; Roman et al., 2020). However, sequencing demonstrated usefulness as a second-tier test to reduce false-positive results and facilitate informed decisions about the infant's care, and, in some cases, enabled the identification of infants with nonclassical forms of NBS conditions that were missed with conventional screening (Adhikari et al., 2020; Ceyhan-Birsoy et al., 2019; Woerner et al., 2021). Studies highlighted the breadth of parental and clinical perspectives on sequencing healthy newborns, including interest in the potential of sequencing to uncover actionable health insights and apprehension about receiving ambiguous or uncertain results.

Many parents chose not to participate in these studies, citing concerns about privacy and insurance discrimination (Genetti et al., 2019). Ultimately, members of the NSIGHT Ethics and Policy Advisory Board published a Hasting Centers Report in which they recommended that targeted sequencing may be appropriate "as a primary test to screen for conditions that meet existing NBS criteria, where sequencing is either the more appropriate or only method for screening for that particular condition." Members of the board recommended strongly against the integration of genomic sequencing to return results that would expand the scope of public health newborn screening beyond conditions that are serious, urgent, and actionable (Johnston et al., 2018, p. S6).[2]

Since the ending of NSIGHT's funding, several large-scale research programs have continued to explore how genomic sequencing could be integrated into public health newborn screening and its potential ethical ramifications (see Box 5-2). The International Consortium of Newborn

---

[2] NSIGHT did not make a position statement on the use of genomic sequencing in public health newborn screening.

BOX 5-2
Ongoing Newborn Sequencing Studies

Researchers around the world are independently studying the usefulness and effectiveness of genome sequencing of healthy newborns. Ongoing studies have varied designs and return different information to newborns and their families. Here is a list of a few such studies conducted in the United States:

BabySeq Project is a randomized controlled trial designed to rigorously assess the medical, social, and psychosocial effects of genome sequencing in healthy newborns (Holm et al., 2018). Families of newborns randomized to the sequencing arm receive information that extends beyond the risk for actionable childhood-onset conditions to include pathogenic[a] and likely pathogenic variants (including carrier status) in more than 4,300 genes associated with childhood-onset and actionable adult-onset conditions (Ceyhan-Birsoy et al., 2019; Smith et al., 2024). Ongoing work aims to characterize the outcomes of genome sequencing in a larger, more representative cohort of infants (Smith et al., 2024).

BeginNGS is an international precompetitive public–private consortium that aims to implement a system for screening newborns for genetic diseases, diagnostic confirmation, implementation of effective treatment, and acceleration of drug development. BeginNGS is recruiting from study sites across the United States and internationally with the goal of more representative inclusion of different ancestries. Results will be reported for approximately 400 early-onset, actionable genetic conditions (Kingsmore, 2022; Rady Children's Institute for Genomic Medicine, 2025a). Pathogenic and likely pathogenic variants will be reported (Rady Children's Institute for Genomic Medicine, 2025b). The primary study endpoints are clinical usefulness and cost-effectiveness of BeginNGS versus standard-of-care testing determined at 1 year of age (Kingsmore, 2022).

Early Check is a statewide, consented NBS pilot study conducted in North Carolina that aims to understand the acceptability, feasibility, implementation, and effect of integrating genomic sequencing into public health newborn screening (Bailey et al., 2019). Participants are offered screening for a panel of 178 pediatric-onset, actionable genetic conditions, as well as a second panel of 29 less actionable conditions. Only pathogenic and likely pathogenic variants are reported (Cope et al., 2024). Early Check is assessing the recruitment, education, and consent approaches and evaluating genetic counseling, confirmatory testing, and follow-up protocols across a state with representation from many different ancestral groups (Cope et al., 2023; Kucera et al., 2021; Paquin et al., 2021; Peay et al., 2022).

Genomic Uniform-screening Against Rare Disease in All Newborns (GUARDIAN) study is a multisite, single-group, prospective, observational investigation assessing the implementation of genomic sequencing to assess the feasibility of population-based screening of newborns for early-onset genetic conditions. Two panels of genetic conditions are assessed: (1) 327 early-onset genetic conditions with interventions that prevent or lessen symptoms, and (2) 142 infant or childhood-onset disorders for which medical treatment of epilepsy is effective but medication only partially treats the condition (GUARDIAN Study, n.d.). Pathogenic

> **BOX 5-2 Continued**
>
> and likely pathogenic variants are reported, with variants of unknown significance only reported if they co-occur with a pathogenic or likely pathogenic variant for recessive conditions. A recent report of interim findings from this study discusses the feasibility of this approach, and the need for more studies to understand its effect on clinical management and health outcomes (Ziegler et al., 2024).
>
> ---
>
> [a] A pathogenic variant is a genomic variant that may increase a person's risk of developing a condition, disorder, or disease (NHGRI, 2025).

Sequencing (ICoNS) was recently established to convene experts in this field and harmonize and aggregate data across newborn sequencing projects. ICoNS aims to offer evidence-based resources to inform clinical and public health research and implementation.[3]

Public Health Feasibility Studies

In September 2024 a new initiative was announced at the National Institutes of Health (NIH) Council of Councils meeting: the Newborn Screening by Whole-Genome Sequencing (NBSxWGS) Collaboratory. The goal of the initiative is to demonstrate feasibility for public health newborn screening by whole genome sequencing through a collaborative model with public health programs (Sheely, 2024). The initiative is intended to enable the early identification of infants at risk for serious, but treatable, genetic conditions. A transparent informed consent process will be implemented, and public perception of genomic sequencing as part of public health newborn screening will be assessed.[4] Many other details of the NBSxWGS Collaboratory have yet to be announced, including how conditions will be selected for inclusion, which conditions will be included, which variants will be reported, and how results will be communicated to families.

CONSIDERATIONS FOR INCORPORATING GENOMIC SEQUENCING INTO PUBLIC HEALTH NEWBORN SCREENING

> *"We can reuse these core [genomic] technologies for this very, very different application of screening healthy newborns as opposed to testing affected individuals with a high pretest probability of genetic disease. However, there are some substantial differences, which make this a complex problem to solve"* – Newborn Sequencing Researcher

---

[3] See https://www.iconseq.org/the-consortium (accessed March 4, 2025).
[4] See https://commonfund.nih.gov/venture/nbsxwgs (accessed December 19, 2024).

Decisions around the inclusion of any given technology—including genomic sequencing—require the same level of scrutiny, analysis, and alignment with vision and ethical principles as other decisions that affect the practice of public health newborn screening. Genomic sequencing opens the possibility and opportunity of screening for all genetic diseases that meet the criteria for inclusion on the NBS panel by using a single platform as an initial step (Berg et al., 2017; Ziegler et al., 2024). Applying this technology could also afford greater flexibility to add new conditions and variants as knowledge and new treatments emerge. However, considering the application of genomic sequencing in public health newborn screening raises specific challenges and considerations. This section discusses these considerations and presents key areas and selected questions that must be addressed if genomic sequencing were ever to be applied to public health newborn screening.

Ethical Considerations

Technological advances will provide increasingly detailed health information that may not be clinically actionable (Jameson and Longo, 2015). Different philosophies conflict on how society should approach the development and adoption of such technologies, particularly in the face of uncertainty and risk. Among these philosophies, the *technological imperative* reflects the notion that if a technology can be developed, its development and implementation are inevitable and obligatory (Koenig, 1988). In contrast, the *precautionary principle* argues against implementing a technology until there is a fulsome understanding of its potential risks and impact (COMEST, 2005). The tension between these philosophies arises from their conflicting priorities and assumptions—with the technological imperative prioritizing potential rewards over risks and assuming the inevitability of adoption, and the precautionary principle prioritizing evidence of safety over potential progress.

When applied to public health newborn screening, the technological imperative would favor maximizing the use of available screening technologies and using the technologies' capabilities to drive decision making (Moyer et al., 2008; Pereira and Clayton, 2018). Alternatively, the precautionary principle would advocate for a more cautious approach, emphasizing the need to fully understand the potential benefits, risks, and ethical implications before widespread implementation. In practice, decision making about new applications of genomic sequencing in public health newborn screening can balance these competing views by doing the following:

- Remain grounded in public health ethical principles and values (see Chapter 3) (APHA, 2019).

- Draw on existing frameworks for implementing biomedical technologies (NASEM, 2019).
- Incorporate public engagement to ensure alignment with societal views (APHA, 2019; Mori et al., 2024).
- Reflect a robust review of the evidence and a high standard of evidence (Moyer et al., 2008).
- Incorporate data collected through consented research studies that allow for real-world learning while minimizing risks.

Methodological Considerations

This section briefly describes the opportunities and shortcomings presented by different approaches for genomic sequencing and data analysis. Strategies are considered through the lens of their potential application to public health newborn screening.

Generating exome or genome sequences requires DNA, which can be isolated from newborn dried blood spots (Ziegler et al., 2024). Sequencing methods include short-read sequencing that generates sequence fragments of 150 base pairs or so, and long-read sequencing, which generates sequence lengths of 10,000–100,000 base pairs. Generating long-read sequence data from dried blood spots is currently more difficult and expensive than generating short-read sequence data. Some genomic sequencing methods can also assess methylation-based epigenetic changes (Goodwin et al., 2016). Regardless of what sequence data are generated, analysis can be limited to a prespecified set of genes and/or variants, and analysts can be blinded to data that do not map to the target areas of reporting. This testing strategy of selective analysis is currently employed by many genetic testing laboratories in the context of clinical care with panels of genes in genetic testing (Jezkova et al., 2022).

What to include in the target for sequencing is a balance between the cost of sequencing and data storage and longer-term flexibility to add conditions for analysis without the need to revalidate the test. Test revalidation will become increasingly costly, time-consuming, and complicated with the proposed new Food and Drug Administration (FDA) regulations that reclassify laboratory-derived tests as medical devices/in vitro diagnostic tests and subject them to the entire FDA approval process (Willmarth, 2015).[5] Therefore, whole genome sequencing with analysis limited to a prespecified set of genes and/or variants may afford the greatest flexibility to efficiently add variants and/or conditions as knowledge of disease-causing variants and genes evolves and as treatments

---

[5] https://www.federalregister.gov/documents/2023/10/03/2023-21662/medical-devices-laboratory-developed-tests (accessed March 24, 2025).

become available. However, privacy concerns raised by sequencing may be exacerbated when more sequencing data are collected than are analyzed (Tarini and Goldenberg, 2012).

Sequence data must be aligned to the reference genome, and variants must be called. Variant calling is the process of identifying sequence differences between an individual's sequence data with respect to a reference genome (Olson et al., 2023). Most single nucleotide variants can be readily called. With short-read data, small insertions and deletions (<10 base pairs) are generally called correctly, large deletions and duplications (3 or more exons and 500,000 base pairs or more) are reliably called, and many triplet repeats can be correctly sized with appropriate algorithms. There are significant limitations to short-read data for deletions, duplications, and insertions between 10 and 500,000 base pairs and for variants in complex repetitive regions of the genome. Long-read data have the advantage of being able to correctly call more complex variant types, methylation status, and phase variants for recessive conditions; however, the cost of generating long-read data is currently significantly higher than that of short-read data (Goodwin et al., 2016; Olson et al., 2023).

Because of the extensive experience validating the presence of genetic variants from next-generation sequencing data, most single nucleotide variants do not require confirmation by another method (Beck et al., 2016). However, copy number variants are not as reliably called and often require orthogonal confirmation by quantitative PCR, digital droplet PCR, or an array-based assay (Rajagopalan et al., 2020; Teo et al., 2012). DNA from dried blood spots may not be sufficient for these assays and may therefore require contacting the family and obtaining an additional sample for variant confirmation.

Condition Considerations

Public health newborn screening must remain focused on conditions that are serious, urgent, and treatable to align with public health ethical principles (Chapter 3). Which conditions to include in public health newborn screening must be guided by these criteria rather than the scope of conditions any given technological tool might enable.

Genomic sequencing generates tremendous amounts of data, and much of that should not be the focus of public health newborn screening. For example, all individuals are carriers for multiple autosomal recessive conditions, and being a carrier has no immediate clinical usefulness for the newborn (Clayton, 2010; Fridman et al., 2021; Gao et al., 2015). This information should not be analyzed or returned as part of the public health NBS program both because it does not align with the goals of the program and because of the enormous infrastructure that would be required to support returning this information (see Chapter 3 for further discussion). As described in the methodological considerations section, bioinformatics pipelines may be developed to avert findings related to carrier status when screening for a particular condition. Similarly, data that lead to information that is not medically actionable until adulthood should not be analyzed to become reportable information (hereditary cancer risk such as *BRCA1/BRCA2* or Huntington disease) as it is beyond the scope of the public health program.

Serious conditions that are genetic and amenable to detection by genomic sequencing methods, for which there is an available, effective intervention with proven benefit, and for which individuals are routinely symptomatic at a young age, should all be routinely considered for public health newborn screening even if the condition is rare. Birth prevalence is not a critical factor since the marginal cost of adding a condition once the platform is in use would be minimal. There is a need for ongoing research outside of public health feasibility studies that generates scientific and programmatic evidence to inform decisions about whether to include additional conditions for which treatment is available but not completely effective, for lethal/severe conditions with open clinical trials, and for conditions with gene variants that may or may not result in diseases.

Some conditions require early recognition and treatment and have a readily detectable biomarker with well-established reference ranges (e.g., maple syrup urine disease and galactosemia) (Ding and Han, 2022). It is likely that metabolites and enzyme activities will continue to be the first-tier test and will not be soon supplanted by genomic sequencing unless and until the turnaround time and predictive value of sequencing matches that of metabolite and enzyme activities screening (Bick et al., 2022; Friedman et al., 2017; Tarini and Goldenberg, 2012). Further, some conditions do not have a known genetic cause of all cases and therefore biochemical screening is appropriate (e.g., congenital hypothyroidism) (Persani et al., 2018). On the other hand, given the evolving gene-editing methods that require precise information about the DNA variants causing disease, molecular confirmation of the condition could act as an orthogonal confirmation and determine eligibility for gene therapy (Henderson et al., 2024).

Variant Interpretation and Inclusion Considerations

Currently, NBS tests are designed to identify nearly all affected infants (high sensitivity) but may have a high rate of false positives (lower specificity). For biochemical tests, this paradigm determines how cutoff values are set for biochemical markers (Moyer et al., 2008). For DNA-based screens, which variants to include is also determined based on a balance of sensitivity and specificity. Variants are interpreted and categorized as either pathogenic, likely pathogenic, uncertain significance, likely benign, and benign based on the American College of Medical Genetics and Genomics (ACMG) guidelines (Richards et al., 2015).[6] Variants of uncertain significance (VUS) are challenging when considering what to report as part of public health newborn screening as they could potentially be biologically deleterious (Burke et al., 2022). However, with thousands of VUS, extending the current paradigm of high sensitivity, lower specificity to genome-based screens could risk overwhelming public health programs, clinical care, and families with too many false positives and too much ambiguity (Woerner et al., 2021).

Variant interpretation is not currently accurate across all populations based on the representation of different genetic ancestries in genomic and clinical databases (Gudmundsson et al., 2021; Manrai et al., 2016; Petrovski and Goldstein, 2016). For instance, there is a significant bias toward individuals of European ancestry in ClinVar[7] (Naslavsky et al., 2021). Therefore, variant interpretation pipelines that filter in only pathogenic and likely pathogenic variants may lead to underreporting of disease-causing variants for individuals who are not of European ancestry (Mori et al., 2024). Conversely, if all rare variants were filtered in for manual review, many variants that are rare or absent in the Genome Aggregation Database (gnomAD)[8] (Figure 5-2) yet common in some part of the world would be at greater risk for misclassification (Shah et al., 2018), potentially leading to prognostic odysseys and taxing both public health and clinical care systems (Friedman et al., 2017).

Challenges posed by variant interpretation replicate other challenges that arise in public health newborn screening based off limited knowledge. Sequencing across a population invariably reveals new information beyond what has been learned through clinical populations. Such information could change the interpretation of a particular variant or the understanding of that variant's phenotypic penetrance, among other factors. Therefore, continued research with nonclinical populations and across different ancestral groups is critical to improve variant interpretation.

Given the many genetic ancestries of people born in the United States (Bryc et al., 2015), a more comprehensive understanding of variants and

---

[6] Updated standards for sequence variant classification will be released by ACMG in the spring of 2025.
[7] ClinVar is a public archive of human genetic variants and their relationships to disease and drug responses maintained by the NIH. See https://www.ncbi.nlm.nih.gov/clinvar/ (accessed March 6, 2025).
[8] gnomAD is a publicly available collection of human genetic data developed by an international coalition of investigators with the goal of aggregating and harmonizing both exome and genome sequencing data from across the world. See https://gnomad.broadinstitute.org/ (accessed March 6, 2025).

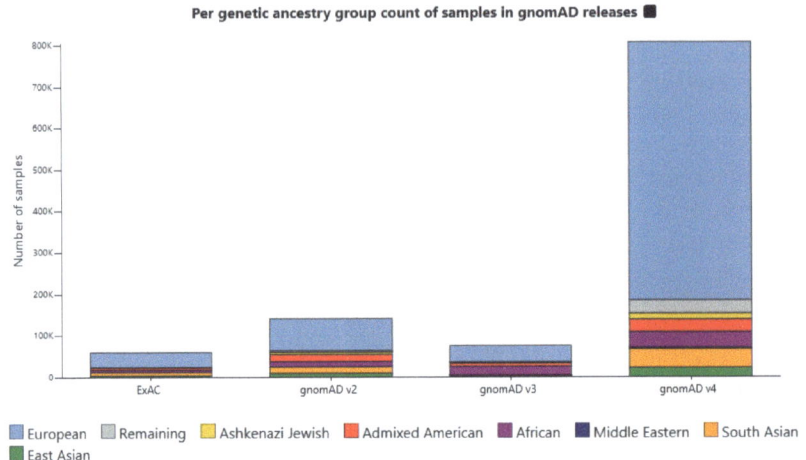

FIGURE 5-2 Composition of ancestral groups included in gnomAD.
SOURCE: Genome Aggregation Database (gnomAD); https://gnomad.broadinstitute.org/stats#diversity (accessed March 11, 2025).

their pathogenicity across ancestral groups is essential. Current challenges to this goal include inadequate representation of genetic ancestries in genomic databases (Corpas et al., 2025), lack of standardized data formats across global large-scale sequencing studies (Abdelhalim et al., 2022), and insufficient information about the pathogenicity of VUS (Burke et al., 2022). Continued actions are needed to address these issues with the goal of improving variant interpretation across all populations. Large-scale sequencing research studies (e.g., All of Us,[9] H3Africa,[10] GenomeAsia 100K[11]) can continue expanding representation of ancestral groups from across the globe through thoughtful community engagement, among other approaches (Lemke et al., 2022, NASEM, 2018, 2024). These studies can also collaborate on standardizing data formats to enable data integration across studies. Data can be shared with a central resource, such as gnomAD, which is currently the largest and most widely used publicly available collection of population variation from harmonized sequencing data (Gudmundsson et al., 2021). Functional studies in animal models can also begin to unravel the pathogenicity of VUS (Yamamoto et al., 2024). Continued research in these areas is crucial for high-quality variant interpretation across the population of the United States.

---

[9] See https://allofus.nih.gov/ (accessed February 13, 2025).
[10] See https://h3africa.org/ (accessed February 13, 2025).
[11] See https://www.genomeasia100k.org/ (accessed February 13, 2025).

If genomic sequencing were incorporated into public health newborn screening, strategies would be needed for interpreting and reporting variants that consider the limitations described above. A balance could be struck by returning only a subset of VUS based on the probability that the variant is truly deleterious determined by a predefined threshold of computational predictions along with availability of inexpensive orthogonal confirmatory assays and an effective treatment, as well as the severity of the clinical consequences of missing a treatment window. Employing confirmatory assays, for example biochemical assays that confirm reduced levels of a certain metabolite, would be essential for restricting reporting to relevant variants. With time, the sensitivity of screening for a condition using sequencing could increase as variant interpretation for the causative gene improves. However, incorporating genomics into public health newborn screening may necessitate a shift toward accepting more false negatives in favor of fewer false positives initially to avoid reporting unclear and unactionable information to parents (Gelb, 2024). This initial practice would be improved over time with knowledge growth about variants across ancestral groups (as indicated in Figure 5-2) and can be mitigated by including only a subset of VUS that can be orthogonally confirmed as pathogenic. Further research is needed to address variant interpretation accuracy across all ancestral populations and how to navigate this issue in a transparent and trustworthy manner.

Data Considerations

"Blood spots contain genetic material that is intensely personal." – Parent

Ensuring data privacy and security would be a challenge to implementing genomic sequencing in public health newborn screening. Ethicists, data privacy advocates, and others have raised concerns about the loss of genetic privacy that could be furthered by sequencing healthy newborns (NASEM, 2023). Unethical uses of genetic information would also be possible in the absence of appropriate regulations. For example, law enforcement could misuse genetic data, mirroring prior seizures of newborn dried blood spots as part of a criminal investigation, if protections are not put in place (Grant, 2022, 2023; Ram, 2022). Parents have expressed concerns about genetic information leading to insurance or employment discrimination (Genetti et al., 2019). Although the Genetic Information Nondiscrimination Act provides protections against health insurance and employment discrimination,[12] it does not provide federal protections against genetic discrimination by life, long-term care, or

---

[12] The Genetic Information Nondiscrimination Act of 2008, P.L. 110-233, 122 Stat. 881.

disability insurers nor does it apply to private companies with fewer than 15 employees, the U.S. military health system, the Indian Health Service, and others (Laboratory, 2023). Beyond these factors, sequencing generates tremendous amounts of data that could challenge public health storage capacities if raw sequence data were stored.

If genomic sequencing were applied to public health newborn screening, privacy concerns must be addressed at several stages including methodological design, storage, governance, and disposition. Methodological design would need to be responsive to concerns about data privacy and only analyze, report, and potentially store sequences relevant to the conditions screened (Tarini and Goldenberg, 2012). Strict governance about who can access the data and under what circumstances would need to be established to ensure trustworthiness. For example, law enforcement would need to be barred from access to NBS samples or the associated data at least for the purposes of prosecution (Grant, 2022, 2023; Ram, 2022; Suter, 2022).[13] Robust encryption and security protocols would be needed, and capacity to store such data would need to be built.

Options for data destruction after a period of time (e.g., after diagnosis or a set number of years), at the request of the individual or their parents, or with sensitivity to local, community, and cultural contexts would need to be considered (Fleskes et al., 2022; Lewis, 2019; NASEM, 2023). Existing frameworks can guide the ethical stewardship of samples or data generated through public health newborn screening at each of these steps (see Box 5-3) (NASEM, 2023; WHO, 2024). See Chapter 4 for an exploration of the complicated landscape of policies and ligation concerning residual dried blood spots and data derived from public health newborn screening, including areas of consideration for genomic data.

Implementation and Scaling Considerations

If genomic sequencing were to be implemented at scale, sufficient and sustainable funding would be necessary to meet the technical and workforce needs and to avert straining a resource-constrained environment (Andrews et al., 2022; Currier, 2022; NASEM, 2023). The cost of the sequence data generation and interpretation depends on the scale since there is an economy

---

[13] A thornier issue is whether exceptions could be made for using a dried blood spot to identify a missing or deceased child. See https://www.babysfirsttest.org/newborn-screening/what-happens-to-the-blood-sample#:~:text=The%20dried%20blood%20spots%20can,child%20at%20the%20parent's%20request (accessed January 16, 2025).

> **BOX 5-3**
> **Frameworks for Ethical Genomics Data Use and Sharing**
>
> Ethical stewardship of samples and data generated through newborn screening, both in research and public health contexts, is vital. Extensive work has been conducted to build frameworks that enhance ethical genomics data use and sharing, particularly for research (Atutornu et al., 2022; Claw et al., 2018; WHO, 2024). These frameworks can be drawn on when considering governance for genomics data generated through newborn sequencing research and if genomic sequencing were ever applied to public health newborn screening. Many of these frameworks concern principles for ethical engagement with groups, including Indigenous communities, who are underrepresented in genomic databases, and thus, are less likely to benefit from genomics and precision medicine (Claw et al., 2018).
>
> The World Health Organization (WHO) recently released guidance for human genome data collection, access, use, and sharing to inform policy makers, researchers, clinicians, and others on handling human genome data in a manner that "advances genomics for individual and population health, protects individual and collective rights and interests, and fosters public trust" (WHO, 2024, p. iv) The guidance aims to (1) promote social and cultural inclusiveness, equity, and justice; (2) promote trustworthiness within the data life cycle; (3) foster integrity and good stewardship; (4) promote communal and personal benefits; and (5) promote the use of common principles in laws, policies, frameworks, and guidelines, within and across countries and contexts. Refer to the WHO guidance for additional details (WHO, 2024).

of scale. Costs include (1) DNA extraction; (2) sequence generation; (3) computational costs for sequence alignment as well as variant filtering and interpretation, data storage, and confirmatory testing; and (4) capital costs for equipment, reagents, and personnel. Sequencing costs have fallen below $1000 per genome (NHGRI, 2023), with variation depending on the test run and the scale at which the tests are performed. These costs are comparatively higher than current fees associated with public health newborn screening, which range from $30 dollars to $258 per test.[14] Over time, costs associated with genomic sequencing could decrease as improvements in efficiency and automation of data generation and variant interpretation occur. In addition to sequencing-related costs, investing in the development of the public health workforce would be needed to ensure the appropriate expertise and skills to support sequencing, variant interpretation, and following up on those results (NASEM, 2023).

---

[14] See https://www.newsteps.org/data-resources/reports/nbs-fees-report (accessed February 11, 2025) for up-to-date information on each state and territorial NBS program's associated fees. Five programs do not charge a fee.

It would likely be unnecessary for all programs to perform their own sequencing and interpretation. Instead, scaling could be achieved in part by the regionalization of sequencing and/or interpretation either initially or long term as state-run programs consider their approach (Andrews et al., 2022). Efforts would be needed to ensure that the application of sequencing does not drive further geographic disparities between the services provided by different state-run programs. Such strategies could include establishing technical support centers, providing additional funding, and developing distributed systems of clinical expertise (see Chapter 4). With appropriate supports, implementation of genomic sequencing could reduce variations in conditions screened across NBS programs by increasing the efficiency of adding new conditions.

Extensive infrastructure would be required for genomic sequencing to be a first-tier test for public health newborn screening. A harmonized infrastructure within public health or referral/regional laboratories would be necessary for DNA extraction, sequence data generation, and variant interpretation. Variant interpretation would need to be rapid, automated, scalable, accurate, and equitable—with flexibility for manual curation as needed; this could be done in part with artificial intelligence, and would improve with more data and experience. Laboratory information management systems would need to be modernized to accommodate sequence interpretation and reporting with the appropriate security features. Data retention and use policy must be developed, and data storage capacity and security must be sufficient.

Clear and effective communication would be needed to inform, educate, and empower the public, parents, and care providers (APHA, 2019; Johnston et al., 2018; WHO, 2024). A workforce of clinicians would be needed to discuss results with families, confirm the diagnoses, and initiate appropriate care and surveillance (Friedman et al., 2017; NASEM, 2023). A data track in ClinVar would be necessary to share variant interpretations and tag the source as that of newborn screening. Ideally, a federated national infrastructure would be needed to track the clinical outcomes of the newborns identified through sequencing-based public health newborn screening to iteratively improve the process including accurate interpretation of variants, disease penetrance, and effectiveness and timing of treatment (see Chapter 6 for information about long-term follow-up).

At this stage, genomic sequencing is not yet ready for implementation at scale in public health programs outside of a consented research study context. More research is needed to address the scientific, technical, ethical, and practical challenges before genomic sequencing could be considered for implementation in the United States. Box 5-4 presents key areas and selected questions that need to be addressed.

BOX 5-4
Selected Questions to Address Before Considering Applying Genomic Sequencing to Public Health Newborn Screening

Findings from ongoing newborn sequencing studies indicate the potential usefulness of genomic sequencing in public health newborn screening. However, many questions remain about how it could be implemented responsibly, whether it is acceptable to the public, what protections might be needed, how to ensure access and accurate interpretation across all populations, whether it is economically and practically feasible, and more. In addition to scientific and technical research, social and behavioral science research will be needed to address these questions. Although not an exhaustive list, here are key areas and selected questions that must be addressed when considering the potential application of genomic sequencing to public health newborn screening.

Scientific and Technical Questions

- What sequence should be generated, what sequence/variants should be analyzed, and what results should be returned?
- What method is most appropriate to generate the target sequence?
- How should the inclusion of conditions be handled when performing population-wide screening may reveal more nuanced symptomatology than initially understood?
- How should variants to report be chosen when population-wide screening may reveal variable penetrance or different symptomatology?
- What strategies are necessary to address accurate variant interpretation across all ancestral populations?
- Will the turnaround time be sufficiently fast while maintaining accuracy to meet timeliness standards?

Ethical, Legal, and Social Issues (ELSI) Questions

- What are public attitudes concerning the application of genomic sequencing into public health newborn screening as a first-tier screening tool?
- What are public attitudes about the role of consent in newborn screening, and how does changing the consent model affect who receives screening?
- What data should be stored after screening, if any, and how will the privacy of genetic data be protected?
- Should stored genomic data be allowed to be used clinically beyond the initial NBS result, if a child becomes symptomatic and could use the data to diagnose a genetic condition not included in newborn screening?
- What considerations should guide any nonclinical secondary uses of stored genomic data, including in research?

Feasibility Questions

- Is genomic sequencing as a first-tier screening methodology cost-effective?
- If public health newborn screening moved toward a consent model, how would informed consent be obtained from parents? Is collection of informed consent feasible?

> **BOX 5-4 Continued**
>
> - What funding, resource sharing, and/or distributed system of clinical expertise would be necessary and effective to support capacity across NBS programs to employ genomic sequencing as a first-tier tool in a high-quality manner across all populations?
> - How would genomic sequencing be integrated with current screening tools?
> - What training is needed for health care providers to interpret DNA-based NBS results and provide guidance to families?

CONCLUSIONS

Conclusion 5-1: Decisions on the inclusion of emerging technologies need to be guided by what is the most suitable tool available to screen for conditions that meet inclusion criteria for public health newborn screening, and such decisions need to be consistent with the core principles of these programs.

Conclusion 5-2: Genomic sequencing that collects and returns results beyond the scope of conditions that are serious, urgent, and treatable is not consistent with the public health focus of newborn screening. Consented research and clinical care can be appropriate venues to attain such information.

Conclusion 5-3: Although genomic sequencing for a targeted panel of genes has the potential to be useful, important technical, ethical, psychosocial, and implementation questions need to be addressed to fully understand the anticipated and unanticipated consequences before its application can be considered for public health newborn screening.

Conclusion 5-4: A more comprehensive understanding of genetic variants and their relationship to disease for many ancestral groups is essential to ensure accurate variant interpretation across the population of infants born in the United States.

REFERENCES

Abdelhalim, H., A. Berber, M. Lodi, R. Jain, A. Nair, A. Pappu, K. Patel, V. Venkat, C. Venkatesan, R. Wable, M. Dinatale, A. Fu, V. Iyer, I. Kalove, M. Kleyman, J. Koutsoutis, D. Menna, M. Paliwal, N. Patel, T. Patel, Z. Rafique, R. Samadi, R. Varadhan, S. Bolla, S. Vadapalli, and Z. Ahmed. 2022. Artificial intelligence, healthcare, clinical genomics, and pharmacogenomics approaches in precision medicine. *Frontiers in Genetics* 13:929736.

ACHDNC (Advisory Committee on Heritable Disorders in Newborns and Children). 2011. *Newborn screening for severe combined immunodeficiency disorder.* https://www.hrsa.gov/sites/default/files/hrsa/advisory-committees/heritable-disorders/reports-recommendations/newborn-screening-scid-report.pdf (accessed December 18, 2024).

Adhikari, A. N., R. C. Gallagher, Y. Wang, R. J. Currier, G. Amatuni, L. Bassaganyas, F. Chen, K. Kundu, M. Kvale, S. D. Mooney, R. L. Nussbaum, S. S. Randi, J. Sanford, J. T. Shieh, R. Srinivasan, U. Sunderam, H. Tang, D. Vaka, Y. Zou, B. A. Koenig, P.-Y. Kwok, N. Risch, J. M. Puck, and S. E. Brenner. 2020. The role of exome sequencing in newborn screening for inborn errors of metabolism. *Nature Medicine* 26(9):1392-1397.

Almannai, M., R. Marom, and V. R. Sutton. 2016. Newborn screening: A review of history, recent advancements, and future perspectives in the era of next generation sequencing. *Current Opinion in Pediatrics* 28(6):694-699.

Andrews, S. M., K. A. Porter, D. B. Bailey, and H. L. Peay. 2022. Preparing newborn screening for the future: A collaborative stakeholder engagement exploring challenges and opportunities to modernizing the newborn screening system. *BMC Pediatrics* 22(1):90.

APHA (American Public Health Association). 2019. *Public health code of ethics.* https://www.apha.org/-/media/files/pdf/membergroups/ethics/code_of_ethics.ashx (accessed December 18, 2024).

Atutornu, J., R. Milne, A. Costa, C. Patch, and A. Middleton. 2022. Towards equitable and trustworthy genomics research. *eBioMedicine* 76:103879.

Bailey, D. B., Jr., L. M. Gehtland, M. A. Lewis, H. Peay, M. Raspa, S. M. Shone, J. L. Taylor, A. C. Wheeler, M. Cotten, N. M. P. King, C. M. Powell, B. Bieseker, C. E. Bishop, B. L. Boyea, M. Duparc, B. A. Harper, A. R. Kemper, S. N. Lee, R. Moultrie, K. C. Okoniewski, R. S. Paquin, D. Pettit, K. A. Porter, and S. J. Zimmerman. 2019. Early check: Translational science at the intersection of public health and newborn screening. *BMC Pediatrics* 19(1):238.

Beck, T. F., J. C. Mullikin, and L. G. Biesecker. 2016. Systematic evaluation of Sanger validation of next-generation sequencing variants. *Clinical Chemistry* 62(4):647-654.

Berg, J. S., P. B. Agrawal, D. B. Bailey, Jr., A. H. Beggs, S. E. Brenner, A. M. Brower, J. A. Cakici, O. Ceyhan-Birsoy, K. Chan, F. Chen, R. Currier, D. Dukhovny, R. Green, J. Harris-Wai, I. Holm, B. Iglesias, G. Joseph, S. F. Kingsmore, B. Koenig, P.-Y. Kwok, J. Lantos, S. J. Leeder, M. A. Lewis, A. McGuire, L. Milko, S. Mooney, R. Parad, S. Pereira, J. Petrikin, B. Powell, C. Powell, J Puck, H. Rehm, N. Risch, M. Roche, J. T. Shieh, N. Veeraraghavan, M. S. Watson, L. Willig, T. Yu, T. Urv, and A. L. Wise. 2017. Newborn sequencing in genomic medicine and public health. *Pediatrics* 139(2):e20162252.

Bick, D., A. Ahmed, D. Deen, A. Ferlini, N. Garnier, D. Kasperaviciute, M. Leblond, A. Pichini, A. Rendon, A. Satija, A. Tuff-Lacey, and R. H. Scott. 2022. Newborn screening by genomic sequencing: Opportunities and challenges. *International Journal of Neonatal Screening* 8(3):40.

Bryc, K., E. Y. Durand, J. M. Macpherson, D. Reich, and J. L. Mountain. 2015. The genetic ancestry of African Americans, Latinos, and European Americans across the United States. *American Journal of Human Genetics* 96(1):37-53.

Burke, W., E. Parens, W. K. Chung, S. M. Berger, and P. S. Appelbaum. 2022. The challenge of genetic variants of uncertain clinical significance: A narrative review. *Annals of Internal Medicine* 175(7):994-1000.

CDC (Centers for Disease Control and Prevention). 2024. Figure used as part of "A Partnership to Expand and Enhance Newborn Screening in New York State—The GUARDIAN Study," presented at International Consortium of Newborn Sequencing (ICoNS) conference, October 9, 2024.

Ceyhan-Birsoy, O., J. B. Murry, K. Machini, M. S. Lebo, T. W. Yu, S. Fayer, C. Genett, T. Schwartz, P. Agrawal, R. Parad, I. Holm, A. McGuire, R. Green, H. Rehm, and A. Beggs. 2019. Interpretation of genomic sequencing results in healthy and ill newborns: Results from the BabySeq project. *American Journal of Human Genetics* 104(1):76-93.

Claw, K. G., M. Z. Anderson, R. L. Begay, K. S. Tsosie, K. Fox, and N. A. Garrison. 2018. A framework for enhancing ethical genomic research with indigenous communities. *Nature Communications* 9(1):2957.

Clayton, E. W. 2010. Currents in contemporary ethics: State run newborn screening in the genomic era, or how to avoid drowning when drinking from a fire hose. *Journal of Law, Medicine & Ethics* 38(3):697-700.

COMEST (World Commission on the Ethics of Scientific Knowledge and Technology). 2005. *The precautionary principle.* Paris: United Nations Educational, Scientific and Cultural Organization.

Cope, H., B. Lincoln-Boyea, A. Y. Gwaltney, B. B. Biesecker, R. Moultrie, A. A. Alexander, N. King, J. Check, A. Corbo, J. Tzeng, K. Porter, and H. L. Peay. 2023. Use of a web-based portal to return normal individual research results in early check: Exploring user behaviors and attitudes. *Clinical Genetics* 103(6):672-680.

Cope, H. L., L. V. Milko, E. R. Jalazo, B. G. Crissman, A. K. M. Foreman, B. C. Powell, N. deJong, J. Hunter, B. Boyea, A. Forsythe, A. Wheeler, R. Zimmerman, S. Suchy, A. Begtrup, K. Langley, K. Monaghan, C. Kraczkowski, K. Hruska, P. Kruszka, K. Kucera, J. Berg, C. Powell, and H. L. Peay. 2024. A systematic framework for selecting gene-condition pairs for inclusion in newborn sequencing panels: Early check implementation. *Genetics in Medicine* 26(12):101290.

Corpas, M., M. Pius, M. Poburennaya, H. Guio, M. Dwek, S. Nagaraj, C. Lopez-Correa, A. Popejoy, and S. Fatumo. 2025. Bridging genomics' greatest challenge: The diversity gap. *Cell Genomics* 5(1):100724.

Currier, R. J. 2022. Newborn screening is on a collision course with public health ethics. *International Journal of Neonatal Screening* 8(4):51.

Ding, S., and L. Han. 2022. Newborn screening for genetic disorders: Current status and prospects for the future. *Pediatric Investigation* 6(4):291-298.

Fleskes, R. E., A. C. Bader, K. S. Tsosie, J. K. Wagner, K. G. Claw, and N. A. Garrison. 2022. Ethical guidance in human paleogenomics: New and ongoing perspectives. *Annual Review of Genomics and Human Genetics* 23:627-652.

Fridman, H., H. G. Yntema, R. Mägi, R. Andreson, A. Metspalu, M. Mezzavilla, C. Tyler-Smith, Y. Xue, S. Carmi, E. Levy-Lahad, C. Gilissen, and H. G. Brunner. 2021. The landscape of autosomal-recessive pathogenic variants in european populations reveals phenotype-specific effects. *American Journal of Human Genetics* 108(4):608-619.

Friedman, J. M., M. C. Cornel, A. J. Goldenberg, K. J. Lister, K. Sénécal, D. F. Vears, and the Global Alliance for Genomics and Health Regulatory and Ethics Working Group Paediatric Task Team. 2017. Genomic newborn screening: Public health policy considerations and recommendations. *BMC Medical Genomics* 10(1):9.

Furnier, S. M., M. S. Durkin, and M. W. Baker. 2020. Translating molecular technologies into routine newborn screening practice. *International Journal of Neonatal Screening* 6(4):80.

Gao, Z., D. Waggoner, M. Stephens, C. Ober, and M. Przeworski. 2015. An estimate of the average number of recessive lethal mutations carried by humans. *Genetics* 199(4):1243-1254.

Gelb, M. 2024. *Expansion of newborn screening by consolidated biomarker assays and genomic sequencing to find highly penetrant genotypes.* Presented at Newborn Screening: Current Landscape and Future Directions: Meeting 3. https://www.nationalacademies.org/event/42550_05-2024_newborn-screening-current-landscape-and-future-directions-meeting-3 (accessed January 22, 2025).

Genetti, C. A., T. S. Schwartz, J. O. Robinson, G. E. VanNoy, D. Petersen, S. Pereira, S. Fayer, H. Peoples, P. Agrawal, W. Betting, I. Holm, A. McGuire, S. Waisbren, T. Yu, R. Green, A. Beggs, R. Parad, and T. W. Yu. 2019. Parental interest in genomic sequencing of newborns: Enrollment experience from the BabySeq project. *Genetics in Medicine* 21(3):622-630.

Goodwin, S., J. D. McPherson, and W. R. McCombie. 2016. Coming of age: Ten years of next-generation sequencing technologies. *Nature Reviews Genetics* 17(6):333-351.

Grant, C. 2022. *Police are using newborn genetic screening to search for suspects, threatening privacy and public health.* https://www.aclu-nj.org/en/news/police-are-using-newborn-genetic-screening-search-suspects-threatening-privacy-and-public (accessed July 23, 2024).

Grant, C. 2023. *Widespread newborn DNA sequencing will worsen risks to genetic privacy.* https://www.aclu.org/news/privacy-technology/widespread-newborn-dna-sequencing-will-worsen-risks-to-genetic-privacy (accessed January 20, 2025).

GUARDIAN Study. n.d. *Conditions screened.* https://guardian-study.org/conditions-screened/ (accessed January 20, 2025).

Gudmundsson, S., M. Singer-Berk, N. A. Watts, W. Phu, J. K. Goodrich, M. Solomonson, Genome Aggregation Database Consortium, H. L. Rehm, D. G. MacArthur, and A. O'Donnell-Luria. 2021. Variant interpretation using population databases: Lessons from gnomAD. *Human Mutation* 43:1012-1030.

Henderson, M. L., J. K. Zieba, X. Li, D. B. Campbell, M. R. Williams, D. L. Vogt, C. Bupp, Y. Edgerly, S. Rajasekaran, N. Hartog, J. Prokop, and J. M. Krueger. 2024. Gene therapy for genetic syndromes: Understanding the current state to guide future care. *BioTech* 13(1):1.

Holm, I. A., P. B. Agrawal, O. Ceyhan-Birsoy, K. D. Christensen, S. Fayer, L. A. Frankel, C. A. Genetti, J. B. Krier, R. C. LaMay, H. L. Levy, A. McGuire, R. B. Parad, P. J. Parker, S. Pereira, H. L. Rehm, T. S. Schwartz, S. E. Waisbren, T. W. Yu, BabySeq Project Team, R. C. Green, and A. Beggs. The BabySeq Project. 2018. The BabySeq project: Implementing genomic sequencing in newborns. *BMC Pediatrics* 18(1):225.

Jameson, J. L., and D. L. Longo. 2015. Precision medicine—Personalized, problematic, and promising. *New England Journal of Medicine* 372(23):2229-2234.

JAX Clinical Education 2023. *Genetic information nondiscrimination act (GINA).* The Jackson Laboratory. https://www.jax.org/education-and-learning/clinical-and-continuing-education/clinical-topics/gina-overview# (accessed January 20, 2025).

Jezkova, J., S. Shaw, N. V. Taverner, and H. J. Williams. 2022. Rapid genome sequencing for pediatrics. *Human Mutation* 43(11):1507-1518.

Johnston, J., J. D. Lantos, A. Goldenberg, F. Chen, E. Parens, B. A. Koenig, and members of the NSIGHT Ethics and Policy Advisory Board. 2018. Sequencing newborns: A call for nuanced use of genomic technologies. *Hastings Center Report* 48(S2):S2-S6.

Kingsmore, S. F. 2022. Dispatches from biotech beginning BeginNGS: Rapid newborn genome sequencing to end the diagnostic and therapeutic odyssey. *American Journal of Medical Genetics Part C: Seminars in Medical Genetics* 190(2):243-256.

Kingsmore, S. F., R. Nofsinger, and K. Ellsworth. 2024. Rapid genomic sequencing for genetic disease diagnosis and therapy in intensive care units: A review. *npj Genomic Medicine* 9(1):17.

Koenig, B. A. 1988. The technological imperative in medical practice: The social creation of a "routine" treatment. In *Biomedicine Examined*, edited by M. Lock and D. Gordon. Dordrecht, The Netherlands: Springer Netherlands. Pp. 465-496.

Kraszewski, J. N., D. M. Kay, C. F. Stevens, C. Koval, B. Haser, V. Ortiz, A. Albertorio, L. Cohen, R. Jain, S. P. Andrew, S. D. Young, N. LaMarca, D. De Vivo, M. Caggana, and W. K. Chung. 2018. Pilot study of population-based newborn screening for spinal muscular atrophy in New York State. *Genetics in Medicine* 20(6):608-613.

Kucera, K. S., J. L. Taylor, V. R. Robles, K. Clinard, B. Migliore, B. L. Boyea, K. C. Okoniewski, M. Duparc, C. Rehder, S. Shone, Z. Fan, M. Raspa, H. Peay, A. Wheeler, C. Powell, D. Bailey, Jr., and L. M. Gehtland. 2021. A voluntary statewide newborn screening pilot for spinal muscular atrophy: Results from early check. *International Journal of Neonatal Screening* 7(1):20.

Lemke, A. A., E. D. Esplin, A. J. Goldenberg, C. Gonzaga-Jauregui, N. A. Hanchard, J. Harris-Wai, J. E. Ideozu, R. Isasi, A. P. Landstrom, A. E. R. Prince, E. Turbitt, M. Sabatello, S. A. S. Vergano, M. R. G. Taylor, J. Yu, K. B. Brothers, and N. A. Garrison. 2022. Addressing underrepresentation in genomics research through community engagement. *American Journal of Human Genetics* 109(9):1563-1571.

Lewis, D. 2019. Australian biobank repatriates hundreds of 'legacy' Indigenous blood samples. *Nature News.* https://www.nature.com/articles/d41586-019-03906-5 (accessed December 30, 2024).

Manrai, A. K., B. H. Funke, H. L. Rehm, M. S. Olesen, B. A. Maron, P. Szolovits, D. M. Margulies, J. Loscalzo, and I. S. Kohane. 2016. Genetic misdiagnoses and the potential for health disparities. *New England Journal of Medicine* 375:655-665.

Minear, M. A., M. N. Phillips, A. Kau, and M. A. Parisi. 2022. Newborn screening research sponsored by the NIH: From diagnostic paradigms to precision therapeutics. *American Journal of Medical Genetics Part C: Seminars in Medical Genetics* 190(2):138-152.

Mori, M., B. P. Chaudhari, M. A. Ream, and A. R. Kemper. 2024. Promises and challenges of genomic newborn screening (NBS) – Lessons from public health NBS programs. *Pediatric Research* 97:1327-1336.

Moyer, V. A., N. Calonge, S. M. Teutsch, J. R. Botkin, and USPSTF. 2008. Expanding newborn screening: Process, policy, and priorities. *Hastings Center Report* 38(3):32-39.

NASEM (National Academies of Sciences, Engineering, and Medicine). 2018. *Understanding disparities in access to genomic medicine: Proceedings of a workshop.* Washington, DC: The National Academies Press.

NASEM. 2019. *Framework for addressing ethical dimensions of emerging and innovative biomedical technologies: A synthesis of relevant national academies reports.* Edited by L. Rand and N. Dickert. Washington, DC: The National Academies Press.

NASEM. 2023. *The promise and perils of next-generation DNA sequencing at birth: Proceedings of a workshop – in brief.* Washington, DC: The National Academies Press.

NASEM. 2024. *Sustaining community engagement in genomics research: Proceedings of a workshop – in brief.* Washington, DC: The National Academies Press.

Naslavsky, M. S., M. O. Scliar, K. Nunes, J. Y. T. Wang, G. L. Yamamoto, H. Guio, E. Tarazona-Santos, Y. Duarte, M. R. Passos-Bueno, D. Meyer, and M. Zatz. 2021. Biased pathogenic assertions of loss of function variants challenge molecular diagnosis of admixed individuals. *American Journal of Medical Genetics Part C: Seminars in Medical Genetics* 187(3):357-363.

NHGRI (National Human Genome Research Institute). 2023. *DNA sequencing costs: Data.* https://www.genome.gov/about-genomics/fact-sheets/DNA-Sequencing-Costs-Data (accessed January 20, 2025).

NHGRI. 2025. *Pathogenic variant.* https://www.genome.gov/genetics-glossary/Pathogenic-Variant (accessed March 7, 2025).

NIH (National Insitutes of Health). 2022. *Newborn sequencing in genomic medicine and public health (NSIGHT).* https://www.genome.gov/Funded-Programs-Projects/Newborn-Sequencing-in-Genomic-Medicine-and-Public-Health-NSIGHT (accessed December 30, 2024).

Olson, N. D., J. Wagner, N. Dwarshuis, K. H. Miga, F. J. Sedlazeck, M. Salit, and J. M. Zook. 2023. Variant calling and benchmarking in an era of complete human genome sequences. *Nature Reviews Genetics* 24:464-483.

Paquin, R. S., M. A. Lewis, B. A. Harper, R. R. Moultrie, A. Gwaltney, L. M. Gehtland, H. Peay, M. Duparc, M. Raspa, A. Wheeler, C. Powell, N. King, S. Shone, and D. B. Bailey, Jr. 2021. Outreach to new mothers through direct mail and email: Recruitment in the early check research study. *Clinical and Translational Science* 14(3):880-889.

Peay, H. L., A. Y. Gwaltney, R. Moultrie, H. Cope, B. L. Boyea, K. A. Porter, M. Duparc, A. Alexander, B. Biesecker, A. Isiaq, J. Check, L. Gehtland, D. Bailey, Jr., and N. M. P. King. 2022. Education and consent for population-based DNA screening: A mixed-methods evaluation of the early check newborn screening pilot study. *Frontiers in Genetics* 13:891592.

Pereira, S., and E. W. Clayton. 2018. Commercial interests, the technological imperative, and advocates: Three forces driving genomic sequencing in newborns. *Hastings Center Report* 48(S2):S43-S44.

Persani, L., G. Rurale, T. de Filippis, E. Galazzi, M. Muzza, and L. Fugazzola. 2018. Genetics and management of congenital hypothyroidism. *Best Practice & Research Clinical Endocrinology & Metabolism* 32(4):387-396.

Petrovski, S., and D. B. Goldstein. 2016. Unequal representation of genetic variation across ancestry groups creates healthcare inequality in the application of precision medicine. *Genome Biology* 17(1):157.

Rady Children's Institute for Genomic Medicine. 2025a. *Begin NGS newborn genomic sequencing.* https://radygenomics.org/begin-ngs-newborn-sequencing/ (accessed February 11, 2025).

Rady Children's Institute for Gneomic Medicine. 2025b. *For providers: What you need to know.* https://radygenomics.org/begin-ngs-newborn-sequencing/for-providers/#instructions (accessed February 11, 2025).

Rajagopalan, R., J. R. Murrell, M. Luo, and L. K. Conlin. 2020. A highly sensitive and specific workflow for detecting rare copy-number variants from exome sequencing data. *Genome Medicine* 12(1):14.

Ram, N. 2022. America's hidden national DNA database. *Texas Law Review* 100(7):1253-1325.

Retterer, K., J. Juusola, M. T. Cho, P. Vitazka, F. Millan, F. Gibellini, A. Vertino-Bell, N. Smaoui, J. Neidich, K. Monaghan, D. McKnight, R. Bai, S. Suchy, B. Friedman, J. Tahiliani, D. Pineda-Alvarez, G. Richard, T. Brandt, E. Haverfield, W. Chung, and S. Bale. 2016. Clinical application of whole-exome sequencing across clinical indications. *Genetics in Medicine* 18(7):696-704.

Richards, S., N. Aziz, S. Bale, D. Bick, S. Das, J. Gastier-Foster, W. W. Grody, M. Hegde, E. Lyon, E. Spector, K. Voelkerding, and H. L. Rehm. 2015. Standards and guidelines for the interpretation of sequence variants: A joint consensus recommendation of the American College of Medical Genetics and Genomics and the Association for Molecular Pathology. *Genetics in Medicine* 17(5):405-424.

Roman, T. S., S. B. Crowley, M. I. Roche, A. K. M. Foreman, J. M. O'Daniel, B. A. Seifert, K. Lee, A. Brandt, C. Gustafson, D. M. DeCristo, N. T. Strande, L. Ramkissoon, L. V. Milko, P. Owen, S. Roy, M. Xiong, R. S. Paquin, R. M. Butterfield, M. A. Lewis, K. J. Souris, D. B. Bailey, Jr., C. Rini, J. K. Booker, B. C. Powell, K. E. Weck, C. M. Powell, and J. S. Berg. 2020. Genomic sequencing for newborn screening: Results of the NC nexus project. *American Journal of Human Genetics* 107(4):596-611.

Shah, N., Y.-C. C. Hou, H.-C. Yu, R. Sainger, C. T. Caskey, J. C. Venter, and A. Telenti. 2018. Identification of misclassified ClinVar variants via disease population prevalence. *American Journal of Human Genetics* 102(4):609-619.

Sheely, D. 2024. *Common fund venture program update.* Presentation to NIH Council of Councils Meeting, September 13, 2024. https://dpcpsi.nih.gov/sites/default/files/2024-09/Day-2-1105AM-CF-Venture-Update-Sheeley-508.pdf (accessed December 30, 2024).

Smith, H. S., B. Zettler, C. A. Genetti, M. R. Hickingbotham, T. F. Coleman, M. Lebo, A. Nagy, H. Zouk, L. Mahanta, K. D. Christensen, S. Pereira, N. D. Shah, N. B. Gold, S. Walmsley, S. Edwards, R. Homayouni, G. P. Krasan, H. Hakonarson, C. R. Horowitz, B. D. Gelb, B. R. Korf, A. L. McGuire, I. A. Holm, and R. C. Green. 2024. The BabySeq project: A clinical trial of genome sequencing in a diverse cohort of infants. *American Journal of Human Genetics* 111(10):2094-2106.

Suter, S. 2022. Mission creep in newborn screening and DNA forensics. *Texas Law Review* 101.

Tarini, B. A., and A. J. Goldenberg. 2012. Ethical issues with newborn screening in the genomics era. *Annual Review of Genomics and Human Genetics* 13(1):381-393.

Teo, S. M., Y. Pawitan, C. S. Ku, K. S. Chia, and A. Salim. 2012. Statistical challenges associated with detecting copy number variations with next-generation sequencing. *Bioinformatics* 28(21):2711-2718.

WHO (World Health Organization). 2024. *Guidance for human genome data collection, access, use and sharing.* Geneva: World Health Organization. https://www.who.int/publications/i/item/9789240102149 (accessed January 20, 2025).

Willig, L. K., J. E. Petrikin, L. D. Smith, C. J. Saunders, I. Thiffault, N. A. Miller, S. E. Soden, J. A. Cakici, S. M. Herd, G. Twist, A. Noll, M. Creed, P. M. Alba, S. L. Carpenter, M. A. Clements, R. T. Fischer, J. A. Hays, H. Kilbride, R. J. McDonough, J. L. Rosterman, S. L. Tsai, L. Zellmer, E. G. Farrow, and S. F. Kingsmore. 2015. Whole-genome sequencing for identification of Mendelian disorders in critically ill infants: A retrospective analysis of diagnostic and clinical findings. *Lancet Respiratory Medicine* 3(5):377-387.

Willmarth, K. 2015. The FDA and genetic testing: Improper tools for a difficult problem. *Journal of Law and the Biosciences* 2(1):158-166.

Woerner, A. C., R. C. Gallagher, J. Vockley, and A. N. Adhikari. 2021. The use of whole genome and exome sequencing for newborn screening: Challenges and opportunities for population health. *Frontiers in Pediatrics* 9:663752.

Yamamoto, S., O. Kanca, M. F. Wrangler, and H. J. Bellen. 2024. Integrating non-mammalian model organisms in the diagnosis of rare genetic diseases in humans. *Nature Reviews Genetics* 25:40-60.

Yang, Y., D. M. Muzny, J. G. Reid, M. N. Bainbridge, A. Willis, P. A. Ward, A. Braxton, J. Beuten, F. Xia, Z. Niu, M. Hardison, R. Person, M. R. Bekheirnia, M. S. Leduc, A. Kirby, P. Pham, J. Scull, M. Wang, Y. Ding, S. E. Plon, J. R. Lupski, A. L. Beaudet, R. A. Gibbs, and C. M. Eng. 2013. Clinical whole-exome sequencing for the diagnosis of Mendelian disorders. *New England Journal of Medicine* 369(16):1502-1511.

Ziegler, A., C. Koval-Burt, D. M. Kay, S. F. Suchy, A. Begtrup, K. G. Langley, R. Hernan, L. M. Amendola, B. M. Boyd, J. Bradley, T. Brandt, L. L. Cohen, A. J. Coffey, J. M. Devaney, B. Dygulska, B. Friedman, R. L. Fuleihan, A. Gyimah, S. Hahn, S. Hofherr, K. S. Hruska, Z. Hu, M. Jeanne, G. Jin, D. A. Johnson, H. Kavus, R. L. Leibel, S. J. Lobritto, S. McGee, J. D. Milner, K. McWalter, K. G. Monaghan, J. S. Orange, N. Pimentel Soler, Y. Quevedo, S. Ratner, K. Retterer, A. Shah, N. Shapiro, R. J. Sicko, E. S. Silver, S. Strom, R. I. Torene, O. Williams, V. D. Ustach, J. Wynn, R. J. Taft, P. Kruszka, M. Caggana, and W. K. Chung. 2024. Expanded newborn screening using genome sequencing for early actionable conditions. *JAMA* 333(3):232-240.

6

The Research Enterprise Relevant to Newborn Screening

"Can we identify all these different assets to see if there's a [way to have] a coordinated effort opposed to a very sequential path? . . . How can we collaborate together to have a coordinated effort?" – Newborn screening researcher

From its inception, public health newborn screening (NBS) has relied on evidence to make programmatic and policy decisions (AAP, 1967). As a public health service, decision makers must maximize public trust in newborn screening through assurances that decisions are based on solid evidence that is accurate, valid, reproducible, informative, and minimally biased (APHA, 2019; USPSTF, 2018). Virtually every aspect of public health newborn screening relies on research to generate evidence for a range of complicated questions, such as assessing which conditions to include; considering the responsible implementation of emerging technologies and updates to existing technology; navigating complex ethical and social issues; and identifying effective health service delivery practices in such areas as results communication, education and training, health outcomes, and economic evaluation. Complicating matters, most conditions considered for inclusion in newborn screening are rare and each state and territory sets its own NBS policies and practices. Thus, gathering enough standardized data to reach an acceptable evidence threshold is arduous and costly, compromising the nation's ability to make evidence-based decisions about public health newborn screening expeditiously and soundly (Minear et al., 2022).

This chapter outlines critical categories of research needed to inform public health newborn screening; it then provides an overview of the current landscape and challenges for evidence generation. The chapter closes by discussing the need for a national plan and the research infrastructure to ensure that NBS research is strategic, systematic, coordinated, nimble, and sufficiently resourced to provide the evidence needed for public health newborn screening to adjust to a rapidly changing landscape and ensure that children and their families receive the high-quality, timely care they need.

THE IMPORTANCE OF RESEARCH TO INFORM NEWBORN SCREENING

NBS research encompasses the study of methods, technologies, policies, and outcomes related to population-based screening of newborns for health conditions shortly after birth. Such research also includes studies to better understand the full range of a condition, which can only be revealed through population-level screening. Ultimately, decision makers need answers to a wide range of questions to inform the policy and practice of public health newborn screening. In general, these questions fall into four broad categories:

1. Defining conditions to guide screening, diagnosis, and treatment;
2. Applying laboratory testing and emerging technologies;
3. Understanding ethical, legal, and social issues; and
4. Investigating public health practice, feasibility, and impact.

Defining Conditions to Guide Screening, Diagnosis, and Treatment

Newborn screening has a special obligation for ensuring that screening is based on solid evidence of net benefit as a public health program that generally operates under the assumption that early screening and treatment of a serious health condition is sufficiently urgent that a state can screen babies without parental consent (Currier, 2022; Faden et al., 1982; King and Smith, 2016). To maintain public acceptance, decisions about what and when to screen must be consistently based on solid and compelling evidence (see Chapter 3 for a discussion of ethical principles and values informing decision making in public health newborn screening).

When considering a condition nominated for newborn screening, the Advisory Committee on Heritable Disorders in Newborns and Children focuses on several questions (see Chapter 2), including those related to understanding the disease proposed to be screened. Such questions include: Is the nominated condition medically serious? Are the condition's case definition and spectrum well described? Can the case definition predict the phenotype or range of symptoms in newborns and children who will be identified through population-based screening? (HRSA, 2022a). Although seemingly simple questions, underlying each are many different topics that must be addressed. Consider, for example, *case definition*. Evidence may be available that indicates that a condition can result in death or impairment; however, this may not provide a complete picture of phenotypes that could arise for a condition in population screening (Lloyd-Puryear et al., 2019). Screening of the general population reveals a condition's broader and complex phenotype and natural history that lays hidden in everyday clinical medicine where only the most severe and homogeneous cases are identified and aggregated.

A useful analogy is to picture screening for any given condition as an iceberg (Figure 6-1) (Last, 2014; Last and Adelaide, 2013). Individuals with the condition who present clinically comprise the tip of the iceberg; these tend to be the most severe cases or those with resources to access clinical care. This tip represents all the data and information that would be known about a condition before population-based screening. Screening will reveal the hidden cases of conditions—the portion of the iceberg located beneath the surface of the water. The submerged portion of the

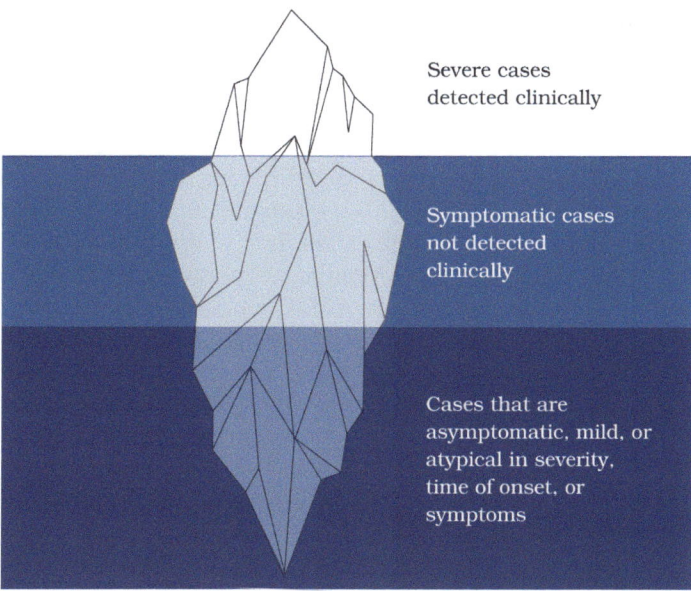

FIGURE 6-1 NBS iceberg.
NOTE: NBS = newborn screening.

iceberg is composed of cases that have evaded clinical detection because they are asymptomatic, mild, or atypical in severity, time of onset, or symptoms.

Because of this, newborn screening faces a "chicken or the egg" dilemma: how to obtain critical population-based data about the full spectrum of a condition without adding it to a mandated NBS panel. For public health newborn screening to add conditions in a manner that is ethical and evidence based, research that reveals the totality of the screening iceberg is essential because it will allow for precise characterization of prospective conditions and inform the development of more effective testing and treatment strategies. For example, if a condition has effects ranging from asymptomatic to severe, it would be important to know if the screening test or the diagnostic procedure could tell the difference, to inform treatment planning and avoid providing a risky treatment (e.g., stem cell transplant) for a child who does not actually need it (e.g., differentiating between infantile and late-onset Krabbe disease) (Guenzel et al., 2020; New York State Krabbe Disease Consortium, 2016). In the absence of population-based screening research, public health newborn screening has to grapple with these decisions in real time with real children who are left to wait and see if they develop signs or symptoms of disease (Kwon and Steiner, 2011; Timmermans and Buchbinder, 2010).

Developing Laboratory Testing and Applying Emerging Technologies

Newborn screening relies on laboratory tests. Without an accurate test that can be performed at scale in a public health laboratory, there is no newborn screening (HRSA, 2022b). Some research questions focus on developing biochemical or molecular tests for first-tier screening; some focus on second-tier screens to provide more sensitivity following an out-of-range screening result (Chen, 2012; Furnier et al., 2020). Implementing screening tests at scale also involves research to appropriately set cutoff values for what results are considered in range and out of range, among other questions that must be addressed (Chen, 2012). Each state and territorial NBS program sets its own cutoff values,[1] complicating research activities across programs (Minear et al., 2022).

Beyond these essential questions, there is also ongoing research about incorporating emerging technologies into newborn screening. Chapter 5 expands on the opportunities, challenges, and considerations for responsible application of emerging technologies, with a focus on genomic sequencing, including the research landscape and outstanding

---

[1] See https://dshs.texas.gov/laboratory-services/programs-laboratories/newborn-screening-laboratory/newborn-screening-faqs (accessed March 20, 2025).

questions. However, genomic sequencing is not the only technology that could impact the future of public health newborn screening. Research is also investigating the utility of other platform technologies, including proteomics approaches. First-tier public health newborn screening currently uses different biochemical approaches, several of which could be consolidated by employing liquid chromatography mass tandem spectrometry (LC-MS/MS) (Gelb, 2024). LC-MS/MS permits screening for more biomarkers than flow-injection analysis tandem mass spectrometry, a common approach used currently (Gelb et al., 2022). LC-MS/MS could potentially save both time and money while continuing to screen for conditions with high specificity and sensitivity (Gelb, 2024; Gelb et al., 2022). However, this approach has a limit on the number of conditions it can detect compared to genomics-based approaches (Gelb, 2024). Beyond platform technologies, researchers are also investigating potential applications of artificial intelligence and machine learning (AI/ML) for public health newborn screening (Peng et al., 2020; Zaunseder et al., 2022; Zhou et al., 2022), which are discussed in Box 6-1.

Understanding Ethical, Legal, and Social Issues

Ethical, legal, and social issues loom large in newborn screening—including the lack of reliable evidence to inform policy and practice decisions; whether parental consent is necessary; and the cost, storage, and reuse of blood spots (Baily, 2023). Data are needed to demonstrate the magnitude of a range of benefits and harms to inform policy decisions, but weighing both to determine net benefit is not easily quantifiable (Goldenberg et al., 2016; President's Council on Bioethics, 2008). For example, screening could identify late-onset or milder forms of a condition, potentially leading to "patients in waiting," anxiety, and uncertainty for families (New York State Krabbe Disease Consortium, 2016; Timmermans and Buchbinder, 2010). Some treatment regimens can be quite lengthy and painful for patients and families (Ledford, 2024). Gene therapy is expensive and offered by a limited number of medical centers, and some families may not be able to access these treatments due to cost, distance, family commitments, or other barriers (Allen et al., 2023; Levins, 2024; Peterson, 2024; Vokinger et al., 2023). A treatment might prevent death, but the child may still have severe disability (Brick et al., 2020; Larcher et al., 2015; Weise et al., 2017). Long-term outcomes of treatments or harms are often unknown, at least initially (Duncan et al., 2024). Prematurely expanding screening could exacerbate health disparities for underserved groups (Sobotka and Ross, 2023). Complex research designs are needed to address these issues, and too frequently the most critical data are missing.

> **BOX 6-1**
> **Areas of Research for Artificial Intelligence and**
> **Machine Learning in Newborn Screening**
>
> Artificial intelligence and machine learning (AI/ML) tools are being developed for a variety of applications in medicine and public health. AI/ML can be used to find patterns in large datasets that may not be detected through other computational methods or human expertise. Additionally, large language models (LLMs), a subset of AI, can process inputs and produce outputs in natural human language, facilitating non-expert interaction and streamlining communication in a range of contexts. Research is needed to better understand whether such AI capabilities could be applied to public health newborn screening in a manner that maximizes benefits while minimizing risks. Two potential applications are discussed briefly here.
>
> *Enhancing Screening Accuracy*
>
> Improving screening accuracy remains an important challenge for public health newborn screening. Emerging evidence indicates that supervised machine learning tools can be used to reduce false positives for metabolic disorders without changing a test's sensitivity. However, training these tools requires large datasets, especially for detecting rare diseases, which may necessitate new infrastructure and data sharing among different research initiatives or potentially NBS programs. In addition, ensuring the effectiveness of these models would require continuous validation and monitoring.
>
> *Support Patient Communication*
>
> LLM-based tools have been developed and deployed to support patient communication and access to care. One tool, Med-PaLM 2, accurately answers medical questions, and clinicians rated its answers to be as safe as a physician's answers. In another example, interacting with an AI chatbot for genetic counseling resulted in patient satisfaction and comprehension comparable to those for in-person services. Both examples highlight how LLMs could support NBS communication.
>
> Although LLMs can reduce administrative burdens and help to compress information to make it more digestible, they can also produce wrong answers, perpetuate biases, and produce responses that are too general to be useful for specific patient situations. Given these strengths and weaknesses, along with important ethical considerations, LLMs are generally seen as tools to assist human experts but not replace them. Further research is needed to assess whether and how these tools can be effectively and ethically applied to newborn screening.
>
> SOURCES: Al Hilli et al., 2023; Mak et al., 2023; Peng et al., 2020; Scharfe, 2024; Singhal et al., 2025; Thirunavukarasu et al., 2023.

Many ethical and social concerns about the practice of newborn screening are framed through normative arguments, when they could in fact be addressed empirically through research. Distinguishing the normative argument[2] with empirical observations provides a more robust understanding of an issue and clarifies trade-offs to enable better-informed decision making. For example, some contend that requiring consent for newborn screening could negatively affect participation rates, particularly for underserved communities, and thus, newborn screening ought to remain an opt-out program. This concern can be addressed empirically to understand whether consent might alter participation rates, and if so, whether it could disproportionately affect certain populations. Engagement as well as survey research are essential to understand public and parental attitudes about these issues and more. Such information gaps signal a need for public health ethics research to gather evidence that informs ethical decision making in this space.

Similarly, legal epidemiology—the study of law as a factor in the cause, distribution, and prevention of disease and injury in a population—can offer valuable, empirical insights into how policies influence public health (Burris et al., 2016). For example, many people express concerns about variable outcomes between states and territories with different screening panels or different levels of funding (Susanna Haas Lyons Engagement Consulting, 2024). These "natural experiment" studies could address whether health outcomes vary between states with different screening panels, or whether funding levels influence the timeline to adoption of RUSP conditions. Legal epidemiological studies could also investigate the effects of religious or cultural exemption policies on participation rates and health outcomes in different jurisdictions. Such studies would require more robust and standardized data collection and sharing by NBS programs, as well as improved long-term follow-up infrastructure.

Investigating Public Health Practice, Feasibility, and Impact

Assessing the nationwide impact of public health newborn screening and its benefits is challenging due to limited coordinated data collection efforts (Watson et al., 2022). Directly linking public health newborn screening to long-term benefits or cost savings at the population level is particularly difficult, though some evidence is available for specific conditions (Grosse, 2015; Van Vliet and Grosse, 2021). Coordinated efforts to collect such data are needed to enable research that investigates how policies and practices affect the delivery, quality, cost, and outcomes of newborn screening as an essential public health service. Conducting

---

[2] Normative arguments are based on value judgments.

successful research in these areas requires multidisciplinary teams that include, but are not limited to, experts in communication, decision analysis, systems engineering, economics, and health services. Such information can inform the development of evidence-based practices and be used to ensure that newborn screening iteratively improves. Prior work includes effort toward (1) identifying how to efficiently and effectively communicate with parents about NBS results to ensure optimal screening outcomes; (2) understanding the costs and health outcomes associated with screening for a condition or adopting a technology can help decision makers make effective use of limited resources; and (3) identifying ways to streamline the delivery of services from specimen collection to results reporting (Cochran et al., 2018; Farrell et al., 2011; Grosse and Van Vliet, 2020; La Pean et al., 2013; Simon et al., 2020).

Long-term follow-up is a critical missing piece of the puzzle needed to understand the effect of newborn screening on population health outcomes (Kellar-Guenther et al., 2024; Kemper et al., 2008). Given that long-term follow-up is outside of the scope of many state and territorial-run programs (see Chapter 4), coordination among researchers, NBS programs, and clinical care may be needed to address this complicated, but important, endeavor. Long-term follow-up, its challenges, and potential paths forward are discussed later in this chapter.

See Box 6-2 for selected questions to address as part of NBS research.

THE INTERSECTION OF NBS RESEARCH AND RARE DISEASE RESEARCH

Population-based newborn screening provides an invaluable tool for understanding the genetic causes and full spectrum of symptomatology for many rare conditions. Without such an approach, only the most severe cases are identified (Figure 6-1). Screening allows for the identification of subclinical or mild forms of a condition, which is essential for understanding the range of potential outcomes, informing individual care decisions for identified patients, and advancing research on diagnosis and treatment.

NBS research and rare disease research can sometimes be conflated, but each area has unique, albeit complementary, scopes. Although NBS research can inform rare disease research, it is not limited to conditions that are rare. The scope of rare disease research extends beyond what can be learned through newborn screening (e.g., pathophysiology and therapeutic development). Rare disease research also addresses a much wider spectrum of diseases that may not be detectable at birth or have no immediate treatments available for infants.

Ultimately, NBS research and rare disease research can inform and complement each other with knowledge gained from one field driving

BOX 6-2
Selected Questions to Address as Part of NBS Research

The list of questions that could be considered when making decisions about NBS policy and practice is a long one. A list of selected questions to address as part of NBS research includes the following:

Defining Conditions to Guide Screening, Diagnosis, and Treatment
- What is the natural history of a condition(s) being considered for newborn screening, either currently or in the foreseeable future?
- What variations exist in the phenotypic expression of various conditions, and what are the resulting implications for screening or treatment decisions?

Developing Laboratory Testing and Applying Emerging Technologies
- What are the comparative advantages, costs, disadvantages between different screening methods, laboratory cutoff values, etc.?
- How well can screening and/or subsequent diagnostic confirmation strategies determine phenotypic subtypes so parents will have a better understanding of potential future health outcomes and clinicians will be able to make more informed decisions about who needs which treatment(s) and when?

(See Chapter 5 for questions related to applying genomic sequencing to public health newborn screening.)

Understanding on Ethical, Legal, and Social Issues
- What are the benefits and harms of screening?
- What is the public perception and acceptability of screening for conditions with a range of outcomes (e.g., a few children have substantial benefit, whereas others have modest, minimal, or no benefit)?
- How do parents and clinicians deal with uncertainty?
- Would a consented approach to newborn screening affect participation rates, and if so, would it do so differently across different populations?
- Would screening for an expanded set of conditions via informed consent affect opt-out newborn screening, and, if so, how?
- How do policies related to NBS practices affect health outcomes?

Investigating Public Health Practice, Feasibility, and Impact
- What are the long-term, longitudinal (5–10 years) outcomes of screening for children and families?
- What is the comparative efficacy of various surveillance strategies for conditions in which timing of treatment is unknown (or is not immediately needed until some other signs are observed)?
- What are the best strategies for helping parents coping with diagnoses and distress about future outcomes?
- How can the delivery of services within the NBS system be optimized for efficiency and quality?
- What outcomes do families experience after receiving NBS results, both short term and long term?

progress in the other. Rare disease research can advance efforts to develop therapies, expand precision medicine, provide global frameworks for classifying diseases and linking them to health information, among others. Each of these aims can support both NBS research and decision making about public health newborn screening, more broadly. Conversely, NBS research to understand the natural history of conditions can inform the development of therapeutics and NBS pilot studies can permit researchers to identify potential presymptomatic participants for clinical trials, accelerating treatment pipelines.

NBS and rare disease research efforts also have a history of working synergistically that could be further leveraged through increased coordination. For example, an infant identified as at risk for spinal muscular atrophy (SMA) through a pilot NBS study was subsequently enrolled in a presymptomatic clinical trial for a gene therapy for SMA. These coordinated efforts demonstrated the feasibility of population-wide screening and treatment effectiveness for SMA and ultimately informed its inclusion on the RUSP (Evidence-based Review Group, 2018; Kraszewski et al., 2018).

However, a distinction must be drawn between public health newborn screening and NBS or rare disease research. Routine public health newborn screening performed without explicit consent cannot be used to conduct research.

THE LANDSCAPE OF NBS RESEARCH

The current NBS research landscape generates valuable tools, technologies, discoveries, and insights for newborn screening. However, these discoveries frequently focus on a single disease, are funded and completed too late to inform programmatic and policy decision making, and are often not responsive to the immediate needs and priorities related to public health newborn screening. This reduces the effectiveness and timeliness of NBS research—especially given a funding environment in which newborn screening must compete for resources with research on more common pediatric conditions such as asthma and obesity. This section provides an overview of prior and ongoing research related to newborn screening and its effect on the field.

NBS Translational Research Network

Prior calls for increased NBS research infrastructure prompted the National Institutes of Health (NIH) to create the Newborn Screening Translational Research Network (NBSTRN). The goal of NBSTRN was to develop and share resources and infrastructure to support NBS researchers (Lloyd-Puryear et al., 2019). NBSTRN was active for 15 years and received over $35 million in funding from the *Eunice Kennedy Shriver* National Institute of Child Health and Human Development (NICHD), making it among the largest investments into NBS research by NIH).[3]

Major contributions by NBSTRN include data tools developed to support NBS research such as the Longitudinal Pediatric Data Resource (LPDR) and the Virtual Repository of Dried Blood Spots (VRDBS) (Chan et al., 2023; Lloyd-Puryear et al., 2019). The LPDR is a database for genomic and phenotypic information collected over the lifespan of newborns identified as at risk through screening to facilitate the understanding of genetic disease and assess the effect of early identification and treatment. Case-level, deidentified datasets from the LPDR are available for secondary research and data mining. As part of this effort, NBSTRN used a consensus-based process with clinical care experts to develop common data elements and then built those into the LPDR (Brower et al., 2021). Promoting the standardization of data elements through the LPDR is recognized as a key contribution of NBSTRN among those in the field (HRSA, 2018).

NBSTRN also created the VRDBS—a web-based tool that allows investigators to access a catalog of dried blood spots from NBS programs that may be available for use in research and NBS program development (Lloyd-Puryear et al., 2019). In addition to data tools, NBSTRN developed resources related to ethical, legal, and social issues (ELSI), including guidelines for parental permission for pilot testing NBS research and a survey to gather input on ELSI needs in NBS research (Botkin et al., 2014; Unnikumaran et al., 2024).

Although NBSTRN created several tools and shared resources, there was limited uptake by the research community and little evidence that these resources facilitated evidence generation to inform policy decisions. For example, the committee identified only two citations that used data from the LPDR to perform secondary research (Hartnett et al., 2022; Wilhelm et al., 2022). Similarly, one published study seemed to use the VRDBS to perform secondary research (on prenatal alcohol exposure) (Baldwin, 2015), and only a handful of investigators submitted protocols (Lloyd-Puryear et al., 2019). Both of these resources relied heavily on public health personnel to input data, and then, for the VRDBS, to facilitate use of the resource (Lloyd-Puryear et al., 2019), which ultimately put a strain on programs rather than adding resources to support their mission. Finally, NBSTRN was likely

---

[3] See https://www.usaspending.gov/award/CONT_AWD_HHSN275200800001C_7529_-NONE-_-NONE- (accessed January 17, 2025); https://www.usaspending.gov/award/CONT_AWD_75N94018C00005_7529_-NONE-_-NONE- (accessed January 17, 2025); https://www.usaspending.gov/award/CONT_AWD_HHSN275201300011C_7529_-NONE-_-NONE- (accessed January 17, 2025).

hampered from setting priorities and stimulating research because of funding constraints and limited authority to guide research.

NICHD recently terminated this initiative after performing a landscape analysis of investments in NBS research. NBSTRN-related responsibilities have been shifted to the National Center for Advancing Translational Sciences (NCATS) in the context of the Rare Disease Clinical Research Network (RDCRN).[4] However, the recent request for applications for new RDCRN centers did not have a requirement for NBS-related research.[5]

NSIGHT and Other Large Programs

Recent advances in genome sequencing technology—including developments that have decreased cost—have attracted large-scale research investment to determine the usefulness and acceptability of genomic sequencing in newborns (Minear et al., 2022). The Newborn Sequencing in Genomic Medicine and Public Health (NSIGHT) program was a research initiative jointly funded by the National Human Genome Research Institute (NHGRI) and NICHD from 2013 to 2019, with an initial funding commitment totaling $25 million (NIH, 2022).[6] Through NSIGHT, four centers investigated genomic sequencing in newborns within different contexts, including the clinical diagnosis of sick newborns in intensive care units and the screening of healthy newborns at birth. Each center used different approaches with minimal coordination and had a sequencing project, a clinical project, and an ethics project. Several major findings were published because of this investment (see Chapter 5), and many more questions were raised (Minear et al., 2022).

With the ending of NSIGHT's funding, several large-scale research programs continue to focus on how genomic sequencing could be integrated into newborn screening and its potential ethical ramifications (see Chapter 5 for information about these ongoing projects). None of these programs rely exclusively on federal funding or a single source of support, seeking money from industry, foundations, and advocacy groups. However, a new initiative was recently announced at an NIH Council of Councils meeting: the Newborn Screening by Whole-Genome Sequencing initiative, which will be solely supported through Common Fund venture support. The initiative will disperse $5 million annually for 3 years with the goal of demonstrating the feasibility of a collaborative model for newborn screening by whole genome sequencing (Sheely, 2024).

---

[4] See https://grants.nih.gov/grants/guide/notice-files/NOT-HD-23-012.html (accessed January 16, 2025).

[5] See https://grants.nih.gov/grants/guide/pa-files/PAR-24-206.html (accessed January 16, 2025).

[6] See https://grants.nih.gov/grants/guide/rfa-files/RFA-HD-13-010.html for initial funding details (accessed January 16, 2025).

Grants, Small Business Agreements, and Contracts Awarded by NIH

NICHD has a suite of grants, small business awards, and contracts specifically addressing NBS-related research. There are currently four program announcements related to NBS research;[7] however, these opportunities do not have promised funds nor are they reviewed through a dedicated study section. Few grants have been funded through these program announcements in recent years (Minear et al., 2022; NICHD, 2024). For investigator-initiated grants, the research focus is typically on a single condition and not necessarily responsive to priorities of public health newborn screening. Small business awards or small business technology transfers awarded by NIH are issued to commercial entities for projects that have the ultimate goal of commercialization; for example, such an award helped fund the development of a microfluidics platform for a panel of four lysosomal storage disorders that was eventually used by NBS programs (Millington et al., 2018). NICHD also contracts task orders to prequalified entities to pilot test conditions considered for inclusion in public health NBS panels. However, these conditions do not necessarily meet the priorities of the system; for example, task orders totaling $750,000 were issued in 2017 for a spinal muscular atrophy pilot study[8] when a large pilot study had just been completed, and the condition was already under consideration for the RUSP (Cure SMA, 2017; Kraszewski et al., 2018; Minear et al., 2022).

Other Federal Research Initiatives Related to Newborn Screening

The Centers for Disease Control and Prevention (CDC), the Health Resources and Services Administration (HRSA), and the Agency for Healthcare Research and Quality (AHRQ) also support research efforts related to newborn screening (see Chapter 2). Briefly, CDC contributes to long-term follow-up efforts, screening tool validation, and population-wide pilot studies (Brosco, 2024). Although HRSA does not fund research grants per se, some of its grants support initiatives that collect data to inform the provision of this public health service, such as long-term follow-up.[9] Since 2018, AHRQ has not awarded any grants that contain the term "newborn screening" in the abstract;[10] however, previously funded studies have investigated cost-effectiveness and health outcomes related to newborn screening (Richardson et al., 2021). More broadly, AHRQ

---

[7] See https://grants.nih.gov/grants/guide/notice-files/NOT-HD-22-042.html (accessed January 16, 2025).

[8] See https://www.highergov.com/vehicle/newborn-screening-pilot-studies-idiq-2276 for funding amounts (accessed January 27, 2025).

[9] See https://www.hrsa.gov/grants/find-funding/HRSA-24-052 (accessed January 27, 2025).

[10] See AHRQ grants by state from 2018 to the present here: https://www.ahrq.gov/funding/grant-mgmt/grants-by-state.html (accessed January 27, 2025).

supports research that may be relevant to the broader NBS ecosystem such as health IT infrastructure research and health services research related to children with medical complexity, rare diseases, care coordination, continuity of care, and developmental screening.[11]

CHALLENGES IN THE EVIDENCE-GENERATION PROCESS

Evidence is essential to inform federal and state or territorial decision makers and advisory bodies as they develop policy and guidance on newborn screening and its implementation. Yet the generation, interpretation, and compilation of the necessary evidence can involve inherent challenges that burden partners across the NBS ecosystem, complicate decision making, and contribute to disparities.

Funding Landscape

It is difficult to capture a complete picture of the NIH's NBS research portfolio as funding is distributed across several institutes and centers, including NCATS, NICHD, NHGRI, the National Institute of Diabetes and Digestive and Kidney Diseases, the National Institute of Neurological Disorders and Stroke, the National Heart, Lung, and Blood Institute, and the National Institute of General Medical Sciences (Minear et al., 2022). NBS-related research is not indexed in the Research, Condition, and Disease Categorization (RCDC) system (NIH, 2024); this system is instrumental for public reporting on the totality of funding for a particular category of research and allows for accurate funding analyses and increased transparency. The RCDC system also provides opportunities for more strategic alignment and coordination of research across institutes and centers. In addition to limited coordination across NIH institutes and centers, there is limited input from the broader NBS ecosystem, including state and federal health partners, on how to best prioritize research questions and most effectively deploy available funds.

Beyond government support, funding for research related to newborn screening is heavily reliant on advocacy and, therefore, susceptible to both perpetuating and exacerbating disparities in research investment (Halley et al., 2022). Patient advocacy organizations work tirelessly to raise funds, build awareness, and promote greater research investment for their condition (Bailey, 2022). On an individual level, advocacy efforts are often deeply personal and rooted in a search for answers to save the

---

[11] See https://www.ahrq.gov/ncepcr/research/health-it/index.html (accessed January 10, 2025).

lives of themselves, loved ones, and/or others affected by a particular condition (Halley, 2021). However, on a systems level, the prominent role of advocacy makes rare disease research investment vulnerable to the identifiable victim effect, or the tendency to offer help to the loudest and most recognizable voices, and not necessarily those with the greatest need (Largent and Pearson, 2012).

Conditions that affect families with the social and financial capital to effectively advocate for research tend to attract the most attention and resources, whereas conditions that affect populations that are smaller, more diffuse, or historically marginalized are more likely to be left behind (Largent and Pearson, 2012). This process places undue burden on all patient communities, and particularly those that may have less resources. Directing resources based on an advocacy model does not support systematic or strategic investment to inform decision making about public health newborn screening.

Industry also plays a role in driving research. The global NBS market was valued at over $3 billion in 2024 and is expected to reach nearly $6 billion by 2032 (Towards Healthcare, 2023). This growth potential has attracted industry investment into technological advancements related to screening, including genome sequencing, in addition to developing new diagnostic tools as well as drugs and other treatments for congenital disorders. Beyond their own investments, industry also supports research initiatives, which tend to be focused on their priorities and not those of the NBS system (Bailey, 2022).

Together, this funding landscape does not promote strategic and coordinated investments to support timely, evidence-based decision making related to public health newborn screening based on the perspectives of the many partners in the NBS ecosystem. A coordinated, planned, and nimble funding strategy for NBS research is critical to ensure that research dollars generate insights that are informative, useful, and timely.

Burden on Public Health Programs

"[Pilot studies] illustrate the importance of collaborations between public health systems and external partners, and the unique and specialized contributions of each." – NBS public health professional

The highest priority of NBS programs must be to screen infants born in their respective jurisdictions in a timely manner and connect infants identified as at risk with confirmatory diagnosis and clinical care. However, there has been an increasing reliance on programs to provide resources and generate the evidence base for inclusion of new conditions, incorporation of novel technologies, and more. Some of this is born out of necessity, as NBS programs are the only source for some data and the specimens needed for relevant research. Researchers rely on public health programs to access deidentified blood spots to develop screening assays, determine condition prevalence, and more, including prospective population-wide pilot studies.[12]

As previously described, newborn screening faces a "chicken or the egg" dilemma: to be included in public health newborn screening, a condition must have a prospective population-wide pilot study, but population-wide pilot studies are best conducted by or in partnership with public health programs to yield a sufficiently large, representative sample (HRSA, 2016). For pilot studies, public health programs may be responsible for scaling a validated screening method and coordinating follow-up for any identified infants; these tasks may raise both foreseeable and unanticipated issues but generally fall within the scope of work performed by programs. However, pilot studies also require educating and recruiting participants, which is not typical for public health personnel. External collaborators are vital to conduct these activities (Kay, 2024).

Past research infrastructure has *drawn* on NBS program staff and resources rather than *added* to their arsenal. For example, NBSTRN created a VRDBS that included dried blood spots from several state programs to serve as a resource for the research community. However, NBS program personnel rather than NBSTRN staff were ultimately responsible for providing researchers with information about the required processes for material transfer agreements, assisting with specific study-related questions, and other tasks that might have been addressed by individuals outside of NBS programs (Lloyd-Puryear et al., 2019). With existing constraints on staff and resources, programs cannot shoulder demands to generate evidence and provide resources without increased funding, personnel, partnerships, and infrastructure. The legal landscape and rising public concerns around the storage and secondary reuse of dried blood spots for research continue to be difficult for both public health personnel and researchers to navigate (Lloyd-Puryear et al., 2019; Therrell et al., 2011).

Long-Term Follow-Up

"We need a national system to track patients and follow-up." – Medical geneticist

NBS longitudinal follow-up refers to the tracking and monitoring of newborns over time. Follow-up from screening to communication of results or confirmatory testing is referred to as short-term follow-up; this responsibility sits within the purview of state- and territorial-run NBS

---

[12] In some jurisdictions, dried blood spots collected through newborn screening are deidentified and available for secondary research.

programs (see Chapter 4). Long-term follow-up in the context of newborn screening generally refers to the surveillance after confirmatory testing is completed. Essentially, it begins with a baby's transition into clinical care and can continue for years to decades (Hinton et al., 2014; Kemper et al., 2008). Despite persistent calls to collect long-term follow-up information, efforts to gather such data have been limited and sporadic at best (Hoff and Hoyt, 2006). The ownership of the responsibility to collect and analyze long-term follow-up data has previously been ill defined, and this diffused accountability has limited efforts (Kellar-Guenther et al., 2024). The types of data pertinent to NBS long-term follow-up are largely beyond the purview of NBS programs or other state- or territorial-run public health programs, falling more within clinical data and large-scale public health surveillance (see Chapter 4), which given the nature of the U.S. health system provides a fragmented and disjointed dataset. However, long-term follow-up provides critical evidence on the health effects of newborn screening and the performance of NBS programs and the system at large.

To support long-term follow-up goals, an ideal strategy would include effective mechanisms for collecting, storing, and sharing data both across public health and clinical care as well as across state lines. Attributes of an ideal long-term follow-up scenario for newborn screening could include

- *Harmonization and interoperability of electronic datasets: Electronic submission of data is critical to limit data silos.* Robust systems for data governance, privacy, and security to ensure appropriate protections when sharing and accessing data across systems would be needed.
- *Standardized NBS templates and data elements:* National standards for patient, laboratory, and genomic data would enable consistency in data collection, which is particularly important when dealing with small sample sizes.
- *Data support for care teams:* Bidirectional links are needed between existing data systems to provide care teams with all the data they need, provide a record of family communication, and support shared case management among different providers and organizations, including NBS programs, pediatric care, primary care providers, and rare disease specialists.
- *Tools for families to engage meaningfully*: Patients need to understand the ways their data might be used, provide informed consent as appropriate, and access their results and records in line with the 21st Century Cures Act.[13]
- *Strategies to ensure data quality, including mechanisms to address gaps or systemic problems.*

---

[13] 21st Century Cures Act, P.L. 114-255.

There are significant barriers to achieving such a scenario. Different NBS programs and clinical care systems employ an incredibly broad array of approaches to collect and handle NBS data, from electronic health records and portals to handwritten notes and faxes. Datasets are often siloed or inaccessible, and even when they can be shared or combined, inconsistencies in nomenclature and data formats limit interoperability and the ability to extract insights. Finally, the infrastructure required for data collection, storage, use, and sharing is costly and requires ongoing maintenance, which can pose a barrier for sustaining systems in the long run. Despite these challenges, there are opportunities to make progress toward a more cohesive system for handling and sharing long-term follow-up data related to newborn screening.

An important first step toward developing a robust national system is aligning partners to define the goals of long-term follow-up efforts. Goals could include identifying particular outcomes to track, such as survival, or particular problems to solve, such as disparities in connection to a specialist. Kellar-Guenther et al. (2024) outline three core long-term follow-up outcomes for a year after birth:

1. Is the child still alive?
2. Did the child have contact with a specialist?
3. Did the child receive appropriate care specific to their diagnosis within 1 year?

Kellar-Guenther et al. also state that a set of minimal data elements is critical for tracking those outcomes as a foundation for understanding the effects of newborn screening within and across programs (Kellar-Guenther et al., 2024). Additional lessons on identifying key metrics and practical data-collection strategies that enable information exchange between private and public health sectors can be gleaned from previous HRSA-supported research initiatives on quality measures for long-term follow-up (HRSA, 2018; Lloyd-Puryear and Brower, 2010). Once a minimal dataset is consistently collected, efforts could be expanded to include more outcome measures or tackle additional problems.

Another critical step is to identify the key players and delineate who has the responsibility and authority to collect, store, and share what data and with whom. Given that this responsibility is outside of the scope for most state- and territorial-run NBS programs (see Chapter 4), it is important to take an expansive view of the key players and data sources involved.

An approach is needed to navigate collecting data across the decentralized NBS programs and health care systems. One approach could be to focus on improving linkages and data sharing among existing disparate systems with the aim of greater interoperability and harmonization.

Another option is to establish a more central screening registry. In either case, starting small and building upon existing resources—including using existing partnerships within and among organizations such as HRSA, CDC, the Association of Public Health Laboratories, and the Council of State and Territorial Epidemiologists, as well as existing registries[14]—is likely to make for a more feasible and sustainable path forward.

Many well-designed data systems exist that could provide a basis for establishing standardized definitions, templates, and data models to support consistency and interoperability among datasets relevant to longitudinal follow-up for newborn screening. The USCDI+ initiative, which supports the development of domain-specific data element lists to advance the use of interoperable data elements among federal and industry partners, could provide a framework for the NBS community to coalesce around shared data elements and harmonize data standards and taxonomies.[15] In addition, Fast Healthcare Interoperability Resources, a standard for the exchange of health care data, could support linkages among disparate systems, potentially with an implementation guide specifically for newborn screening.[16] Health information exchanges (HIEs) may also serve as a repository for long-term follow-up data within each state or territory. Some states have very robust HIEs; for example, the Indiana Health Information Exchange connects data from hospitals, laboratories, state-run public health programs, and other health care entities.[17] Ongoing work by the Trusted Exchange Framework and Common Agreements to support standardizing formats for HIE interoperability nationally could also enable more efficient exchange of information across HIEs.[18] Systems such as electronic case reporting, which automates the exchange of data between electronic health records and public health agencies, provide another useful model that could be built upon for sharing data on NBS follow-up.[19]

Electronic health record (EHR) vendors could collaborate with researchers and others to set up disease-specific templates and collect standardized data elements for long-term follow-up. If Epic, Oracle Cerner, and Meditech participated, it is estimated that 75 percent of hospitals in the United States would be covered (Bruce, 2023). The template could integrate quality of life or other patient-reported metrics

---

[14] Some conditions screened through newborn screening have robust registries coordinated by foundations. For example, 36,518 individuals participated in the Cystic Fibrosis Foundation Patient Registry in 2020 (Cromwell et al., 2023).
[15] See https://www.healthit.gov/topic/interoperability/uscdi-plus (accessed March 6, 2025).
[16] See https://hl7.org/fhir/ (accessed March 6, 2025).
[17] See https://www.ihie.org/ (accessed March 6, 2025).
[18] See https://www.healthit.gov/topic/interoperability/policy/trusted-exchange-framework-and-common-agreement-tefca (accessed March 6, 2025).
[19] See https://www.cdc.gov/ecr/php/about/index.html (accessed March 6, 2025).

(Azad et al., 2016). Such IT infrastructure would avoid attrition by individuals who move across states lines, so long as they continued to be seen at a hospital using the same EHR vendor. A dashboard component embedded in the EHR that permitted easy access to—and visualization of—patient data might also encourage patient participation. This option would align with the 21st Century Cures Act, which includes measures to make research data more accessible to participants and to improve transparency.[20] Combining this approach with electronic case-reporting tools could enable interaction between many components across the NBS ecosystem.

EHR dashboards have been employed by the Connecticut Department of Health in partnership with the Connecticut NBS Network to establish registries for long-term follow-up of patients identified through newborn screening. This effort may serve as a model for applying population health tools to track care delivery and quickly fill identified care gaps; preliminary results indicate this approach can lead to improvements in the percentage of visits up-to-date and condition-specific performance metrics for patients identified through newborn screening. Limitations of this approach include the need for an analyst with specialized training in EHR systems to implement and optimize the dashboard, interpret data, and identify areas for continuous improvement in clinical care. Comprehensive training for the clinical care teams is also necessary to ensure successful implementation of the dashboard and meaningful improvements in care management (Raboin et al., 2024).

Gathering information at a national level will ultimately require national coordination and the investment into a national data infrastructure. The current landscape of long-term follow-up is fractured and ad hoc: some NBS programs have begun engaging in long-term follow-up, particularly those with support from HRSA Propel and Co-Propel grants, and others have also made initial investments in this space (HRSA, 2024a,b; Kellar-Guenther et al., 2024; Raboin et al., 2024). The long-term follow-up challenge can be best addressed by thinking beyond NBS programs to include other partners in the NBS ecosystem and taking a national view of data collection and infrastructure.

Challenges Related to Rare Disease

Another tension in the evidence-generation process for newborn screening reflects inherent challenges with studying rare diseases more broadly. The rarity of these conditions makes it difficult to generate the data needed, particularly for population-level insights (Belter et al.,

---

[20] 21st Century Cures Act, P.L. 114-255.

2024; Venugopal et al., 2024). Before population-based pilot studies are conducted, most of the data available on these conditions reflect individuals who are symptomatic or clinically affected, potentially missing those who have not developed symptoms or received a diagnosis (Lloyd-Puryear et al., 2019). It often takes large screening studies or population-wide screening to accurately estimate the prevalence of a disease in a population, but without some understanding of the prevalence it can be difficult to generate the funding and research interest required to conduct these studies (Belter et al., 2024; Venugopal et al., 2024). Since these conditions are rare, coordination across multiple sites and complex data sharing and aggregation efforts may be necessary to achieve sufficient statistical power for studies, including those to estimate prevalence in the population and within different subgroups (Belter et al., 2024; Venugopal et al., 2024).

ADDRESSING UNMET NEEDS IN NBS RESEARCH

Research is essential to provide the information required to make informed decisions about NBS policy and practice. No formal infrastructure or program currently exists to gather this information in a coordinated or expeditious fashion. There is a need for strategic, systematic, nimble, and sufficiently funded research to provide the evidence necessary for newborn screening to adjust to a rapidly changing landscape of new technologies and new treatments. Several mechanisms could be considered to advance NBS research, each of which has its own set of trade-offs.

Options to Address Research Needs Related to Newborn Screening

Substantially Increase Funding for Investigator-Initiated Research

Most NIH funding is currently dispersed to NBS-related research through investigator-initiated grants. However, investigators historically have not been incentivized to include NBS-related questions in their research as there is not a set-aside study section for grant review. Few grants have been funded through previous NBS program announcements (Minear et al., 2022; NICHD, 2024).

Increasing NIH funding for investigator-initiated grants would prompt researchers to focus on newborn screening. Grants awarded with these funds would need to be reviewed by a separate study section comprising reviewers familiar with newborn screening to allow for an accurate assessment of the overall effect and significance of the proposed research. There would almost certainly be a substantial increase in strong research proposals given the increased amount of funding available and the opportunity to be reviewed by those who understand the importance of certain kinds of studies (e.g., natural history) to the NBS evidence base.

Establish NBS Research Centers

Research centers, or centers of excellence, are a common model employed by NIH to support and promote interdisciplinary research with a unifying focus. Centers operate independently and may collaborate but typically do not. Centers often have larger budgets than individual research projects and require increased overall investment by NIH. For example, grants to fund the recently established Autism Centers of Excellence, composed of nine centers, total an estimated $100 million, which will be distributed over a period of 5 years—with each center ultimately receiving just over $2 million per year (NICHD, 2022). Usually, centers consist of several projects supported by specialized cores that provide services to promote research. Different centers have different cores depending on the strengths of the institution (e.g., biostatistics, genomics, pathology).

This model has been employed previously to study the implications of genome sequencing with both healthy and symptomatic newborns through the NSIGHT program. Funded under a cooperative agreement, there was some effort to organize meetings involving all four centers, but, ultimately, there was little research collaboration. By working independently, centers were able to develop and investigate different approaches, and ultimately their collective research led to major findings that pushed the field forward (see Chapter 5).

Each prospective academic center would apply in partnership with an NBS public health program. Partnerships between public health NBS programs and academic institutions have already proven highly successful at expeditiously generating evidence to inform policy decisions. Several features would be needed to establish a rigorous research enterprise that does not strain the partner public health program—adding rather than detracting resources to support its mission. Appropriate staffing and training by the academic center would be necessary to avoid drawing on existing public health personnel who already have limited bandwidth. Certain agreements (e.g., business associate agreement, memorandum of understanding) would be needed to enable the recruitment of infants within the jurisdiction, to allow data sharing of protected health information with consent, and to gain access to deidentified dried blood spots as appropriate,[21] among other logistical hurdles (Bailey et al., 2019).

---

[21] See Chapter 7 for an exploration of the issues surrounding deidentified dried blood spots in secondary research.

Preestablishing partnerships and data-sharing agreements would reduce administrative burden of both the researchers and public health professionals, and thus, ought to be required criteria for centers.

Establish a Coordinated Network of NBS Research Centers

Research networks are a model used by NIH to create a more efficient and responsive research ecosystem that can address complex research questions through increased coordination (e.g., neonatal research network) (Watterberg et al., 2022). A network of research centers could be established with each center expected to work in a coordinated and nimble fashion to address timely issues related to newborn screening. Centers would develop their own research questions and would also work together to generate evidence to address high-priority issues in the field. Centers in the network would work in partnership with NBS public health programs with appropriate safeguards to protect strained public health resources and agreements in place to reduce administrative burden, as described for the research center model. A data-coordinating center and a decision-making body (involving all the centers) would provide the central glue to facilitate coordinated and strategic research to inform policy in a timely manner.

Investigating conditions considered for screening, which tend to be rare, often requires coordination across multiple sites with complicated data sharing and aggregation efforts to achieve sufficient statistical power. Further, generating data for population-level insights to inform decisions about newborn screening also likely requires large-scale, multisite studies. A research network could facilitate such coordinated research, and a data coordination center (DCC) would be instrumental to accomplish this goal. Across the network, the DCC would ensure data quality and consistency, provide statistical support for study design, collect and manage data, analyze data, and manage centralized databases and data sharing, among other tasks. Ultimately, the DCC would ensure consistency, efficiency, and scientific rigor across participating centers and would be necessary to address the key challenges in NBS research (see Box 6-3).

The network would be guided by a steering committee to identify high-priority questions for the centers to align on gathering evidence. Reflecting the systems-level research needs of newborn screening, the committee would involve members representing different sectors, including representatives from each center, public health, the medical community, and researchers outside the centers. The steering committee would draw on federal perspectives to identify high-priority research questions that must be addressed quickly. The research network would also involve patient advocacy groups using the Coalition of Patient Advocacy Groups

> **BOX 6-3**
> **Examples of NBS-Related Studies Enabled by a Coordinated Research Network**
>
> **Natural history studies**—Conducting natural history studies across multiple sites would ensure access to a larger pool of potential participants, enable recruitment of enough patients for statistical power, and capture a more representative patient population.
>
> **Comparison studies**—Coordination across multiple sites would allow for studies comparing the outcomes of different informed consent approaches for expanded screening, or the sensitivity and specificity of different screening approaches, among other comparisons.
>
> **Expanded DNA sequencing studies**—Studies that incorporate DNA-based screening across multiple sites would enable continued inclusion of representative ancestral populations in genomic databases and a fuller understanding of the implications of applying this technology to screen healthy newborns.

(PAGs) model, or similar, employed by the Rare Disease Clinical Research Network (Merkel et al., 2016). PAGs would advise researchers and facilitate bilateral communication about perspectives, needs, and interests of patients with rare disease.

Trade-Offs

Increased investment into investigator-initiated grants—with a set-aside study section for review—would provide broad access to newly infused resources into the NBS research space. This mechanism would also enable bottom-up communication of avenues for inquiry. However, investigator-initiated grants would not systematize coordination across multiple sites, which can be critical to achieve statistical power, nor would this mechanism enable investigators to quickly address questions informed by national research priorities. Therefore, greatly expanding investigator-initiated projects alone would not solve the problem of a coordinated system and would be quite slow in producing evidence to address problems for which a solution is urgently needed.

Establishing NBS research centers could stimulate research on a broad range of topics related to newborn screening and involve teams of investigators. However, without some sort of coordinating mechanism and mandate, centers tend to work independently and not necessarily in accordance with public need. Therefore, the center model would likely limit coordination and strategy to address questions in a timely manner based on national priorities.

Research networks are designed to enable investigators to coordinate and answer questions quickly with increased access to resources, but generally this occurs at the expense of a fairer allocation of available resources. This mechanism can also create an information bubble in which the same set of individuals sets priorities and allocates resources according to what they consider important without knowledge of, or maybe consideration for, the interests of the broader research community or those with lived experience.

However, there are several strategies that may prove useful to combat these potential pitfalls. Research network resources could be made available to outside investigators (this is already common, though such use is typically more expensive). A hub-and-spoke approach could be used where the research center serves as the hub that provides resources or technological support through its specialized cores to investigators at spoke institutions. Creating a multistakeholder steering committee, or having routinized avenues to gather multistakeholder input, would help avoid creating an echo chamber concerning research priorities. It would be particularly important to ensure that interests of researchers that are not part of the network are represented on the committee.

CONCLUSIONS

Conclusion 6-1: Research is critical to inform evidence-based decisions about newborn screening policies and practice. There are gaps in these essential areas: defining conditions to guide screening, diagnosis, and treatment; applying laboratory testing and emerging technologies; understanding ethical, legal, and social issues; and investigating public health practice, feasibility, and impact.

Conclusion 6-2: Linking public health newborn screening to long-term health outcomes is difficult with existing data. Coordinated efforts to collect long-term follow-up data are needed. Such data would better support research on the effect of newborn screening on population health outcomes and guide policies and practices for public health newborn screening.

Conclusion 6-3: The full breadth of investment in newborn screening research by the federal government, advocacy, and industry is difficult to assess. Indexing newborn screening in the Research, Condition, and Disease Categorization system would help clarify at least the National Institutes of Health's portfolio of investments in newborn screening.

Conclusion 6-4: Newborn screening (NBS) research studies can strain public health resources. Gaining a population-level understanding of the rare congenital conditions included or considered for newborn screening often requires researchers to draw on resources embedded in NBS programs, including accessing dried blood spots or conducting population-wide pilot studies on the feasibility and effectiveness of screening for the condition through newborn screening. However, sharing these resources, or embedding research within the public health sphere, burdens public health programs. Mechanisms are needed to ensure that research infrastructure does not detract from public health bandwidth.

Conclusion 6-5: More robust, coordinated newborn screening (NBS) research infrastructure would enable strategic evidence generation that is responsive to high-priority questions. Existing mechanisms to perform research and gather data to support NBS are scattered, uncoordinated, and nonstrategic. The current landscape is overly reliant on investigator-initiated research and research driven by advocacy and industry, which do not necessarily reflect systems-level needs or priorities. Further, overreliance on advocacy places undue burden on patient communities, particularly those that are ultrarare or underresourced, to drive research. There is a need to strategically prioritize questions with input from partners in the NBS ecosystem.

REFERENCES

AAP (American Academy of Pediatrics). 1967. Statement on compulsory testing of newborn infants for hereditary metabolic disorders. *Pediatrics* 39(4):623-624.

Al-Hilli, Z., R. Noss, J. Dickard, W. Wei, A. Chichura, V. Wu, K. Renicker, H. J. Pederson, and C. Eng. 2023. A randomized trial comparing the effectiveness of pre-test genetic counseling using an artificial intelligence automated chatbot and traditional in-person genetic counseling in women newly diagnosed with breast cancer. *Breast Oncology* 30: 5990-5996.

Allen, J., D. Berry, F. Cook, A. Hume, R. Rouce, A. Srirangam, J. Wellman, and C. McCombs. 2023. Medicaid coverage practices for approved gene and cell therapies: Existing barriers and proposed policy solutions. *Molecular Therapy Methods and Clinical Development* 29:513-521.

APHA (American Public Health Association). 2019. *Public health code of ethics.* https://www.apha.org/-/media/files/pdf/membergroups/ethics/code_of_ethics.ashx (accessed January 18, 2025).

Azad, T. D., M. Kalani, T. Wolf, A. Kearney, Y. Lee, L. Flannery, D. Chen, R. Berroya, M. Eisenberg, J. Park, L. Shuer, A. Kerr, and J. K. Ratliff. 2016. Building an electronic health record integrated quality of life outcomes registry for spine surgery. *Journal of Neurosurgery: Spine SPI* 24(1):176-185.

Bailey, D. B., Jr. 2022. A window of opportunity for newborn screening. *Molecular Diagnosis & Therapy* 26(3):253-261.

Bailey, D. B., Jr., L. M. Gehtland, M. A. Lewis, H. Peay, M. Raspa, S. M. Shone, J. L. Taylor, A. C. Wheeler, M. Cotten, N. M. P. King, C. M. Powell, B. Biesecker, C. E. Bishop, B. L. Boyea, M. Duparc, B. A. Harper, A. R. Kemper, S. N. Lee, R. Moultrie, K. C. Okoniewski, R. S. Paquin, D. Pettit, K. A. Porter, and S. J. Zimmerman. 2019. Early Check: Translational science at the intersection of public health and newborn screening. *BMC Pediatrics* 19(1):238.

Baily, M. A. 2023. *Newborn screening. Bioethics Briefings.* The Hastings Center for Bioethics. https://www.thehastingscenter.org/briefingbook/newborn-screening/ (accessed November 8, 2024).

Baldwin, A. 2015. Retrospective assessment of prenatal alcohol exposure by detection of phosphatidylethanol in stored dried blood spot cards: An objective method for determining prevalence rates of alcohol consumption during pregnancy. *International Journal of Alcohol and Drug Research* 4(2):131-137.

Belter, L., J. L. Taylor, E. Jorgensen, J. Glascock, S. M. Whitmire, J. J. Tingey, and M. Schroth. 2024. Newborn screening and birth prevalence for spinal muscular atrophy in the US. *JAMA Pediatrics* 178(9):946-949.

Botkin, J. R., M. H. Lewis, M. S. Watson, K. J. Swoboda, R. Anderson, S. A. Berry, N. Bonhomme, J. P. Brosco, A. M. Comeau, A. Goldenberg, E. Goldman, B. Therrell, J. Levy-Fisch, B. Tarini, and B. Wilfond. 2014. Parental permission for pilot newborn screening research: Guidelines from the NBSTRN. *Pediatrics* 133(2):e410-e417.

Brick, C., G. Kahane, D. Wilkinson, L. Caviola, and J. Savulescu. 2020. Worth living or worth dying? The views of the general public about allowing disabled children to die. *Journal of Medical Ethics* 46(1):7-15.

Brosco, J. P. 2024. *Perspectives from federal NBS partners: HRSA*. Presented at webinar on perspectives from federal NBS partners. https://www.nationalacademies.org/event/42199_03-2024_newborn-screening-current-landscape-and-future-directions-webinar-on-perspectives-from-federal-nbs-partners (accessed January 24, 2025).

Brower, A., K. Chan, M. Hartnett, and J. Taylor. 2021. The longitudinal pediatric data resource: Facilitating longitudinal collection of health information to inform clinical care and guide newborn screening efforts. *International Journal of Neonatal Screening* 7(3):37.

Bruce, G. 2023. EHR vendor market share in the US. *Becker's Health IT*. https://www.beckershospitalreview.com/ehrs/ehr-vendor-market-share-in-the-us.html (accessed January 18, 2025).

Burris, S., M. Ashe, D. Levin, M. Penn, and M. Larkin. 2016. A transdisciplinary approach to public health law: The emerging practice of legal epidemiology. *Annual Review of Public Health* 37:135-148.

Chan, K., Z. Hu, L. W. Bush, H. Cope, I. A. Holm, S. F. Kingsmore, K. Wilhelm, C. Scharfe, and A. Brower. 2023. NBSTRN tools to advance newborn screening research and support newborn screening stakeholders. *International Journal of Neonatal Screening* 9(4):63.

Chen, B. 2012. Good laboratory practices for biochemical genetic testing and newborn screening for inherited metabolic disorders. *Morbidity and Mortality Weekly Report* 61(RR-2):1-44.

Cochran, A. L., B. A. Tarini, M. Kleyn, and G. Zayas-Cabán. 2018. Newborn screening collection and delivery processes in Michigan birthing hospitals: Strategies to improve timeliness. *Maternal and Child Health Journal* 22(10):1436-1443.

Cromwell, E. A., J. S. Ostrenga, J. V. Todd, A. Elbert, A. W. Brown, A. Faro, C. H. Goss, and B. C. Marshall. 2023. Cystic fibrosis prevalence in the United States and participation in the Cystic Fibrosis Foundation Patient Registry in 2020. *Journal of Cystic Fibrosis* 22(3):436-442.

Cure SMA. 2017. *RUSP nomination for SMA accepted into evidence review*. http://www.curesma.org/rusp-nomination-for-sma-accepted-into-evidence-review/ (accessed January 27, 2025).

Currier, R. J. 2022. Newborn screening is on a collision course with public health ethics. *International Journal of Neonatal Screening* 8(4):51.

Duncan, C. N., J. R. Bledsoe, M. Grzywacz, A. Beckman, M. Bonner, F. S. Eichler, J.-S. Kühl, M. H. Harris, S. Slauson, R. A. Colvin, V. K. Prasad, G. F. Downey, F. J. Piercey, M. A. Kenney, M. Foos, A. Lodaya, N. Floro, G. Parsons, A. C. Dietz, A. O. Gupta, P. J. Orchard, H. L. Thakar, and D. A. Williams. 2024. Hematologic cancer after gene therapy for cerebral adrenoleukodystrophy. *New England Journal of Medicine* 391(14):1287-1301.

Evidence-based Review Group. 2018. *Evidence-based review of newborn screening for spinal muscular atrophy (SMA): Final report*. https://www.hrsa.gov/sites/default/files/hrsa/advisory-committees/heritable-disorders/reports-recommendations/sma-final-report.pdf (accessed March 5, 2025).

Faden, R. R., N. A. Holtzman, and A. J. Chwalow. 1982. Parental rights, child welfare, and public health: The case of PKU screening. *American Journal of Public Health* 72(12):1396-1400.

Farrell, M. H., S. A. Christopher, A. Tluczek, K. Kennedy-Parker, A. La Pean, K. Eskra, J. Collins, G. Hoffman, J. Panepinto, and P. M. Farrell. 2011. Improving communication between doctors and parents after newborn screening. *WMJ* 110(5):221-227.

Furnier, S. M., M. S. Durkin, and M. W. Baker. 2020. Translating molecular technologies into routine newborn screening practice. *International Journal of Neonatal Screening* 6(4):80.

Gelb, M. 2024. *Expansion of newborn screening by consolidated biomarker assays and genomic sequencing to find highly penetrant genotypes*. Presented at Newborn Screening: Current Landscape and Future Directions: Meeting 3. https://www.nationalacademies.org/event/42550_05-2024_newborn-screening-current-landscape-and-future-directions-meeting-3 (accessed January 22, 2025).

Gelb, M. H., K. Basheeruddin, A. Burlina, H. Chen, Y. Chien, G. Dizikes, C. Dorley, R. Giugliani, A. Hietala, X. Hong, S. Kao, H. Khaledi, T. Klug, F. Kubaski, H. Liao, M. Martin, A. Manning, J. Orsini, Y. Peng, E. Ranieri, A. Rohrwasser, N. Szabo-Fresnais, C. T. Turgeon, F. M. Vaz, L. Wang, and D. Matern. 2022. Liquid chromatography–tandem mass spectrometry in newborn screening laboratories. *International Journal of Neonatal Screening* 8(4):62.

Goldenberg, A. J., A. M. Comeau, S. D. Grosse, S. Tanksley, L. A. Prosser, J. Ojodu, J. R. Botkin, A. R. Kemper, and N. S. Green. 2016. Evaluating harms in the assessment of net benefit: A framework for newborn screening condition review. *Maternal and Child Health Journal* 20(3):693-700.

Grosse, S. D. 2015. Showing value in newborn screening: Challenges in quantifying the effectiveness and cost-effectiveness of early detection of phenylketonuria and cystic fibrosis. *Healthcare* (Basel) 3(4):1133-1157.

Grosse, S. D., and G. Van Vliet. 2020. Challenges in assessing the cost-effectiveness of newborn screening: The example of congenital adrenal hyperplasia. *International Journal of Neonatal Screening* 6(4):82.

Guenzel, A. J., C. T. Turgeon, K. K. Nickander, A. L. White, D. S. Peck, G. B. Pino, A. L. Studinkski, V. K. Prasad, J. Kurtzberg, M. L. Escolar, M. L. D. Lasio, J. E. Pellegrino, A. Sakonju, R. E. Hickey, N. M. Shallow, M. A. Ream, J. J. Orsini, M. H. Gelb, K. Raymond, D. K. Grabrilov, D. Oglesbee, P. Rinaldo, S. Totorelli, and D. Matern. 2020. The critical role of psychosine in screening, diagnosis, and monitoring of Krabbe disease. *Genetics in Medicine* 22(6):1108-1118.

Halley, M. C. 2021. From "ought" to "is": Surfacing values in patient and family advocacy in rare diseases. *American Journal of Bioethics* 21(12):1-3.

Halley, M. C., H. S. Smith, E. A. Ashley, A. J. Goldenberg, and H. K. Tabor. 2022. A call for an integrated approach to improve efficiency, equity and sustainability in rare disease research in the United States. *Nature* 54:219-222.

Hartnett, M. J., M. A. Lloyd-Puryear, N. P. Tavakoli, J. Wynn, C. L. Koval-Burt, D. Gruber, T. Trotter, M. Caggana, W. K. Chung, N. Armstrong, and A. M. Brower. 2022. Newborn screening for Duchenne muscular dystrophy: First year results of a population-based pilot. *International Journal of Neonatal Screening* 8(4):50.

Hinton, C. F., C. T. Mai, S. K. Nabukera, L. D. Botto, L. Feuchtbaum, P. A. Romitti, Y. Wang, K. N. Piper, and R. S. Olney. 2014. Developing a public health-tracking system for follow-up of newborn screening metabolic conditions: A four-state pilot project structure and initial findings. *Genetics in Medicine* 16(6):484-490.

Hoff, T., and A. Hoyt. 2006. Practices and perceptions of long-term follow-up among state newborn screening programs. *Pediatrics* 117(6):1922-1929.

HRSA (Health Resources and Services Administration). 2016. *Report and recommendations to the pilot studies workgroup*. https://www.hrsa.gov/sites/default/files/hrsa/advisory-committees/heritable-disorders/2016-05-09-botkin-pilot-study.pdf (accessed January 18, 2025).

HRSA. 2018. *The role of quality measures to promote long-term follow-up of children identified by newborn screening programs.* https://www.hrsa.gov/sites/default/files/hrsa/advisory-committees/heritable-disorders/reports-recommendations/role-quality-measures-nbs-sept2018-508c.pdf (accessed January 18, 2025).

HRSA. 2022a. *Key questions considered by the committee.* https://www.hrsa.gov/advisory-committees/heritable-disorders/key-questions (accessed January 18, 2025).

HRSA. 2022b. *Nominating a condition for the Recommended Uniform Screening Panel for newborn screening: Frequently asked questions and other guidance.* https://www.hrsa.gov/advisory-committees/heritable-disorders/frequently-asked-questions (accessed July 31, 2024).

HRSA. 2024a. *State newborn screening system priorities (NBS Propel) program.* https://mchb.hrsa.gov/programs/newborn-screening-propel (accessed March 5, 2025).

HRSA. 2024b. *Cooperative newborn screening system priorities (NBS Co-Propel) program.* https://mchb.hrsa.gov/programs/cooperative-newborn-screening-system-priorities (accessed September 26, 2024).

Kay, D. 2024. *Lessons learned from coordination between research, public health and newborn screening programs.* Presented at Newborn Screening: Current Landscape and Future Directions: Meeting 3. https://www.nationalacademies.org/event/42550_05-2024_newborn-screening-current-landscape-and-future-directions-meeting-3 (accessed January 22, 2025).

Kellar-Guenther, Y., L. Barringer, K. Raboin, G. Nichols, K. Y. F. Chou, K. Nguyen, and M. K. Sontag. 2024. Defining the minimal long-term follow-up data elements for newborn screening. *International Journal of Neonatal Screening* 10(2):37.

Kemper, A. R., C. A. Boyles, J. Aceves, D. Dougherty, J. Figge, J. L. Fisch, A. R. Hinman, C. L. Greene, C. A. Kus, J. Miller, D. Robertson, B. Therrell, M. Lloyd-Puryear, P. C. van Dyck, and R. R. Howell. 2008. Long-term follow-up after diagnosis resulting from newborn screening: Statement of the U.S. Secretary of Health and Human Services' Advisory Committee on Heritable Disorders and Genetic Diseases in Newborns and Children. *Genetics in Medicine* 10(4):259-261.

King, J. S., and M. E. Smith. 2016. Whole-genome screening of newborns? The constitutional boundaries of state newborn screening programs. *Pediatrics* 137(Suppl 1):S8-S15.

Kraszewski, J. N., D. M. Kay, C. F. Stevens, C. Koval, B. Haser, V. Ortiz, A. Albertorio, L. L. Cohen, R. Jain, S. P. Andrew, S. D. Young, N. M. LaMarca, D. C. De Vivo, M. Caggana, and W. K. Chung. 2018. Pilot study of population-based newborn screening for spinal muscular atrophy in New York State. *Genetics in Medicine* 20(6):608-613.

Kwon, J. M., and R. D. Steiner. 2011. "I'm fine; I'm just waiting for my disease": The new and growing class of presymptomatic patients. *Neurology* 77(6):522-523.

La Pean, A., M. H. Farrell, K. L. Eskra, and P. M. Farrell. 2013. Effects of immediate telephone follow-up with providers on sweat chloride test timing after cystic fibrosis newborn screening identifies a single mutation. *Journal of Pediatrics* 162(3):522-529.

Larcher, V., F. Craig, K. Bhogal, D. Wilkinson, and J. Brierley. 2015. Making decisions to limit treatment in life-limiting and life-threatening conditions in children: A framework for practice. *Archives of Disease in Childhood* 100(Suppl 2):s1.

Largent, E. A., and S. D. Pearson. 2012. Which orphans will find a home? The rule of rescue in resource allocation for rare diseases. *Hastings Center Report* 42(1):27-34.

Last, J. M. 2014. Commentary: The iceberg revisited. *International Journal of Epidemiology* 42(6):1613-1615.

Last, J., and M. B. Adelaide. 2013. The iceberg: 'Completing the clinical picture' in general practice. *International Journal of Epidemiology* 42(6):1608-1613.

Ledford, H. 2024. Doctors cured her sickle-cell disease. So why is she still in pain? *Nature* 633:501-511.

Levins, H. 2024. *Sustainable funding and equitable access for multimillion dollar gene therapies: Penn LDI panel unpacks barriers and options for change.* https://ldi.upenn.edu/our-work/research-updates/sustainable-funding-and-equitable-access-for-multi-million-dollar-gene-therapies/ (accessed February 5, 2025).

Lloyd-Puryear, M. A., and A. Brower. 2010. Long-term follow-up in newborn screening: A systems approach for improving health outcomes. *Genetics in Medicine* 12:S256-S260.

Lloyd-Puryear, M., A. Brower, S. A. Berry, J. P. Brosco, B. Bowdish, and M. S. Watson. 2019. Foundation of the newborn screening translational research network and its tools for research. *Genetics in Medicine* 21(6):1271-1279.

Mak, J., G. Peng, A. Le, N. Gandota, G. M. Enns, C. Scharfe, and T. M. Cowan. 2023. Validation of a targeted metabolomics panel for improved second-tier newborn screening. *Journal of Inherited Metabolic Disease* 46(2):194-205.

Merkel, P. A., M. Manion, R. Gopal-Srivastava, S. Groft, H. A. Jinnah, D. Robertson, J. P. Krischer, and Rare Diseases Clinical Research Network. 2016. The partnership of patient advocacy groups and clinical investigators in the rare diseases clinical research network. *Orphanet Journal of Rare Diseases* 11(1):66.

Millington, D., S. Norton, R. Singh, R. Sista, V. Srinivasan, and V. Pamula. 2018. Digital microfluidics comes of age: High-throughput screening to bedside diagnostic testing for genetic disorders in newborns. *Expert Review of Molecular Diagnostics* 18(8):701-712.

Minear, M. A., M. N. Phillips, A. Kau, and M. A. Parisi. 2022. Newborn screening research sponsored by the NIH: From diagnostic paradigms to precision therapeutics. *American Journal of Medical Genetics C: Seminars in Medical Genetics* 190(2):138-152.

New York State Krabbe Disease Consortium. 2016. Newborn screening for Krabbe disease in New York State: The first eight years' experience. *Genetics in Medicine* 18(3):239-248.

NICHD (*Eunice Kennedy Shriver* National Institute of Child Health and Human Development). 2022. *Release: NIH awards $100 million for autism centers of excellence program.* https://www.nichd.nih.gov/newsroom/news/090622-NIH-awards-ACE-program (accessed January 18, 2025).

NICHD. 2024. *202410 natural history of disorders screenable in the newborn period.* https://www.nichd.nih.gov/about/advisory/council/archive/202410/history-disorders-IDDB (accessed January 22, 2025)

NIH (National Institutes of Health). 2022. *Newborn Sequencing in Genomic Medicine and Public Health (NSIGHT).* https://www.genome.gov/Funded-Programs-Projects/Newborn-Sequencing-in-Genomic-Medicine-and-Public-Health-NSIGHT (accessed January 18, 2025).

NIH. 2024. *About research, condition, and disease categorization.* https://report.nih.gov/funding/categorical-spending/rcdc (accessed January 18, 2025).

Peng, G., Y. Tang, T. M. Cowan, G. M. Enns, H. Zhao, and C. Scharfe. 2020. Reducing false-positive results in newborn screening using machine learning. *International Journal of Neonatal Screening* 6(1):16.

Peterson, E. 2024. The thorny ethical conundrums of time-limited gene therapies for rare pediatric neuromuscular disorders. *Neurology Today* 24(5):1-35.

President's Council on Bioethics. 2008. *The changing moral focus of newborn screening: An ethical analysis by the President's Council on Bioethics.* https://bioethicsarchive.georgetown.edu/pcbe/reports/newborn_screening/ (accessed January 18, 2025).

Raboin, K., D. Ellis, G. Nichols, M. Hughes, M. Brimacombe, and K. Rubin. 2024. Advancing newborn screening long-term follow-up: Integration of EPIC-based registries, dashboards, and efficient workflows. *International Journal of Neonatal Screening* 10(2):27.

Richardson, J. S., A. R. Kemper, S. D. Grosse, W. K. K. Lam, A. M. Rose, A. Ahmad, A. Gebremariam, and L. A. Prosser. 2021. Health and economic outcomes of newborn screening for infantile-onset Pompe disease. *Genetics in Medicine* 23(4):758-766.

Scharfe, C. 2024. *Artificial intelligence / machine learning.* Presented at Newborn Screening: Current Landscape and Future Directions: Meeting 3. https://www.nationalacademies.org/event/42550_05-2024_newborn-screening-current-landscape-and-future-directions-meeting-3 (accessed January 22, 2025).

Sheely, D. 2024. *Common fund venture program update.* Presented at the National Institutes of Health Council of Councils meeting, Bethesda, Maryland, September 13, 2024. https://dpcpsi.nih.gov/sites/default/files/2024-09/Day-2-1105AM-CF-Venture-Update-Sheeley-508.pdf (accessed January 22, 2025).

Simon, N. J., A. Atkins, C. Yusuf, and B. A. Tarini. 2020. Systems integration: The next frontier in newborn-screening timeliness. *Journal of Public Health Management and Practice* 26(6):E8-E15.

Singhal, K., T. Tu, J. Gottweis, R. Sayres, E. Wulczyn, M. Amin, L. Hou, K. Clark, S. R. Pfohl, H. Cole-Lewis, D. Neal, Q. Mamunur Rashid, M. Schaekermann, A. Wang, D. Dash, J. H. Chen, N. H. Shah, S. Lachgar, P. A. Mansfield, S. Prakash, B. Green, E. Dominowska, B. Agüera y Arcas, N. Tomaškev, Y. Liu, R. Wong, C. Semturs, S. S. Mahdavi, J. K. Barral, D. R. Webster, G. S. Corrado, Y. Matias, S. Azizi, A. Karthikesalingam, and V. Natarajan. 2025. Toward expert-level medical question answering with large language models. *Nature Medicine* 31(3):943-950.

Sobotka, S. A., and L. F. Ross. 2023. Newborn screening for neurodevelopmental disorders may exacerbate health disparities. *Pediatrics* 152(4):e2023061727.

Susanna Haas Lyons Engagement Consulting. 2024. *What we heard: Engagement summary for committee on newborn screening: Current landscape and future directions.* Washington, DC: National Academies of Sciences, Engineering, and Medicine.

Therrell, B. L., Jr., W. H. Hannon, D. B. Bailey, Jr., E. B. Goldman, J. Monaco, B. Norgaard-Pedersen, S. F. Terry, A. Johnson, and R. R. Howell. 2011. Committee report: Considerations and recommendations for national guidance regarding the retention and use of residual dried blood spot specimens after newborn screening. *Genetics in Medicine* 13(7):621-624.

Thirunavukarasu, A. J., D. S. J. Ting, K. Elangovan, L. Gutierrez, T. F. Tan, and D. S. W. Ting. 2023. Large language models in medicine. *Nature Medicine* 29(8):1930-1940.

Timmermans, S., and M. Buchbinder. 2010. Patients-in-waiting: Living between sickness and health in the genomics era. *Journal of Health and Social Behavior* 51(4):408-423.

Towards Healthcare. 2023. *Newborn screening industry analysis and opportunities report.* https://www.towardshealthcare.com/insights/newborn-screening-market-sizing (accessed January 18, 2025).

Unnikumaran, Y., M. Lietsch, and A. Brower. 2024. Charting the ethical frontier in newborn screening research: Insights from the NBSTRN ELSI researcher needs survey. *International Journal of Neonatal Screening* 10(3):64.

USPSTF (United States Preventative Services Task Force). 2018. *Grade definitions.* https://www.uspreventiveservicestaskforce.org/uspstf/about-uspstf/methods-and-processes/grade-definitions#july2012 (accessed March 5, 2025).

Van Vliet, G., and S. D. Grosse. 2021. Newborn screening for congenital hypothyroidism and congenital adrenal hyperplasia: The balance of benefits and costs of a public health success. *Medical Sciences* (Paris) 37(5):528-534.

Venugopal, N., G. Naik, K. Jayanna, A. Mohapatra, F. J. Sasinowski, R. V. Kartha, and H. K. Rajasimha. 2024. Review of methods for estimating the prevalence of rare diseases. *Rare Disease and Orphan Drugs Journal* 3(1):5.

Vokinger, K. N., J. Avorn, and A. S. Kesselheim. 2023. Sources of innovation in gene therapies—Approaches to achieving affordable prices. *New England Journal of Medicine* 388(4):292-295.

Watson, M. S., M. A. Lloyd-Puryear, and R. R. Howell. 2022. The progress and future of US newborn screening. *International Journal of Neonatal Screening* 8(3):41.

Watterberg, K. L., W. A. Carlo, L. P. Brion, C. M. Cotten, and R. D. Higgins. 2022. Overview of the neonatal research network: History, contributions, challenges, and future. *Seminars in Perinatology* 46(7):151634.

Weise, K. L., A. L. Okun, B. S. Carter, C. W. Christian, Committee on Bioethics, Section on Hospice and Palliative Medicine, and the Committee on Child Abuse and Neglect. 2017. Guidance on forgoing life-sustaining medical treatment. *Pediatrics* 140(3):e20171905.

Wilhelm, K., M. J. Edick, S. A. Berry, M. Hartnett, and A. Brower. 2022. Using long-term follow-up data to classify genetic variants in newborn screened conditions. *Frontiers in Genetics* 13:859837.

Zaunseder, E., S. Haupt, U. Mütze, S. F. Garbade, S. Kölker, and V. Heuveline. 2022. Opportunities and challenges in machine learning-based newborn screening—A systematic literature review. *JIMD Reports* 63(3):250-261.

Zhou, M., L. Deng, Y. Huang, Y. Xiao, J. Wen, N. Liu, Y. Zeng, and H. Zhang. 2022. Application of the artificial intelligence algorithm model for screening of inborn errors of metabolism. *Frontiers in Pediatrics* 10:855943.

7

Envisioning the Future of Newborn Screening

Newborn screening (NBS) as a public heath endeavor faces a complex array of needs, competing priorities, and viewpoints. NBS programs, federal agency partners, families, care providers, and many others must address longstanding challenges around the inclusion of conditions on screening panels, difficulties advancing the evidence base in the context of rare diseases, and the lack of awareness about public health newborn screening, while attending to issues on the horizon such as the appropriate use of genome-based screening technologies and continued legal and ethical scholarship around the consent and reuse of blood spot samples. A high-performing NBS system must exemplify excellence, and this chapter focuses on actions essential to not only sustain public health newborn screening but strengthen and prepare it for the future.

Taking a strategic, system-based approach to public health newborn screening is needed to navigate these challenges, bring together the many involved and affected parties, foster proactive recognition of shared challenges and issues, provide clarity and develop guidance, and work collaboratively with partners throughout the NBS system to develop solutions while respecting state and territorial autonomy. Drawing on the information and analyses provided throughout this report, the committee drew two overarching conclusions that informed its recommendations for preserving and strengthening newborn screening:

> *Overarching Conclusion 1: The next era of public health newborn screening needs to effectively use the resources and knowledge of state- and territorial-run public health programs and embrace opportunities for national coordination, strategy, and priority setting. Leadership and coordination at the national level*

are needed to set priorities and maintain high performance while adapting to the longstanding and emerging challenges facing public health newborn screening.

Overarching Conclusion 2: Many perspectives—not only those of decision makers in the federal government—are essential to creating a unified vision for public health newborn screening and a road map to achieve it, but driving this vision forward will require federal leadership, accountability, and coordination.

RECOMMENDATIONS

The nine recommendations below outline a path forward to navigate the tensions and pressures facing public health newborn screening in the United States while preserving and enhancing what is already a valuable and effective public health achievement (Figure 7-1). Collectively, these recommendations call for a more systematic and coordinated approach to align the NBS ecosystem around shared goals, build on the large array of efforts and programs already under way, and support newborn screening as it enters its next era.[1]

Establish National Vision, Coordination, and Leadership

Newborn screening, although fundamentally operated as a state- and territorial-run program, has been searching for a national vision for over

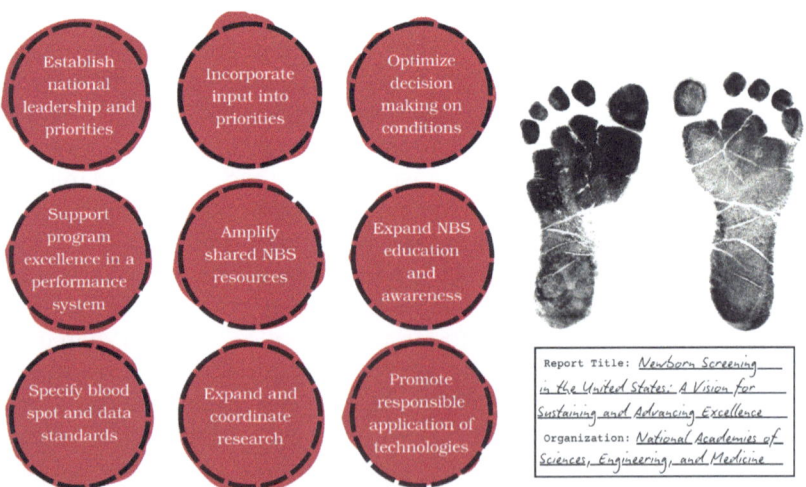

FIGURE 7-1 Summary of recommendations: A road map forward.
NOTE: NBS = newborn screening.

---

[1] The report focuses on critical functions and actions to strengthen public health newborn screening for the future; descriptions of the roles and structures of federal and nonfederal activities relevant to newborn screening are current as of March 24, 2025.

two decades. The American Academy of Pediatrics (AAP), American College of Medical Genetics and Genomics (ACMG), and others have called for increased national coordination and guidance since the late 1990s (AAP Newborn Screening Task Force, 2000; ACMG Newborn Screening Expert Group, 2006; Andrews et al., 2022). Among these reports, the 2006 ACMG report provided recommendations to move "toward a unified screening panel and system" to contend with a similar set of challenges as today. These recommendations served as the basis for establishing the Recommended Uniform Screening Panel (RUSP)—a key piece of national guidance (ACMG Newborn Screening Expert Group, 2006).

Beyond the RUSP, five federal partners—the Health Resources and Services Administration (HRSA), Centers for Disease Control and Prevention (CDC), National Institutes of Health (NIH), Food and Drug Administration (FDA), and Agency for Healthcare Research and Quality (AHRQ)—each provide support, leadership, and guidance for different portions of the NBS landscape (see Chapter 2) (HHS, 2015). However, the totality of newborn screening encompasses processes and priorities that traverse public health, clinical care, and research. Parties across the broader NBS ecosystem have acknowledged that insufficient coordination and communication among federal agencies have previously hampered national data collection and decision making regarding the funding and implementation of newborn screening (Andrews et al., 2022). Greater national leadership can support that goal as well as the accomplishment of others, identified in Box 7-1.

Despite the efforts and progress of the federal agencies and others to bring a more unified vision to the complex landscape of public health newborn screening, the same challenges have persisted—and new ones have arisen. Box 7-2 provides examples of challenges that require national approaches to effectively address.

> **Recommendation 1: Establish national leadership and set priorities. The U.S. Department of Health and Human Services (HHS) should provide unified leadership, accountability, and coordination across government agencies, newborn screening (NBS) programs, and the broader NBS community.**
>
> a. With input from partners (see Recommendation 2), HHS should establish a 10-year strategic plan to implement this report's recommendations and begin to implement them.
> b. HHS should designate a mechanism with appropriate authority, accountability, and resources to facilitate realization of this plan.

Federal leadership, accountability, and coordination are needed to advance this coherent vision for public health newborn screening, enhancing

> **BOX 7-1**
> **Goals to Be Addressed with Increased**
> **National Vision and Coordination**
>
> 1. Create more intentionality and coordination within an ecosystem that has been highly fragmented, particularly on the federal level, ultimately bringing more resources, authority, and capacity to the patchwork quilt of public health newborn screening (NBS).
> 2. Align on a national vision and strategic plan by convening and drawing on perspectives from interested parties across the NBS ecosystem to ensure voices are heard.
> 3. Develop a continuous performance improvement process, together with state and territorial NBS programs, to ensure the highest standards for public health newborn screening across all jurisdictions.
> 4. Enable the collection of timely data to proactively inform policy decisions and act strategically within the entirety of the NBS ecosystem.
> 5. Effectively allocate resources by maximizing their usefulness at a national and state level to address issues within the NBS ecosystem.
> 6. Establish an accountability partner at the federal level for the achievement of goals within the NBS ecosystem.
> 7. Serve as a communication locus for multiple stakeholders and rightsholders across the NBS ecosystem to enhance awareness of needs and opportunities and align efforts.

its impact without diminishing the unique roles and responsibilities of different parties. Although implemented through 56 state and territorial programs, public health newborn screening is buttressed by the contributions not only of federal agencies, but also of laboratory and clinical professional communities, patient groups, researchers from academia and industry, and others (see Chapter 2). All participants in this informal NBS ecosystem are dedicated to excellence within their sphere, but fragmentation and lack of

> **BOX 7-2**
> **Selected Challenges in Public Health Newborn Screening**
> **Requiring National Coordination to Address**
>
> 1. Geographic disparities across state- and territorial-run newborn screening (NBS) programs
> 2. Timely evidence generation to inform the Recommended Uniform Screening Panel
> 3. Effective public communication concerning newborn screening
> 4. Long-term follow-up infrastructure
> 5. National recommended standards for the collection, retention, sharing, and use of newborn dried blood spots

coordination can permit goals and efforts to misalign. Newborn screening needs to embrace opportunities for coordination and priority setting while leveraging and respecting the autonomy and local expertise of state-run programs. Additional federal partners are essential to the success of newborn screening, and their involvement would enhance coordination and impact. For example, the Centers for Medicare & Medicaid Services (CMS) is not a named federal NBS partner (HHS, 2015), but Medicaid covers NBS fees for approximately 40 percent of births annually (CMS, 2024). A coordinated approach, coupled with appropriate resources, authority, and accountability, can better align the efforts of the many partners involved in public health screening and enable each to understand their role in driving a strategic plan forward.

The national vision and coordination called for in this recommendation could be operationalized in different ways, while also recognizing and respecting the autonomy and unique roles of federal and state programs and agencies. Several options are described below.

Increased Interagency Coordination

Effectively using existing practices and authorities, federal agencies could maintain their respective spheres of influence and coordinate through interagency working groups with renewed purpose to develop strategic plans. Additional, relevant federal partners (e.g., CMS) can be brought into these working groups to strengthen coordination. However, such an approach would not permit whole-of-government coordination, nor would it provide a true accountability partner that can give due attention to the totality of public health newborn screening, avert issues related to diffusion of responsibility, and ensure progress on all items in the strategic plan.

Accountability Partner Embedded in an Agency

Another option would be to designate an accountability partner at one of the federal agencies, which could avoid issues related to diffused responsibility for achieving NBS-related goals. However, the five federal agencies that interact in newborn screening each contribute guidance and support (HRSA, CDC, NIH, FDA, and AHRQ) in different spheres, and the entirety of responsibilities would not fit neatly under any one agency.

Private–Public Strategic Council

The Department of Health and Human Services could create a public–private strategic council to establish a vision and set strategic priorities for public health newborn screening. However, executing that vision would be difficult with no oversight authority or budget. The ad hoc nature of many advisory bodies also means that long-term sustainability to monitor progress in achieving priorities or to identify and address issues over time is limited and uncertain. An advisory body would also be limited in its ability to coordinate across the agencies and ensure the most effective and strategic use of resources.

Nonprofit Entity

A separate nonprofit entity could be created to convene partners to establish a national vision, and with appropriate funding, provide resources and supports. A nonprofit entity could excel at building partnerships across the public and private sectors to craft and enact innovative solutions. This model has been effective for the Fund for Public Health NYC, which was established as an independent nonprofit organization to connect the New York City Health Department to private-sector partners and the greater philanthropic communities.[2] However, a primary purpose of a national mechanism would be to have appropriate authority and coordination across the federal agencies. Given that a nonprofit entity is situated outside of the federal government, opportunities to provide oversight and coordinate among the federal agencies would be limited.

Office, Point Person, or Advisor in HHS

An office, point person, or advisor could be designated in the Department of Health and Human Services (HHS) to ensure coordination and a unified plan across the federal government and others, while recognizing and preserving the unique roles and responsibilities of agencies, state-run programs, and other stakeholders and rightsholders. The HHS Office of the Assistant Secretary of Health, which oversees HHS public health efforts, is a potential locus for such accountability.[3] An office, point person, or advisor in HHS could coordinate across agencies, have convening power to solicit input from a wide-ranging set of stakeholders, establish national standards and guidance, and have a dedicated budget to follow through on strategic plans. This mechanism would require an investment of resources and might face scrutiny about government expansion. However, federal offices, point persons, and advisors are designated for many reasons, and often to advise on topics affecting vulnerable populations. Newborns are a large potentially at-risk population in the United States, with nearly 3.6 million babies screened each year, and an investment of resources could be merited to reduce morbidity and mortality across the population.

---

[2] https://fphnyc.org/about/our-story/ (accessed December 12, 2024).
[3] https://www.hhs.gov/ash/index.html (accessed December 18, 2024).

Combined Approaches

Some of the options outlined may be able to be combined to balance trade-offs and maximize benefit. For example, an office, point person, or advisor in HHS could be combined with a nonprofit entity. The position in HHS could provide oversight, accountability, and coordinate across federal agencies, and the nonprofit entity could function as the operational arm.

Incorporate Multistakeholder and Rightsholder Input on Newborn Screening

Creating a unified and strategic plan for newborn screening must draw in many perspectives—not only those of decision makers in the federal government. Representatives of the many groups personally and professionally affected by newborn screening must be engaged in identifying critical issues and potential solutions, developing a unified vision and strategic plan, and continually advancing and implementing this plan.

> **Recommendation 2: Incorporate multistakeholder and rightsholder input into newborn screening priorities.[4] The U.S. Department of Health and Human Services should establish a multistakeholder/rightsholder advisory body to provide input to the national leadership identified in Recommendation 1. This advisory body should identify high-level, cross-agency, cross-state, and cross-system challenges; elevate potential solutions to those challenges; inform the development of a strategic plan; and monitor and advise on progress in its implementation. The advisory body should engage wide-ranging expertise and experiences to inform the strategic plan and enable all partners to understand their role in driving it forward.**

Currently, the discretionary HHS Advisory Committee on Heritable Disorders in Newborns and Children (ACHDNC) provides recommendations to the HHS secretary on newborn and childhood screening, including the appropriate application of tests, technologies, policies, guidelines, and standards to effectively reduce morbidity and mortality in newborns and children with serious disorders (HRSA, 2024b). ACHDNC might seem like a natural fit to take on such a strategic advising task. However, as currently designed, ACHDNC would not

---

[4] The term *rightsholder* is incorporated to recognize use of this term among Native American and Indigenous communities and to reflect their distinct legal and political contexts.

be suitable to take on this function for two reasons. First, although the scope of ACHDNC's mandate is theoretically broad, the committee's attention is primarily directed toward reviewing conditions for potential addition to the RUSP. This emphasis is responsive to the importance of evidence-based decision making for adding conditions to the RUSP, but it limits ACHDNC's capacity to focus on overarching strategy. Second, the current membership of ACHDNC primarily represents federal agencies, state-run programs with a focus on laboratory expertise, and medical professionals.[5] The current ACHDNC does not comprise the full breadth of expertise and experiences that would be necessary for this more strategic advisory mission.

The multistakeholder/rightsholder advisory body called for in Recommendation 2 would focus on high-level, cross-agency, cross-state, and cross-system challenges. Other mechanisms or approaches are needed to address processes associated with the RUSP (see Recommendation 3). The multistakeholder/rightsholder advisory body could be established in different ways, including as a formal federal advisory committee or through other federal or nonfederal convening mechanisms. Regardless of how it might be implemented, a wide range of expertise and perspectives is essential to the success of public health newborn screening and the advisory body would need to include

- members among state/territorial NBS program directors, laboratory experts, and follow-up experts;
- prenatal and birth care providers;
- health care providers such as genetic counselors, pediatricians, and disease specialists;
- members reflecting family and rare disease community organizations and perspectives;
- the multiple federal agencies involved;
- philanthropic organizations active in this area; and
- the private sector.

Newborn screening involves a complex nexus of federal, state, tribal, and private rights and responsibilities. Additional conversations are needed with tribal nations and leaders to understand these intersecting rights and authorities, involve tribal communities in the national vision for newborn screening, and ensure that priorities and solutions meet the needs of Indigenous communities.

---

[5] The current membership roster of ACHNDC is available at https://www.hrsa.gov/sites/default/files/hrsa/advisory-committees/heritable-disorders/achdnc-membership-roster.pdf (accessed December 18, 2024). Public health, medical, or community advocacy organizations may also serve as nonvoting organizational representatives.

Optimizing the RUSP

Prior to the creation of the Recommended Uniform Screening Panel in 2010, there was no national guidance on which conditions to include in state NBS panels, leading to substantial variation in disorders screened from state to state. Although the RUSP is not a mandate, it has helped harmonize the landscape of NBS programs and emphasized the importance and role of rigorous evidence review when making decisions about conditions to include in population-wide screening (See Chapter 2).

Overarching Conclusion 3: The Recommended Uniform Screening Panel (RUSP) remains an important source of evidence-based guidance on which conditions to include in state panels for newborn screening (NBS). Striving for alignment with the RUSP promotes consistency across NBS programs and provides infants born across the United States with an equal opportunity to be screened for these conditions.

However, the process for evaluating or incorporating new conditions on the RUSP is long and burdensome (Andrews et al., 2022; Armstrong, 2024; HRSA, 2024a; Susanna Haas Lyons Engagement Consulting, 2024). This protracted time line is a consequence of multiple inputs spanning evidence generation, nomination, evidence review, decision making in the face of limited and incomplete data, and other associated factors. There are no simple answers to the RUSP. A complete reimagining of the RUSP review process risks exhausting already resource-constrained public health and clinical care systems; however, the process as it currently exists is untenable, burdensome, and frustrating to many.

Addition of a condition to the RUSP also does not translate into uniform screening implementation, or even consideration, across states and territories. Instead, advocates and others must navigate state-by-state processes for adding conditions to NBS panels. Every state or territory needs a mechanism to ensure the systematic consideration of conditions added to the RUSP in a timely manner, even if screening is not ultimately implemented.

Recommendation 3: Optimize decision making on conditions included in newborn screening. The U.S. Department of Health and Human Services (HHS) and state and territorial newborn screening (NBS) programs should optimize the process of considering conditions in public health newborn screening.

a. **HHS leadership should designate a focused committee or mechanism to provide advice on the Recommended Uniform Screening Panel (RUSP), composed of appropriate experts and distinct from the strategic advisory body in Recommendation 2. In addition to advising on nominated**

conditions, this committee should (1) proactively assess which conditions could meet criteria for inclusion on the RUSP; (2) identify specific gaps in evidence necessary for RUSP decision making for conditions identified in this assessment and highlight what strategic research is needed (see Recommendation 8); (3) periodically reassess evidence and consider whether RUSP removal is warranted for any condition based on knowledge gained from its implementation in public health newborn screening.
b. HHS leadership should expand the scientific and technical capacity for reviewing evidence for conditions under consideration for addition to the RUSP, including exploring the applicability of rapid review mechanisms.
c. State and territorial NBS programs should have a mechanism to consider implementation of RUSP conditions within a designated time line.

This recommendation could be achieved by focusing and enhancing the ACHDNC's current mission. In the near term, action is needed to streamline the evidence generation and review processes for the RUSP while maintaining sufficient scientific and technical rigor. A major first step is commissioning a landscaping analysis to understand which conditions could fit inclusion criteria for public health newborn screening, facilitate proactive decision making, and identify gaps in research evidence necessary to inform decision making for RUSP inclusion. Such gaps could inform conditions to include in NBS pilot studies or other research endeavors. This analysis would be critical to enable strategic research investment and timely, evidence-based decision making. Comparisons of gene-condition lists across multiple newborn sequencing research programs focused on serious, urgent, and treatable conditions may inform this work (Downie et al., 2024; Minten et al., 2024). For example, a comparison across 27 programs identified 74 genes included by over 80% of programs (Minten et al., 2024). Of those genes, 58 are associated with conditions already on the RUSP, but other associated conditions could provide a starting point for a landscaping analysis.

In the face of genomic technologies and ongoing therapeutic innovation for rare diseases, groundwork must also be laid for a future where an increased number of conditions that align with the public health goals of newborn screening could be incorporated in screening. Pilot testing the feasibility of adopting more rapid review mechanisms used by consented research studies exploring DNA-based screening in newborns is one avenue to explore. The processes used for condition review and inclusion determinations for consented research studies using genomic sequencing in newborns, such as NC Nexus or Early Check, may be informative as these studies include hundreds of conditions on screening panels (Cope et al., 2024; Milko et al., 2019). However, their primary focus is on whether conditions meet inclusion criteria of being serious, urgent, and actionable; review of implementation data is not included. One study comparing rapid review versus full systematic review mechanisms to assess newborn screening for a single condition found that rapid reviews may be appropriate tools if safeguards are in place (Taylor-Phillips et al., 2017).

Exploring the implications of adopting or adapting rapid review mechanisms for the RUSP may be one first step toward reenvisioning the RUSP process, though careful attention will need to be paid to context as RUSP decisions inform universal public health newborn screening rather than consented research pilots. The process for adding conditions to the RUSP will need to be reexamined periodically, in light of further developments in screening technologies and in the evidence base for diseases that could potentially be included, as well as in the context of the enhanced public health NBS system recommended in this report.

Other actions to enhance the RUSP process include increasing the number of scientific and technical experts involved in evidence review and designating a dedicated or specialized committee or mechanism whose focus is to provide advice on the RUSP. Evidence evaluation for RUSP decision making needs to focus on relevant scientific, clinical, and technical aspects of the condition; its effects and treatments; and its implementation in public health screening. Issues related to individual NBS program operational feasibility are better addressed through supports to state-level programs (see Recommendations 4 and 5).

State and territorial NBS programs may need to work with their legislatures, public health departments, and other involved communities to identify and implement a mechanism to assess conditions as they are added to the RUSP. One mechanism could include a process and time line for considering a newly added RUSP condition by their state's advisory committee (e.g., Washington State).[6] Another would be for a state or territory to enact RUSP alignment laws, which require NBS programs to implement screening for RUSP conditions within a certain time frame. While some states already have these mechanisms in place, others do not.[7] When states or territories do not implement a RUSP condition, some may choose to inform parents of other mechanisms parents could pursue

---

[6] See https://sboh.wa.gov/sites/default/files/2024-11/Tab09a_Cover%20Memo_NBS%20TAC%20Review.pdf (accessed March 6, 2025).

[7] The National Organization for Rare Disorders documents policies for considering and/or implementing RUSP disorders across the United States. See https://rarediseases.org/policy-issues/newborn-screening/#_ftn3 (accessed March 7, 2025) and select appendices to see detailed information about each state.

for screening (e.g., private laboratory testing). Although mechanisms for timely consideration or implementation of RUSP conditions are needed, the successful implementation of high-quality screening across programs will require more robust systems of support, described below.

Establish a System to Support NBS Program Excellence

Public health newborn screening is implemented through 56 NBS programs, which operate independently from each other under a wide range of operational and funding structures and within the different contexts of their local health care systems. Variation in the practice of newborn screening across state- and territorial-run programs is inevitable given these circumstances and can enable programs to address their specific circumstances and populations. However, strengthening the network of NBS programs requires addressing detrimental variability that arises from insufficient resources or support and that can negatively affect health outcomes. Ensuring that all 56 programs have what they need to achieve excellent performance in their essential functions requires more systematic data collection and analysis and more strategic alignment of financial and nonfinancial supports and incentives (see Chapter 4).

Enhanced data collection and analysis efforts can build on the foundation initiated through current, grant-based efforts that rely on voluntary submission from NBS programs, such as the Association of Public Health Laboratories' (APHL's) Newborn Screening Technical assistance and Evaluation Program (NewSTEPs) data repository and resource center, supported by a grant from HRSA.[8] Clarity on common metrics and commitments to collect and use data systematically is needed from NBS programs and federal agencies.

> **Recommendation 4: Support newborn screening (NBS) program excellence in a performance system.** The U.S. Department of Health and Human Services (HHS) leadership (Recommendation 1) and state- and territorial-run NBS program directors should partner to establish a universal performance improvement system. Data collected should enable each program to assess its laboratory and follow-up performance, benchmark with peers, and iteratively improve its processes. To accomplish this the following needs to occur:
>
> a. HHS should incentivize participation from all programs.
> b. HHS should collaborate with state and territorial NBS program directors to identify a common set of performance

---

[8] See https://www.newsteps.org/ (accessed December 18, 2024).

metrics all states will collect to monitor and improve laboratory and follow-up performance.
c. State/territorial-run NBS programs should agree to participate and commit to using collected data to close gaps and pursue excellence.
d. HHS should provide responsive financial investment and technical assistance based on performance assessment.

Several approaches could be taken to establish a universal NBS performance excellence and improvement system. One option could be to augment the existing NewSTEPs or envisioned Enhancing Data-driven Disease Detection in Newborns (ED3N) resources.[9] Currently, data collected through NewSTEPs may not target the most useful metrics, have limited or partial participation from state and territorial NBS programs, and are not analyzed and used in a holistic way to inform responsive or strategic decisions. CDC's ED3N platform, currently in development, aims to serve as a voluntary collection and analysis platform for biochemical and molecular testing data to assist NBS partners to improve screening performance. Potential ED3N modules for clinical or follow-up data analysis have also been envisioned (see Chapter 4).

Strengthening, expanding, and systematizing NewSTEPs and/or ED3N infrastructure to serve as a universal NBS performance improvement system would require coordinated efforts with federal and state agencies, programs, and others to identify and agree on a common set of key performance metrics, incentives for programs to participate, and responsive funding and technical assistance based on performance. Other potential approaches could include establishing an expanded federal cooperative assistance program (such as the CDC Epidemiology and Lab Capacity Program) or other forms of private or nonprofit organization that focus on performance excellence (such as the California Perinatal and Maternal Quality Care Collaboratives) (see Chapter 4). For the approach selected, the HHS leadership mechanism established in Recommendation 1 would need to provide funding (both to support the system itself and to incentivize state and territorial program participation), oversight, guidance, and accountability.

Measuring, documenting and understanding the longer-term effects of newborn screening on the care, services, and health outcomes of infants diagnosed with a screened condition is important for analyzing how well newborn screening programs function and for making decisions about their future. Designing and implementing a mechanism to collect and analyze such long-term follow-up data after newborn

---

[9] https://www.cdc.gov/newborn-screening/php/about/ed3n-project.html (accessed March 4, 2025).

screening remains challenging because it entails information across state public health agencies, medical records housed in varied care settings, public and private insurance records, and other data sources. A universal and strategic NBS performance improvement system might not, at least initially, include metrics related to long-term follow-up. Although long-term follow-up data are critical to understand the public health effect of newborn screening and to strengthen the NBS system, collection of such information requires clinical health and public health partnerships, health information technology infrastructures, and other capacities that are outside the scope and ability of most state and territorial NBS programs. See Chapter 5 for options to address long-term follow-up data collection.

Amplify Program Excellence Through Shared Resources

NBS programs vary in their resources, expertise, and capacities for advanced technical analysis of newborn blood spots, development and implementation of new screening assays, establishing connections with specialized genetic counseling and clinical care communities for screened conditions, and other factors. As described in Chapter 4, available federal resources are often ad hoc or grant based, requiring NBS program staff to identify challenges, locate prospective resources, and prepare competitive grant applications. While helpful, this approach risks exacerbating existing disparities among programs, in which already strong and well-resourced NBS programs are better positioned to apply. Informal "ask a colleague" requests through community forums such as the APHL NewSTEPs discussion board and via personal networks and contacts, as well as formal, individual state-to-state agreements, are other approaches used to supplement NBS programs' capacities.

All programs must achieve and maintain excellence in the core functions necessary to deliver on the promise of universal, at-birth newborn screening. Strengthening the network of 56 NBS programs will require each to have access to the range of resources, capacities, and expertise needed to provide an excellent public health service to all babies. Mechanisms to facilitate sharing across NBS programs will also help maximize and support more efficient use of scarce resources and expertise, such as for capabilities for advanced technical analysis and genetic counseling expertise.

> **Recommendation 5:** Amplify newborn screening (NBS) program excellence through shared resources. The U.S. Department of Health and Human Services (HHS) leadership (Recommendation 1) should foster NBS programs' ability to

efficiently access and use specialized resources and expertise. To achieve this, HHS should survey NBS program directors to identify each program's capacities, strengths, and sources of specialized expertise in both laboratory and follow-up performance; assess this resulting landscape; and establish infrastructure for more systematic and efficient use of shared resources among programs.

A variety of mechanisms and approaches could be used to implement this recommendation. One useful first step is identifying the landscape of strengths, specialized resources, and expertise each NBS program provides, along with major gaps or needs. HHS could develop a centralized repository of such information, establish or designate resource centers to facilitate connections between programs, and provide additional or targeted federal support to enable programs to share these assets and skills. Which resource-sharing agreements would need to be established among states, the benefits and burdens that would pose, and the ability for national templates and federal support to facilitate that process would need to be better understood.

More formalized centers for expertise could also be established at several NBS programs to provide direct services and peer mentorship. Establishing or designating centers for specialized expertise would help provide access to important capacities, although the full implications would need to be further explored as this approach may direct federal resources toward the already strongest programs.

Parents and Providers as Partners in the NBS System

Despite longstanding calls for increased NBS education, particularly during the prenatal period (ACOG Committee on Genetics, 2019; Botkin et al., 2016; Davis et al., 2006; Therrell et al., 2011), current efforts are not effectively engaging all families (see Chapter 4). Many parents are unaware of newborn screening until the moment it occurs, and others do not recall that their infant ever received newborn screening (Campbell and Ross, 2004; Kusyk et al., 2013; Susanna Haas Lyons Engagement Consulting, 2024). Parents and caregivers need more systematic information about the purpose of newborn blood spot screening, when and how it will happen, what to expect after blood spot collection, and parental options—both concerning screening and the retention and reuse of the residual dried blood spot. Education and engagement can take varied forms including printed materials (e.g., pamphlets and posters), electronic resources (e.g., videos, images, and websites), and conversations with care providers and educators. Many NBS educational resources exist, developed by family support and advocacy organizations, professional associations, government agencies, and others.[10] Providers must have sufficient knowledge about the basic practices of newborn screening, how to routinely integrate and disseminate resources on newborn screening into care, and the fundamentals of genetics so they are prepared to engage with patients responsibly about newborn screening.

> **Recommendation 6: Expand public and professional newborn screening (NBS) education and awareness.** Engagement with pregnant individuals, parents, and caregivers should occur at multiple points during the perinatal period. This education should start in the prenatal period and cover the purpose of newborn screening, when and how it will happen, what to expect after blood spot collection, parental options, and communication of the infant's results.
>
> a. All professional associations involved in perinatal and infant care should issue recommendations for communicating about newborn screening with pregnant patients, parents, and/or caregivers and support accurate communication through professional education.
> b. The multistakeholder/rightsholder advisory body described in Recommendation 2 should work with relevant professional societies, patient/family organizations, and experts in effective public communication to design goals and communication approaches that can be adapted to local contexts, drawing on existing materials and research.

Reaching as many parents and caregivers as possible will require disseminating resources at multiple points by multiple actors using a "no wrong door" approach. Key opportunities for communication include prenatal care and prenatal classes, following birth at the point of screening, and during the newborn period as part of pediatric care. Relevant professional societies that must participate in NBS education include, but are not limited to, the American College of Obstetricians and Gynecologists; Association of Women's Health, Obstetric, and Neonatal Nurses; American Association of Birth Centers; American College of Nurse-Midwives; American Academy

---

[10] Links to multiple resources and materials on newborn screening are available through the HRSA's Newborn Screening Resources page (https://newbornscreening.hrsa.gov/about-newborn-screening/newborn-screening-resources; accessed November 27, 2024), through Baby's First Test (https://www.babysfirsttest.org/newborn-screening/resources; accessed November 27, 2024), through Expecting Health (https://expectinghealth.org/programs/newborn-screening-family-education-program; accessed February 4, 2025), and through multiple other sources.

of Pediatrics; American Academy of Family Physicians; National Association of Family Nurse Practitioners; National Association of Pediatric Nurse Practitioners; Society of Pediatric Nurses; and others. Clarifying professional recommendations and clinical practice guidelines for NBS education during the perinatal period, as well as the coding and reimbursement of such services, may be necessary to help support and facilitate widespread adoption.

Specifying Standards for the Retention and Use of Dried Blood Spots

After newborn screening, a portion of the dried blood spot is usually left over. These residual dried blood spots have many important uses that are essential to the core purpose of public health newborn screening, including retesting or second-tier testing if needed, as well as quality control, assurance, and improvement efforts. Residual dried blood spots can also be used for other purposes, including for research or forensics (see Chapter 4). Despite these important potential uses, there are few consistent policies at the federal, state, tribal,[11] or laboratory level setting rules or expectations for NBS dried blood spot retention and use, along with varying parental disclosure or consent policies about what will happen to their child's specimen (Botkin et al., 2013; Ram, 2022).

Stakeholders and rightsholders throughout the NBS system have strong views on the appropriate uses and limitations of these specimens. Concerns about storage and reuse are rising and have only been exacerbated by instances of law enforcement access for the purposes of prosecution. Several court cases have challenged the retention and secondary use of these blood spots as federally unconstitutional under the Fourth Amendment (prohibiting unreasonable searches and seizures) and the Fourteenth Amendment (prohibiting the deprivation of liberty without due process), leading to the destruction of millions of blood spots. Developing clear state standards and protections are necessary to act in trustworthy ways and avoid federal constitutional challenge.

Recommendation 7: Specify standards for the retention, sharing, and use of newborn dried blood spots and derived data.

a. State legislatures should set law and policy for the retention, sharing, and use of newborn dried blood spots and any derived data. These policies and laws should do the following:
    i. Protect the retention of newborn screening (NBS)

---

[11] Additional clarifications may be needed to understand legal authorities over newborn dried blood spots collected in tribal health care settings, jurisdiction of tribal data sovereignty, and applicable state laws governing NBS programs.

dried blood spots for at least a limited period for primary public health screening goals including, but not limited to, retesting samples, quality assessment, and quality improvement.

ii. Set transparent practices for the retention, sharing, and use of dried blood spots for purposes other than those described above, including research.

iii. Allow parents the option to request the destruction of their child's specimen after the limited time period of retention for primary public health screening goals, and allow the dried blood spot contributor the option to request the destruction of their own specimen when they reach the age of 18.

iv. Prohibit the sharing or use of NBS dried blood spots and derived data to conduct criminal, civil, or administrative investigations and/or impose criminal, civil, or administrative liability on the NBS contributor or blood relatives.

b. The U.S. Department of Health and Human Services (HHS) leadership (Recommendation 1) should provide national guidance or recommendations on these standards.

c. HHS leadership and state legislatures should establish additional guidance if NBS programs begin implementing genomic sequencing methods that increase the generation and identifiability of sensitive data.

Courts have pointed to the duration of retention as a critical component of assessing whether the government collection of NBS dried blood spots and associated data is "narrowly tailored" to achieve the public health goals of newborn screening.[12] Courts have also established that written consent for research with dried blood spots collected for public health newborn screening is necessary.[13] However, opt-in approaches for research with residual dried blood spots have been criticized as being too burdensome for hospitals to implement. Concerns arise that hospitals will not ask for consent and therefore limit the supply of dried blood spots for research, even from parents that would otherwise consent (Botkin et al., 2013; Drabiak-Syed, 2011). For example, the comprehensive opt-in approach implemented by the Michigan BioTrust for Health resulted in a reduction in dried blood spots available for research but did not result in an increase in parental refusal for public health newborn screening

---

[12] *Kanuszewski v. Mich. HHS*, 927 F. 3d 396.
[13] *Kanuszewski v. Mich. HHS*, 684 F. Supp. 3d 637, 660 (2023).

itself. The program considered the consequences of this approach, which favors increased transparency, a reasonable public health trade-off (Duquette et al., 2011, 2012; Langbo et al., 2013). Balancing these feasibility, ethical, and legal concerns will require national guidance. Further discussions may be needed as the legal landscape continues to evolve.

National guidance could also include recommendations for how to securely and effectively store NBS dried blood spots, including practices to preserve samples for future use, secure facilities, and label samples.

Strengthening the NBS Research Enterprise

NBS policy and programmatic decisions must be guided by a robust review of the available evidence (see Chapter 5). Research that informs these decisions falls into four major categories:

1. defining conditions to guide screening, diagnosis, and treatment;
2. developing laboratory testing and applying emerging technologies;
3. understanding ethical, legal, and social issues; and
4. investigating public health practice, feasibility, and impacts.

However, robust and timely evidence generation in these areas is complicated by many factors, including the rarity of conditions considered for inclusion in newborn screening and the lack of coordination limiting the ability to draw clear conclusions (Bailey, 2022; Halley et al., 2022; Largent and Pearson, 2012). Furthermore, research funding is not consistently strategic and responsive to pressing needs for public health newborn screening, diminishing the effect of these investments. Therefore, a national plan with associated research infrastructure is needed to ensure that research informing public health newborn screening provides timely evidence to address priorities.

> **Recommendation 8: Expand and coordinate research to inform newborn screening (NBS) policy and practice.** The U.S. Department of Health and Human Services should establish an NBS research network with centers that address system-level research priorities in a coordinated and nimble manner. This network of research centers should operate in partnership with state/territorial NBS public health programs as appropriate to carry out research in the following areas:
>
> a. Defining diseases to guide screening, diagnosis, and treatment.
> b. Developing laboratory tests and applying emerging technologies.

c. Understanding ethical, legal, and social issues.
d. Investigating public health practice, feasibility, and impact.

Centers in this NBS research network should develop their own research questions and work together to generate evidence to address high-priority issues in the areas above. Such studies will help inform analyses and policy decisions affecting the delivery, quality, cost, and health outcomes associated with public health newborn screening. The NBS research network should involve patient advocacy groups in research design to facilitate bidirectional communication about perspectives, needs, and interests. This recommendation is not meant to replace all federally funded investigator-initiated NBS research, which is important to promote creativity and elevate research questions identified among investigators throughout the community.

Investing more systematically and strategically in NBS research would also advance research on rare diseases. NBS research and rare disease research have unique but complementary scopes (see discussion in Chapter 5). Because population-based screening is an important approach for understanding the full phenotypic spectrum for rare diseases and identifying presymptomatic individuals, many are eager for their condition of interest to be added to public health newborn screening. However, NBS research must not be conflated with public health newborn screening, which cannot be used for research purposes. Instead, NBS research provides an important avenue to understand rare diseases and inform the development of treatments and other related priorities. This investment toward NBS research would thus complement but have a distinct focus from other initiatives aimed at advancing rare disease therapies, such as the NIH-funded Rare Diseases Clinical Research Network and FDA's recent establishment of the Rare Disease Innovation Hub.[14]

Applying Technology to Newborn Screening

Decisions around the application of screening technologies require the same level of scrutiny, analysis, and alignment with vision and ethical principles as other decisions that affect the practice of newborn screening. Recent advances in genomic sequencing technology have attracted substantial research investment to determine the usefulness and acceptability of genomic sequencing in newborns (Minear et al., 2022). DNA-based tools, including sequencing of single genes, are

---

[14] See https://www.rarediseasesnetwork.org/ and https://www.fda.gov/industry/medical-products-rare-diseases-and-conditions/fda-rare-disease-innovation-hub (both accessed January 16, 2025).

already used in limited capacities across NBS programs (Furnier et al., 2020). Genomic sequencing could provide the opportunity to screen for all genetic conditions that meet criteria for inclusion on NBS panels using a single platform as a first step. However, many questions remain about how it could be implemented responsibly, whether it is acceptable to the public, what protections might be needed, how to ensure equitable access and accurate interpretation across ancestral populations, whether it is economically and practically feasible, and more (see Chapter 5). Key questions can guide the investments and activities of funders and investigators across government, nonprofit organizations, and industry.

> **Recommendation 9: Promote the responsible application of technologies to newborn screening (NBS).** Funders and investigators of feasibility studies should address the following key scientific, technical, ethical, and implementation questions before considering genomic sequencing for public health newborn screening:
>
> a. What sequence should be generated, what sequence/variants should be analyzed and interpreted, and what results should be returned?
> b. What strategies are necessary to ensure the accuracy of variant interpretation across ancestral populations?
> c. What are public attitudes concerning the application of genomic sequencing into public health newborn screening as a first-tier screening tool?
> d. What data should be stored after screening, if any, and how will the privacy of genomic data be protected given its risk of reidentification?
> e. Is genomic sequencing as a first-tier screening methodology cost-effective?
> f. What funding, resource sharing, and/or distributed system of clinical expertise would be necessary and effective to support employing population-based genomic sequencing as a first-tier tool across NBS programs?

Near-Term Actions to Make Progress Toward This Vision

Accomplishing the nine recommendations presented above entails a long-term vision. However, progress can be made now through multiple actions to advance elements of these recommendations and strengthen public health newborn screening. Box 7-3 highlights examples of achievable starting points.

BOX 7-3
Selected Examples of Starting Points and Near-Term Actions

- Identify each newborn screening (NBS) program's capacities, strengths, and sources of specialized expertise in laboratory operations, follow-up, education, and other areas (state and territorial NBS programs, federal agency partners, and information coordination and repository partners such as the Association of Public Health Laboratories).
- Connect NBS records to vital records that record births. This helps understand whether every baby received newborn screening and informs analysis (NBS programs, working with their state legislatures and public health departments as needed).
- Implement electronic messaging so NBS programs can both receive and transmit electronic messages. This enables rapid communication between NBS programs and health care providers and may support more timely connection to clinical care (NBS programs, working with their state legislatures and public health departments as needed).
- Begin identifying core metrics to understand whether screening assays perform differently among babies from different ancestral backgrounds and to understand whether all at-risk babies received follow-up and a clinical care handoff (NBS programs, working with other state offices, primary and specialty care providers, electronic health record vendors, and other partners).
- Commit to providing existing NBS communication materials (for example, a simple brochure) and engaging in initial conversations about newborn screening with all prospective parents during prenatal visits (prenatal care provider associations, care providers, NBS programs, and NBS education partners such as patient and family organizations).
- Understand each state's current requirements for the collection, retention, sharing, and use of newborn dried blood spots and derived data, and enact protections against law enforcement use of NBS blood spots if not already prohibited (NBS programs, working with other state offices as needed).
- Index newborn screening in the Research, Condition, and Disease Categorization system to provide greater clarity on the scope and range of investigator-initiated research funding addressing NBS (NIH).
- Commission the analysis of conditions to determine which meet inclusion criteria for newborn screening and to identify evidence gaps to guide research (HHS).
- Begin aligning partners to define the goals of a national system for the collection and analysis of long-term follow-up data, including the key questions to be addressed from the resulting data analysis and the associated outcomes to track, such as survival.

REFERENCES

AAP (American Academy of Pediatrics) Newborn Screening Task Force. 2000. *Serving the family from birth to the medical home*. A report from the Newborn Screening Task Force convened in Washington, DC, May 10-11, 1999. *Pediatrics* 106(2 Pt 2):383-427.

ACMG (American College of Medical Genetics) Newborn Screening Expert Group. 2006. Newborn screening: Toward a uniform screening panel and system. *Genetics in Medicine* Suppl 1:1S-252S.

ACOG (American College of Obstetricians and Gynecologists) Committee on Genetics. 2019. Newborn screening and the role of the obstetrician-gynecologist. ACOG Committee Opinion Number 778. *Obstetrics and Gynecology* 133(5):e357-e361.

Andrews, S. M., K. A. Porter, D. B. Bailey, Jr., and H. L. Peay. 2022. Preparing newborn screening for the future: A collaborative stakeholder engagement exploring challenges and opportunities to modernizing the newborn screening system. *BMC Pediatrics* 22(1):90.

Armstrong, N. 2024. *Advocacy perspectives on adding new diseases: Experiences with developing a nomination package*. Presented at Committee on Newborn Screening: Current Landscape and Future Directions Meeting 2. https://www.nationalacademies.org/event/42052_03-2024_newborn-screening-current-landscape-and-future-directions-meeting-2 (accessed January 23, 2025).

Bailey, D. B., Jr. 2022. A window of opportunity for newborn screening. *Molecular Diagnosis & Therapy* 26(3):253-261.

Botkin, J. R., A. J. Goldenberg, E. Rothwell, R. A. Anderson, and M. H. Lewis. 2013. Retention and research use of residual newborn screening bloodspots. *Pediatrics* 131(1):120-127.

Botkin, J. R., E. Rothwell, R. A. Anderson, N. C. Rose, S. M. Dolan, M. Kuppermann, L. A. Stark, A. Goldenberg, and B. Wong. 2016. Prenatal education of parents about newborn screening and residual dried blood spots: A randomized clinical trial. *JAMA Pediatrics* 170(6):543-549.

Campbell, E. D., and L. F. Ross. 2004. Incorporating newborn screening into prenatal care. *American Journal of Obstetrics and Gynecology* 190(4):876-877.

CMS (Centers for Medicare and Medicaid Services). 2024. *2024 Medicaid & CHIP beneficiaries at a glance: Maternal health*. https://www.medicaid.gov/medicaid/benefits/downloads/2024-maternal-health-at-a-glance.pdf (accessed February 19, 2025).

Cope, H. L., L. V. Milko, E. R. Jalazo, B. G. Crissman, A. K. M. Foreman, B. C. Powell, N. A. DeJong, J. E. Hunter, B. L. Boyea, A. N. Forsythe, A. C. Wheeler, R. S. Zimmerman, S. F. Suchy, A. Begtrup, K. G. Langley, K. G. Monaghan, C. Kraczkowski, K. S. Hruska, P. Kruszka, K. S. Kucera, J. Berg, C. M. Powell, and H. L. Peay. 2024. A systematic framework for selecting gene-condition pairs for inclusion in newborn sequencing panels: Early Check implementation. *Genetics in Medicine* 26(12):101290.

Davis, T. C., S. G. Humiston, C. L. Arnold, J. A. Bocchini, Jr., P. F. Bass 3rd, E. M. Kennen, A. Bocchini, P. Kyler, and M. Lloyd-Puryear. 2006. Recommendations for effective newborn screening communication: Results of focus groups with parents, providers, and experts. *Pediatrics* 117(5 Pt 2):S326-S340.

Downie, L., S. E. Bouffler, D. J. Amor, J. Christodoulou, A. Yeung, A. E. Horton, I. Macciocca, A. D. Archibald, M. Wall, J. Caruana, S. Lunke, and Z. Stark. 2024. Gene selection for genomic newborn screening: Moving toward consensus? *Genetics in Medicine* 26(5):101077.

Drabiak-Syed, K. 2011. Legal regulation of banking newborn blood spots for research: How *Bearder* and *Beleno* resolved the question of consent. *Houston Journal of Health Law and Policy* 11:1-46.

Duquette, D., A. P. Rafferty, C. Fussman, J. Gehring, S. Meyer, and J. Bach. 2011. Public support for the use of newborn screening dried blood spots in health research. *Public Health Genomics* 14(3):143-152.

Duquette, D., C. Langbo, J. Bach, and M. Kleyn. 2012. Michigan BioTrust for Health: Public support for using residual dried blood spot samples for health research. *Public Health Genomics* 15(3-4):146-155.

Furnier, S. M., M. S. Durkin, and M. W. Baker. 2020. Translating molecular technologies into routine newborn screening practice. *International Journal of Neonatal Screening* 6(4):80.

Halley, M. C., H. S. Smith, E. A. Ashley, A. J. Goldenberg, and H. K. Tabor. 2022. A call for an integrated approach to improve efficiency, equity and sustainability in rare disease research in the United States. *Nature* 54(3):219-222.

HHS (U.S. Department of Health and Human Services). 2015. *Report to Congress: Newborn screening activities.* https://mchb.hrsa.gov/sites/default/files/mchb/programs-impact/nbs-report.pdf (accessed February 21, 2025).

HRSA (Health Resources and Services Administration). 2024a. *Nominate a condition.* https://www.hrsa.gov/advisory-committees/heritable-disorders/rusp/nominate (accessed December 18, 2024).

HRSA. 2024b. *Charter: Advisory Committee on Heritable Disorders in Newborns and Children.* https://www.hrsa.gov/sites/default/files/hrsa/advisory-committees/heritable-disorders/achdnc-charter.pdf (accessed December 18, 2024).

Kusyk, D., K. Acharya, K. Garvey, and L. F. Ross. 2013. A pilot study to evaluate awareness of and attitudes about prenatal and neonatal genetic testing in postpartum African American women. *Journal of the National Medical Association* 105(1):85-91.

Langbo, C., J. Bach, M. Kleyn, and F. P. Downes. 2013. From newborn screening to population health research: Implementation of the Michigan BioTrust for Health. *Public Health Reports* 128(5):377-384.

Largent, E. A., and S. D. Pearson. 2012. Which orphans will find a home? The rule of rescue in resource allocation for rare diseases. *Hastings Center Report* 42(1):27-34.

Milko, L. V., J. M. O'Daniel, D. M. DeCristo, S. B. Crowley, A. K. M. Foreman, K. E. Wallace, L. F. Mollison, N. T. Strande, Z. S. Girnary, L. J. Boshe, A. S. Aylsworth, M. Gucsavas-Calikoglu, D. M. Frazier, N. L. Vora, M. I. Roche, B. C. Powell, C. M. Powell, and J. S. Berg. 2019. An age-based framework for evaluating genome-scale sequencing results in newborn screening. *Journal of Pediatrics* 209:68-76.

Minear, M. A., M. N. Phillips, A. Kau, and M. A. Parisi. 2022. Newborn screening research sponsored by the NIH: From diagnostic paradigms to precision therapeutics. *American Journal of Medical Genetics Part C: Seminars in Medical Genetics* 190(2):138-152.

Minten, T., N. B. Gold, S. Bick, S. Adelson, N. Gehlenborg, L. M. Amendola, F. Boemer, A. J. Coffey, N. Encina, A. Ferlini, J. Kirschner, B. E. Russell, L. Servais, K. L. Sund, R. J. Taft, P. Tsipouras, H. Zouk, ICoNS Gene List Contributors; D. Bick, R. C. Green, and the International Consortium on Newborn Sequencing (ICoNS). 2024. Data-driven prioritization of genetic disorders for global genomic newborn screening programs. *medRxiv* [Preprint]. https://doi.org/10.1101/2024.03.24.24304797.

Ram, N. 2022. America's hidden national DNA database. *Texas Law Review* 100(7):1253-1325.

Susanna Haas Lyons Engagement Consulting. 2024. *What we heard: Newborn sceening in the United States.* Presented to the Committee on Newborn Screening: Current Landscape and Future Directions at the National Academies of Sciences, Engineering, and Medicine. https://www.nationalacademies.org/documents/embed/link/LF2255DA3DD1C-41C0A42D3BEF0989ACAECE3053A6A9B/file/D35FB72C883DD3F3496A747004FB20B434E54764D1D0?noSaveAs=1 (accessed December 18, 2024).

Taylor-Phillips, S., J. Geppert, C. Stinton, K. Freeman, S. Johnson, H. Fraser, P. Sutcliffe, and A. Clarke. 2017. Comparison of a full systematic review versus rapid review approaches to assess a newborn screening test for tyrosinemia type 1. *Research Synthesis Methods* 8(4):475-484.

Therrell, B. L., Jr., W. H. Hannon, D. B. Bailey, Jr., E. B. Goldman, J. Monaco, B. Norgaard-Pedersen, S. F. Terry, A. Johnson, and R. R. Howell. 2011. Committee report: Considerations and recommendations for national guidance regarding the retention and use of residual dried blood spot specimens after newborn screening. *Genetics in Medicine* 13(7):621-624.

A

Information Sources and Methods

The Committee on Newborn Screening: Current Landscape and Future Directions was tasked with examining the landscape of newborn screening (NBS) systems, processes, and research in the United States and developing recommendations for future improvements that help modernize newborn screening to be adaptable, flexible, coordinated, communicative, capable of efficient and sustainable adoption of screening for new conditions using new technologies, and a public health program from which all infants benefit. The committee was asked to develop a report to provide both short-term options to strengthen existing NBS programs and to establish a vision to be accomplished over the next 5 to 15 years.

COMMISSION COMPOSITION

The National Academies of Sciences, Engineering, and Medicine appointed a committee of 14 experts to undertake the statement of task. The committee was composed of members with expertise in NBS systems, lived and parental experience, bioethical and legal issues, existing and emerging technologies, health systems, health economics, and clinical care disciplines, among other areas. Appendix B provides biographical information for each committee member.

INFORMATION-GATHERING ACTIVITIES

The committee deliberated from approximately January 2024 to December 2024 to gather and discuss information and draft its report.

To address its task, the committee solicited public input online through a questionnaire and several listening sessions, analyzed information obtained from reviewing current literature and other publicly available resources, and undertook information-gathering activities, such as inviting experts and experts by experience to share perspectives during virtual and hybrid public sessions.

Community Input and Engagement

Public participation is a cornerstone value that supports ethical decision making; enhances legitimacy, transparency, and justice; and builds trust. Therefore, providing opportunities for those personally or professionally affected by newborn screening to share their views was essential to ensure that the recommendations developed by the committee were responsive to the needs of the system. To this end, the committee and National Academies staff worked with a civic engagement consultant to design and conduct a process to solicit input from individuals interested in or affected by newborn screening through an online questionnaire and virtual listening sessions.

The questionnaire and listening sessions were promoted to people across the United States. In addition to sharing information about the engagement activities through National Academies communication channels and the study website, the committee and staff reached out to associations, organizations, and other groups interested in or affected by newborn screening. Nearly 30 groups helped share the committee's call for input to their networks. The aim was to obtain input from individuals reflecting a wide range of NBS experiences in the United States.

This multiperspective engagement process enabled the committee to gain insights from parents, parents of children with a rare disease, persons with a rare disease, disease advocates, health administrators, health care providers, health researchers, health industry representatives, NBS laboratory professionals, NBS follow-up professionals, public health professionals, payors, privacy advocates, specific underserved communities, and the general public. A total of 667 participants were involved in the engagement activities.

The committee's core questions to participants were: *How can we strengthen today's NBS system? What changes would you like to see in the future?* Participants shared their perspectives on current NBS strengths and challenges, as well as short-term and long-term opportunities to strengthen newborn screening in the United States. Altogether, the input highlights several tensions and seemingly contradicting positions, reflecting the range of key actors, groups, and communities that have strong stakes in newborn screening, as well as the fact that decisions about the role and operation of newborn screening in the United States involve moral, political, health-related, and practical considerations.

Two key engagement opportunities were undertaken:

- **Questionnaire (April 18–May 26, 2024):** An online questionnaire available in both English and Spanish was open for public input for 38 days. The questionnaire was developed using Alchemer, a feedback and data-collection platform. The questionnaire had general questions on newborn screening, as well as targeted questions depending on the respondent's self-identified connection to newborn screening. Limited demographic questions were asked of respondents at the end of the questionnaire for the purpose of understanding and reporting who participated. All questions, including demographic questions, were optional. A total of 570 questionnaire responses were included in the analysis.
- **Listening Sessions (May 1–June 11, 2024):** Six facilitated virtual listening sessions were held with individuals professionally or personally affected by newborn screening, involving 97 people. Two of these sessions were convened with the assistance of organizations to support participation by groups whose voices might otherwise be less heard.
  - NBS laboratory and follow-up professionals (May 1)
  - Rare disease patients, families, and advocacy organizations (May 5)
  - Health administrators, payors, and health care industry (May 6)
  - Health care providers (May 13)
  - Spanish-speaking parents of rare disease patients (May 23): This session was conducted in Spanish and convened with assistance from the Akari Foundation, which educates and empowers the Hispanic community on rare diseases.
  - Families with children 2 years of age or younger, who are eligible for Medicaid, or lack insurance altogether (June 11): This session was convened with assistance from REACHUP, Inc., a Florida-based organization that advocates for and mobilizes resources to help communities achieve equality in health care and positive health for families.

Each session was up to 2.5 hours long. Most of each session was spent in small group discussion to ensure that participants were able to share their views and hear from others.

Further details on the methodology and analysis, the description of who participated in the questionnaire and listening sessions, and the results can be found in the publicly available paper, *What We Heard:*

Engagement Summary on Newborn Screening in the United States.[1] Findings from the engagement process were integrated into the committee's report.

Literature Review

Members and staff drew on relevant articles from peer-reviewed journals, reports, statements, websites, and other literature sources to complement committee expertise and other sources of information gathering. Strategies to identify literature relevant to the committee's charge included searches of bibliographic databases, including PubMed, Scopus, and ProQuest Research Library, to obtain articles related to newborn screening. Search areas included those related to public health ethics; practices, operations, and guidance around newborn screening; screening technologies; communication, engagement, and education; near-term and longer-term diagnosis and follow-up care; retention and use of NBS dried blood spot samples and data; informed consent; rare disease research; and others. In addition, committee members, speakers, sponsors, and other interested parties identified or submitted articles, reports, and statements on these topics. Committee members and staff also analyzed federal guidance and procedures related to newborn screening from agencies including the Health Resources and Services Administration and the Centers for Disease Control and Prevention. The committee's collection of background and reference information was updated throughout the study process.

Public Meetings and Webinars

Sessions at meetings held over the course of the study enabled the committee to obtain input from a range of additional experts. The committee's first public meeting was held virtually in January 2024 and provided an opportunity for the committee to discuss the focus, goals, and timeline of the study. The committee held public sessions in March, May, and October 2024. Speakers who provided input to the committee are listed below. Sessions with invited speakers and experts included the following:

- Perspectives on the study context and goals from the sponsoring organization, state NBS programs, and child health or rare disease organizations (January 2024)
- Presentation and discussion on the roles and perspectives of federal partners in the NBS system (March 2024)

---

[1] Susanna Haas Lyons Engagement Consulting. 2024. What We Heard: Engagement Summary. Newborn Screening in the United States. The full paper, paper summary in English, and paper summary in Spanish are available at https://www.nationalacademies.org/our-work/newborn-screening-current-landscape-and-future-directions (accessed December 4, 2024).

APPENDIX A   241

- Workshop discussing near-term and fundamental needs and challenges facing the NBS system, with a focus on considerations for adding conditions to public health NBS programs (March 2024)
- Workshop focusing on the forward-looking needs and challenges facing the NBS system, with a focus on new technologies, data collections strategies, and trustworthiness (May 2024)
- Presentation and discussion on the roles and perspectives of health care providers that care for pregnant people, babies, and their families on their role in family education for newborn screening (October 2024)

Consulted Experts

The following individuals were invited speakers at information-gathering sessions of the committee:

Niki Armstrong, Foundation for Angelman Syndrome Therapeutics
Barb Ballard, SCID Angels for Life Foundation
Julie Beans, Southcentral Foundation
Cheryl Bellamy, Henry Ford Hospital
Stanton Berberich, State Hygienic Laboratory at the University of Iowa (retired)
Alisha Blanks, Office on Women's Health, Department of Health and Human Services
Natasha Bonhomme, Expecting Health
Jeffrey Brosco, Health Resources and Services Administration, Department of Health and Human Services
Paula Caposino, U.S. Food and Drug Administration
Kee Chan, ValueMinded LLC
Anne Claiborne, Chan Zuckerberg Initiative
Ellen Wright Clayton, Vanderbilt University Medical Center
Anne Marie Comeau, New England Newborn Screening Program
Carla Cuthbert, U.S. Centers for Disease Control and Prevention
M. Christine Dorley, Tennessee Department of Health
Amy Gaviglio, Connetics Consulting
Michael H. Gelb, University of Washington
Aaron Goldenberg, Case Western Reserve University School of Medicine
Scott Grosse, Centers for Disease Control and Prevention
Sonia S. Hassan, Wayne State University
Eric Hendricks, Michigan Department of Health and Human Services
Allison Herrity, National Organization for Rare Disorders (NORD)
Benjamin Hoffman, Oregon Health and Science University
Debbie Jessup, Sage Femme Strategies
Denise M. Kay, New York State Department of Health

Alex Kemper, Nationwide Children's Hospital
Annie Kennedy, EveryLife Foundation for Rare Diseases
Jeanie Kim, Chan Zuckerberg Initiative
Stephen Kingsmore, Rady Children's Institute for Genomic Medicine
Sylvia Mann, Hawaii State Department of Health
Jerry Menikoff, National University of Singapore [HHS Office for Human Research Protections (retired)]
Kamila Mistry, Agency for Healthcare Research and Quality
Jelili Ojodu, Association of Public Health Laboratories
Melissa Parisi, *Eunice Kennedy Shriver* National Institute of Child Health and Human Development
Marianna Raia, Expecting Health
Natalie Ram, University of Maryland Carey School of Law
Britton Rink, Mount Carmel East Hospital
Lainie Friedman Ross, University of Rochester
Curt Scharfe, Yale University
Jill Simonetti, Minnesota Department of Health
Julia Skapik, National Association of Community Health Centers
Dominic Smith, Michigan Department of Health and Human Services
Heeju Sohn, Emory University
Marci Sontag, Center for Public Health Innovation
Michelle Takemoto, Alliance for Genomic Justice
Susan Tanksley, Texas Department of State Health Services
John Thompson, Washington State Department of Health
Ines Maria Vigil, Independent
Heidi Wallis, Association for Creatine Deficiencies
Melissa Wasserstein, Albert Einstein College of Medicine
Deanna Wathington, American Public Health Association and REACHUP
Michael Watson, Washington University School of Medicine [American College of Medical Genetics (retired)]
Trinisha Williams, Haven Midwifery Birthing Center
Michele Wright, National Organization of African Americans with Cystic Fibrosis
Terry Wright, National Organization of African Americans with Cystic Fibrosis

Website and Communications

To make study activities transparent and accessible, a website hosted by the National Academies was periodically updated to reflect recent and planned committee activities. Study outreach included an email address for comments and questions. A subscription to receive periodic announcements or updates was available to share further information and solicit additional comments and input to the committee.

B

Committee Member and Staff Biographies

COMMITTEE MEMBERS

Jewel Mullen, M.D., M.P.A., M.P.H. (*Chair*), is associate dean for health equity and associate professor of population health and internal medicine at the University of Texas at Austin Dell Medical School where she leads strategies to embed health equity as an operating principle across research, education, and practice. Her previous roles in state government and as the Principal Deputy Assistant Secretary for Health at the Department of Health and Human Services focused on ensuring equitable access to medical and public health services for all people. During her tenure as Commissioner of the Connecticut Department of Public Health, her department built and opened a new public health laboratory and deliberated adding new conditions to its newborn screening panel. Dr. Mullen also collaborated with the Association of Public Health Laboratories to increase overall state laboratory efficiency. In addition to serving on the National Academies of Sciences, Engineering, and Medicine's (the National Academies') Board on Population Health and Public Health Practice, she is a current member of the *Morbidity and Mortality Weekly Report* Editorial Board and the National Vaccine Advisory Committee. Her two most recent National Academies study committees addressed *A Fairer and More Equitable Cost-Effective and Transparent System of Donor Organ Procurement, Allocation, and Distribution,* and *Equitable Allocation of Vaccine for the Novel Coronavirus.* Dr. Mullen received her bachelor's and master of public health degrees from Yale University where she also completed a postdoctoral fellowship in psychosocial epidemiology, her M.D. from the

Mount Sinai School of Medicine, a master in public administration from Harvard's Kennedy School of Government, and a certificate in bioethics from Georgetown's Kennedy Institute of Ethics.

Don Bailey, Ph.D., M.Ed., is a distinguished fellow in the Genomics and Translational Research Center at RTI International. Before joining RTI in 2006, he was on the faculty of the University of North Carolina at Chapel Hill (UNC-CH) for 27 years, where he was a W. R. Kenan, Jr., Distinguished Professor and, for 14 years, Director of the Frank Porter Graham Child Development Institute. Dr. Bailey's research addresses early identification and early intervention for children with disabilities, as well as family adaptation to disability. He has an extensive record of publications on topics related to newborn screening, early intervention, disability, and family support. Currently, his work focuses on the future of newborn screening, family outcomes of newborn screening, and policy considerations when determining net benefit of screening. He is a senior advisor for the Early Check program, a research study offering free additional screening tests to newborns in North Carolina. Early Check has multiple sources of support, including direct funding from the Leona M. and Henry B. Helmsley Charitable Trust, JDRF International (through a collaboration with Janssen Pharmaceuticals), Travere Therapeutics, and Orchard Therapeutics. Early Check previously received donated sequencing services from GeneDx and in-kind contributions from Illumina. Dr. Bailey's work has previously been funded by companies including Asuragen, Janssen Pharmaceuticals, Orchard Therapeutics, Sarepta Therapeutics, Illumina, and Shionogi. Additionally, he has received travel support to present research findings from Travere Pharmaceuticals, PerkinElmer, and Janssen Pharmaceuticals. Dr. Bailey has presented research findings to organizations including the Association of Public Health Laboratories and EveryLife Foundation. From 2011 to 2017, he served as a member of the Department of Health and Human Services' Advisory Committee on Heritable Disorders in Newborns and Children. He holds a B.A. in psychology (Davidson College), an M.Ed. in early childhood special education (UNC-CH), and a Ph.D. in early childhood special education (University of Washington).

Mei Baker, M.D., FACMG, is a professor in the Department of Pediatrics and Director of the Newborn Screening Laboratory at the University of Wisconsin School of Medicine and Public Health. Dr. Baker practiced medicine before being trained in both biochemical and molecular genetics, obtaining a clinical biochemical genetics certification from the American Board of Medical Genetics and Genomics in 2009. She has 20 years of experience in routine newborn screening (NBS) with specific interest in, and a successful track record of, applying emerging technologies to implement new screening tests for disorders and improving ongoing screening tests. She is one of the leading scientists who made Wisconsin the first state in the nation and the world to implement universal newborn screening for severe combined immunodeficiency in 2008. She has developed and implemented cystic fibrosis newborn screening using next-generation sequencing technology in the Wisconsin NBS program. She also implemented the newborn screening for spinal muscular atrophy in Wisconsin with the unique approach of incorporating additional SMN2 copy number assessment. Dr. Baker recently completed a research project supported by Ultragenyx to help develop a screening assay for Angelman syndrome. Dr. Baker's contribution to science has been widely recognized, as evidenced by receiving the Harry Hannon Laboratory Improvement Award in Newborn Screening from the Association of Public Health Laboratories (APHL) in 2014, and Everyday Life Saver in Newborn Screening Award from the APHL in 2022. Dr. Baker served as a member of the Department of Health and Human Services' Advisory Committee on Heritable Disorders in Newborns and Children from 2016 to 2021. She currently serves on the scientific advisory boards for the Global Foundation for Peroxisomal Disorders and the Foundation for Angelman Syndrome Therapeutics.

Wendy K. Chung, M.D., Ph.D. (NAM), is a clinical and molecular geneticist and the Chair of the Department of Pediatrics at Boston Children's Hospital and Harvard Medical School. Dr. Chung leads the GUARDIAN study piloting genome sequencing as a platform for newborn screening, which is funded by private philanthropy, in addition to sequencing services from GeneDx, in-kind contributions from Illumina, and funds for participant recruitment from Sanofi. She has also led previous pilot studies of newborn screening for spinal muscular atrophy. Dr. Chung directs National Institutes of Health–funded research programs in human genetics of pulmonary hypertension, breast cancer, obesity, diabetes, autism, and congenital anomalies including congenital diaphragmatic hernia and congenital heart disease. She is a national leader in the ethical, legal, and social implications of genomics. She was the recipient of the Rare Impact Award from the National Organization of Rare Disorders and is a member of the National Academy of Medicine and the American Academy of Physicians. She serves as a member on the Board of Directors for Prime Medicine, which is developing platform technologies for potential gene therapy applications. Dr. Chung received her B.A. in biochemistry from Cornell University, her M.D. from Cornell University Medical College, and her Ph.D. from the Rockefeller University in genetics.

Titilope A. Fasipe, M.D., Ph.D., is Codirector of the Sickle Cell and Thalassemia Program at Texas Children's Hospital and assistant professor of pediatrics in hematology/oncology at Baylor College of Medicine in Houston, Texas. She is involved in community and policy efforts aimed at improving health outcomes in sickle cell disease. Further, she has the unique perspective of relating to and understanding the need for education, community awareness, support, and medical care as she is a pediatric hematologist as well as an individual with sickle cell disease. Dr. Fasipe has been repeatedly appointed to advisory committees of the Texas Department of State Health Services and currently serves on their Newborn Screening Advisory Committee and chairs the Sickle Cell Task Force. Her professional memberships include the American Academy of Pediatrics, the Heartland-Southwest Sickle Cell Disease Network, the American Society of Hematology, the American Society of Pediatric Hematology/Oncology, and the Global Action Network for Sickle Cell and Other Inherited Blood Disorders. Dr. Fasipe has consulted as a sickle cell disease educator for several pharmaceutical and therapeutic companies, including Forma Therapeutics, Novartis, Global Blood Therapeutics, Bluebird Bio, and Emmaus Medical. Dr. Fasipe received her bachelor of science from the University of Texas at Arlington and graduated from the combined M.D.-Ph.D. program at the University of Texas Medical Branch. She then completed her pediatric residency at Cincinnati Children's Hospital Medical Center and her pediatric hematology/oncology fellowship at Baylor College of Medicine and Texas Children's Hospital.

Faith Fletcher, Ph.D., M.A., is an associate professor in the Center for Medical Ethics and Health Policy at Baylor College of Medicine (BCM). She is also a senior advisor to the Hastings Center and a Hastings Center fellow. Her research program examines the social and structural barriers to scientific research and health care engagement facing traditionally marginalized populations and is grounded in methodological and theoretical approaches from the fields of public health, bioethics, and behavioral science. Her K01 Award funded through the National Human Genomic Research Institute uses a stakeholder engagement approach to develop ethical practices and guidelines for engaging residents of the deep South in genomics research. Dr. Fletcher was recently named to the Greenwall Faculty Scholars Program in Bioethics Class of 2026. In 2017, Dr. Fletcher was named one of the National Minority Quality Forum's 40 under 40 Leaders in Health for her commitment to advancing health equity. She recently received the BCM Women of Excellence Award for her outstanding contributions and accomplishments in advancing health and health care equity as a field leader in alignment with the mission of the college. Dr. Fletcher received her B.S. in biology from Tuskegee

University with concentrations in bioethics and philosophy; her M.A. in bioethics, humanities, and society from Michigan State University; and her Ph.D. in health promotion, education and behavior from the University of South Carolina. Dr. Fletcher also completed a National Cancer Institute R25T-funded postdoctoral fellowship in the Department of Behavioral Science at the University of Texas MD Anderson Cancer Center.

Meghan Halley, Ph.D., M.P.H., is an assistant professor in the Center for Biomedical Ethics at Stanford University. A medical anthropologist by training, her research focuses on ethical and policy issues arising through the introduction of new genomic technologies for the diagnosis and treatment of rare diseases. Her current projects include examining ethical issues related to sustainability and the governance of patient data and relationships when large clinical genomic studies transition to new models of funding; ethnographic work exploring how diverse stakeholders perceive value in the use of genome sequencing for the diagnosis of rare diseases; and the development of new measures for assessing patient-centered outcomes in pediatric rare diseases. In 2021, she was awarded a career development grant from the National Human Genome Research Institute focused on the ethics and economics of genomic sequencing in rare disease. Dr. Halley received her doctorate in anthropology and her master of public health from Case Western Reserve University in Cleveland, Ohio. The parent of a child with a rare disease, she serves as President of the Board of Directors for the Undiagnosed Diseases Network Foundation, a nonprofit with the mission of improving access to diagnosis, research, and care for individuals with undiagnosed and ultra-rare diseases and has written on the parental experience navigating complex medical decisions.

Amanda Ingram, RN, is the Director of the Pediatric Case Management and Newborn Screening Follow-up Program for the Tennessee Department of Health. Before becoming director, Mrs. Ingram served as a Case Manager and the Case Management Coordinator for the program for 1 year each. Mrs. Ingram has been a registered nurse for 25 years and worked as a Neonatal Intensive Care Nurse for 13 years before coming to the Department of Health. As a neonatal nurse, Mrs. Ingram had experiences with receiving newborn screening results, requests for repeat testing, and collection of newborn screening specimens. She is a member of the Association of Public Health Laboratories (APHL) and serves on three APHL workgroups to collaborate with other programs to continue newborn screening awareness and improvement. She was selected to participate on the Krabbe Review Technical Expert Panel that informs the Department of Health and Human Services' Advisory Committee on Heritable Disorders in Newborns and Children. Mrs. Ingram has coauthored and contributed to multiple articles in the newborn screening field and was a contributor to the recently updated Clinical and Laboratory Standards Institute Guidelines for Newborn Screening Follow-up and Education.

José A. Pagán, Ph.D. (NAM), is professor and chair of the Department of Public Health Policy and Management at the School of Global Public Health, New York University. He is also Chair of the Board of Directors of NYC Health + Hospitals, the largest municipal health care system in the United States. He formerly served as Chair of the National Advisory Committee of the Robert Wood Johnson Foundation's Health Policy Research Scholars and was a member of the Board of Directors of the Interdisciplinary Association for Population Health Science and the American Society of Health Economists. He is a member of the National Academy of Medicine. He has led research, implementation, and evaluation projects on the redesign of health care delivery and payment systems. His areas of focus include population health management, health care payment and delivery system reform, and the social determinants of health. Dr. Pagán received his Ph.D. in economics from the University of New Mexico.

Jochen Profit, M.D., M.P.H., is the Wendy J. Tomlin-Hess Endowed Professor of Pediatrics at Stanford University and Co-Principal Investigator and Co-Chair of the California Perinatal Quality Care Collaborative and California Maternal Quality Care Collaborative. Dr. Profit's research focuses on optimizing the quality of neonatal–perinatal health care delivery, with an emphasis on enhancing organizational effectiveness. He is also interested in the use of information technology to support families, care professionals, and policy makers in their efforts to provide optimal care to sick infants. For over a decade, his research has received continuous funding from the National Institutes of Health and other federal, foundation, and intramural sources. Dr. Profit has served on various national scientific and professional organizations, including for the National Institutes of Health. Recently, he served as a member of the National Academies of Sciences, Engineering, and Medicine consensus study committee on Research Issues in the Assessment of Birth Settings. He graduated from the University of Freiburg Medical School in Germany and completed his neonatology and health services research training at Harvard.

Scott M. Shone, Ph.D., HCLD (ABB), is the Director of the North Carolina State Laboratory of Public Health. He received his doctorate in molecular microbiology and immunology from the Johns Hopkins Bloomberg School of Public Health and is a board-certified high-complexity clinical laboratory director. Dr. Shone spent 9 years managing the New Jersey Newborn

Screening (NBS) Laboratory. As a senior research public health analyst at RTI International, he focused on NBS pilot studies such as Early Check as the Clinical Laboratory Improvement Amendments Director. Currently, he leads a team of over 230 staff for the delivery of clinical and environmental laboratory testing, certification, and quality improvement services in North Carolina. Dr. Shone received the Jean Dussault Medal for Young Investigators from the International Society for Neonatal Screening and the Governor's Award for Excellence from the State of North Carolina. Dr. Shone served as a voting member of the Department of Health and Human Services' Advisory Committee on Heritable Disorders in Newborns and Children from 2017 to 2022. Currently, he is the Association of State and Territorial Health Officials organizational representative to this federal advisory committee. He has consulted for the Association of Public Health Laboratories (APHL) to develop contingency plans for NBS programs during states of emergency. He is a member of the editorial board for the *International Journal of Neonatal Screening*, a member of the APHL NBS Committee, and President-elect for APHL.

Kayte Spector-Bagdady, J.D., M.Be., is a lawyer and bioethicist and associate professor of obstetrics and gynecology at the University of Michigan (U-M) Medical School. She also directs the bioethics program for the U-M Center for Bioethics and Social Sciences in Medicine, which won the 2022 American Society for Bioethics & Humanities Cornerstone Award. She is an Associate Editor of *The American Journal of Bioethics* and was the Chair of the American Heart Association's *Principles for Health Information Collecting, Sharing, and Use*. She was an American Society of Law, Medicine & Ethics Health Law Scholar in 2019 and is a current Greenwall Faculty Scholar. Her work has been funded by the National Human Genome Research Institute, the National Center for Advancing Translational Sciences, and the Greenwall Foundation, and her research is on improving the governance of research with health data and specimens with a focus on public–private partnerships. Before joining U-M, she was an Associate Director for President Obama's Presidential Commission for the Study of Bioethical Issues and is a former practicing drug and device attorney. She received her B.A. from Middlebury College, her J.D. and M.Be. from the University of Pennsylvania, and was an empirical bioethics postdoctoral fellow at U-M.

Beth A. Tarini, M.D., M.S., M.B.A., is the Associate Director of the Center for Translational Research at Children's National Hospital. She previously served as the Division Director of General Pediatrics at the University of Iowa. She is a formally trained health services researcher (graduate of the Robert Wood Johnson Clinical Scholars Program) who conducts health services research that focuses on optimizing the delivery of genetic services to children and their families, particularly through newborn screening. Her research has been funded by the National Institutes of Health, the Health Resources and Services Administration, the Robert Wood Johnson Foundation, and the Cystic Fibrosis Foundation. Dr. Tarini is a former president of the Society for Pediatric Research, a fellow of the American Academy of Pediatrics, and a member of the Genomics & Society Working Group of the National Human Genome Research Institute. She has been appointed to and led federal, national, and state committees that provide policy recommendations for genetics services and newborn screening, including the Department of Health and Human Services' Advisory Committee on Heritable Disorders in Newborns and Children. Dr. Tarini received her M.D. from Albert Einstein College of Medicine and her B.A. from Harvard University. She has an M.S. in health services from the University of Washington and an M.B.A. from George Washington University.

Krystal Tsosie (Diné/Navajo Nation), Ph.D., M.P.H., M.A., is an assistant professor at Arizona State University in the School of Life Sciences. She cofounded the first U.S. Indigenous-led biobank, a 501(c)(3) nonprofit research institution called the Native BioData Consortium. Dr. Tsosie's research centers on ethical engagement with Indigenous communities in precision health and genomic medicine. Her areas include genetic epidemiology, bioethics, public health, and community research approaches. She previously patented a combined targeted ultrasound imaging and chemotherapeutic drug delivery device for treating early metastases in cancer. Dr. Tsosie is currently on the Board of Directors for the American Society of Human Genetics, and on the ethics committee of the American Society for Cell and Gene Therapies. Her background includes a master of arts in bioethics for studying genetic controversies in Indigenous communities, a master of public health in genetic epidemiology for studying gene variation related to hypertension and uterine fibroids, and a Ph.D. in genomics and health disparities. She recently served on the National Academies of Sciences, Engineering, and Medicine (the National Academies) consensus study committee, Creating a Framework for Emerging Science, Technology, and Innovation in Health and Medicine and on the National Academies planning committee, Engaging Scientists in Central Asia on Data Governance Principles for Life Science Data. Dr. Tsosie accepted a one-time speaker honorarium from Regeneron for serving as a guest speaker at the DRIFT Symposium in 2022 to inform the company how to improve their interactions with Indigenous communities. In 2024, Dr. Tsosie served as a paid consultant and member of the Clinical Advisory Board for Cache DNA, a company that developed technology that encapsulates and stores nucleic acids without refrigeration to make DNA and RNA isolation more equitable.

STAFF MEMBERS

Katherine Bowman, Ph.D., is a senior program officer with the Board on Health Sciences Policy and staff officer for the ongoing study Newborn Screening: Current Landscape and Future Directions. Her activities often focus on the implications of developments in science and technology, including Toward Equitable Innovation in Health and Medicine: A Framework (2023), Heritable Human Genome Editing with colleagues at the Royal Society (2020), and a recent workshop on scientific, ethical, and regulatory implications of stem cell-derived human gametes. She also directs the Forum on Traumatic Brain Injury and served as director of the report *Traumatic Brain Injury: A Roadmap for Accelerating Progress* (2022). She received her Ph.D. in biomedical engineering from Johns Hopkins University.

Emily Packard Dawson, Ph.D., is a program officer with the Board on Health Sciences Policy and codirector of the study Newborn Screening: Current Landscape and Future Directions. She first joined the National Academies of Sciences, Engineering, and Medicine as a Mirzayan Science and Technology Policy Graduate Fellow. As a fellow, Dr. Packard Dawson supported a workshop on scientific, ethical, and governance implications of in vitro gametogenesis, and drafted the resulting proceedings. Prior to moving into science policy, her postdoctoral and graduate research interests revolved around the specification of the germ cell lineage for sperm and eggs. She earned a Ph.D. in cell and molecular biology from Baylor College of Medicine.

Sarah H. Beachy, Ph.D., PMP, is a senior program officer with the National Academies of Sciences, Engineering, and Medicine. In this capacity, Dr. Beachy serves as director of the Roundtable on Genomics and Precision Health and the Forum on Regenerative Medicine, in addition to leading other projects. In these roles, she has facilitated impactful activities on topics such as Population Descriptors in Genetics/Genomics Research, Improving Diversity of the Genomics Workforce, Changing the Culture of Data Sharing and Management, and An Examination of Emerging Bioethical Issues in Biomedical Research, among others. In 2022, Dr. Beachy was awarded a National Academy of Medicine Cecil Award for Individual Excellence for her contributions to the National Academies. Prior to her time at the National Academies, Dr. Beachy completed an AAAS Science and Technology Policy Fellowship in diplomacy at the U.S. Department of State, working closely with the Office of the Science and Technology Adviser to the Secretary. She was selected as a Mirzayan Science and Technology Policy Fellow at the National Academies in 2011. Prior to moving into science policy, Dr. Beachy was a postdoctoral fellow in the Genetics

Branch at the National Cancer Institute, where she generated and characterized transgenic mouse models of leukemia and lymphoma. She earned her Ph.D. in biophysics from the Roswell Park Cancer Institute Graduate Division at the University at Buffalo.

Emily Backes, J.D., M.A., is deputy board director for the Board on Children, Youth, and Families (BCYF) and the Committee on Law and Justice (CLAJ) in the Division of Behavioral, Social Sciences, and Education at the National Academies of Sciences, Engineering, and Medicine (the National Academies). In her time at the National Academies, she has served as study director for the reports *The Promise of Adolescence: Realizing Opportunity for All Youth; Birth Settings in America: Outcomes, Quality, Access, and Choice; Transforming the Financing of Early Care and Education;* and *Decarcerating Correctional Facilities during COVID-19: Advancing Health, Equity, and Safety.* Emily has also provided analytical and editorial assistance to National Academies projects on child poverty, transforming the pediatric health care system, breastfeeding, child and youth mental and behavioral health, out-of-school time settings for children and youth, science literacy, and science communication. She received an M.A. and B.A. in history from the University of Missouri, specializing in U.S. human rights policy and international law, and a J.D. from the University of the District of Columbia, where she represented clients as a student attorney with the Low-income Taxpayer Clinic and the Juvenile and Special Education Law Clinic.

Michael Berrios, M.A., B.A., is a research associate in the Board on Health Sciences Policy at the National Academies of Sciences, Engineering, and Medicine (the National Academies). In his time at the National Academies, he has worked on projects in several subject areas, from vaccine clinical trials during the 2014–2015 Ebola epidemic in West Africa to medication-assisted therapy for opioid use disorder. He received an M.A. in Asian studies from the George Washington University.

Emily McDowell, M.P.H., is a research associate with the Board on Health Sciences Policy of the National Academies of Sciences, Engineering, and Medicine. Most recently, she assisted with a consensus study, *Advancing Clinical Research in Pregnant and Lactating Populations Overcoming Real and Perceived Liability Risks*, and she has contributed to other projects at the National Academies relating to health equity and policy. She is a M.P.H. graduate from George Washington University concentrating her studies on epidemiology and environmental health. Before joining the National Academies, Ms. McDowell worked for a nonprofit emergency management organization, Healthcare Ready, and assisted with the reauthorization of the Pandemic and All-Hazards Advancing Innovation Act. Her studies at George Washington University concluded with the presentation of her thesis entitled "Microplastics and Human Health: An Inescapable Exposure." Ms. McDowell received her B.S. in community health, concentrating in global health at George Mason University.

Gayatri Somaiya, B.A., is a senior program assistant in the Board on Health Sciences Policy at the National Academies of Sciences, Engineering, and Medicine. They are interested in the societal and legal implications of cognitive psychology research, specifically research in attention and memory. They work on a number of different projects including the study Newborn Screening: Current Landscape and Future Directions and the Forum on Traumatic Brain Injury. Previously, they worked as a paralegal at Healthcare Legal Solutions L.L.C. They graduated from Cornell University, earning their bachelor of arts in biology, concentrating in neuroscience, and political science.

Clare Stroud, Ph.D., is senior board director for the Board on Health Sciences Policy at the National Academies of Sciences, Engineering, and Medicine. In this capacity, she oversees a program of activities aimed at fostering the basic biomedical and clinical research enterprises; addressing the ethical, legal, and social contexts of scientific and technologic advances related to health; and strengthening the preparedness, resilience, and sustainability of communities. Previously, she served as director of the National Academies' Forum on Neuroscience and Nervous System Disorders, which brings together leaders from government, academia, industry, and nonprofit organizations to discuss key challenges and emerging issues in neuroscience research, development of therapies for nervous system disorders, and related ethical and societal issues. She also led consensus studies and contributed to projects on topics such as pain management, medications for opioid use disorder, traumatic brain injury, preventing cognitive decline and dementia, supporting persons living with dementia and their caregivers, the health and well-being of young adults, and disaster preparedness and response. Dr. Stroud first joined the National Academies as a Mirzayan Science and Technology Policy Graduate Fellow. She has also been an associate at AmericaSpeaks, a nonprofit organization that engaged citizens in decision making on important public policy issues. Dr. Stroud received her Ph.D. from the University of Maryland, College Park, with research focused on the cognitive neuroscience of language, and her bachelor's degree from Queen's University in Canada.